# Current Topics in Microbiology and Immunology

# Volume 318

Moses Rodriguez
Editor

# Advances in Multiple Sclerosis and Experimental Demyelinating Diseases

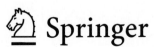 Springer

Moses Rodriguez
Department of Neurology and Immunology
Mayo Clinic, College of Medicine
200 First Street SW, Rochester
MN 55905, USA
e-mail: rodriguez.moses@mayo.edu

*Cover Illustration:* Remyelination-promoting antibodies that bind to oligodenrocytes, from left to right: mouse model, rat model, human

ISBN 978-3-540-73676-9          e-ISBN 978-3-540-73677-6

Current Topics in Microbiology and Immunology ISSN 007-217x

Library of Congress Catalog Number: 72-152360

*Cover design*: WMXDesign GmbH, Heidelberg

Printed on acid-free paper

9 8 7 6 5 4 3 2 1

springer.com

# Preface

There is a need for a paradigm shift in our thinking about the pathogenesis of multiple sclerosis (MS). From the days of Charcot in the 1800s, MS has been pathologically characterized primarily by demyelination; that is, the loss of myelin with the relative preservation of axons. Early manuscripts emphasized the inflammatory component, but in many cases, this was not thought to play a major role in the pathogenesis.

At the present time, the prevailing concept in MS is that the inflammatory response is critically involved in the destruction of the myelin sheath. This is derived from relatively weak data in humans but primarily based on an experimental model of MS known as experimental autoimmune encephalomyelitis (EAE), in which animals are immunized with myelin antigens. These animals usually develop a monophasic disease characterized primarily by inflammation and the relative absence of demyelination. More recently, this experimental model has demonstrated clear evidence of demyelination. This has mostly occurred as a result of the adoptive transfer of antibody directed against one of the myelin-specific proteins, myelin oligodendrocyte glycoprotein (MOG).

However, after more than 100 years of investigation into this disease, there still is no diagnostic clinical test dealing with the immunology of MS to support the autoimmune hypothesis. This is in contrast to a disease related to MS, neuromyelitis optica, in which patients develop an antibody directed against aquaporin 4 (see the chapter by B.G. Weinshenker and D.M. Wingerchuk). In this situation, there is evidence that autoimmunity plays a major role. This is not surprising in that neuromyelitis optica, for a very a long time, has been associated with other autoimmune disorders. Specifically, patients with neuromyelitis optica frequently develop antibodies against native DNA, antinuclear antibodies, and antibodies to other autoantigens. Unfortunately, similar assays done in MS have failed to reveal a specific antibody associated with the disease. Even the most recent attempts to associate antibodies to myelin basic proteins or MOG to disease progression have not been replicated by a number of investigators. MS is not associated with other autoimmune diseases. At this point in time, there is insufficient evidence to consider MS an autoimmune disease.

If the disease is not autoimmune in nature, then what is the basis of its pathogenesis? In an effort to begin to understand this, it is important to go back to the roots of neuropathology. The neuropathology of this disease has been revisited (see the chapter by C.F. Lucchinetti). It is clear that there are different subtypes of MS; at least four have been identified. Two of these are diseases in which myelin appears to be the primary target; in the other two subtypes, the disease appears to be directed against the cells that make the myelin sheaths, the oligodendrocytes. Even in those subtypes in which myelin sheaths are the primary target of injury, there is still loss of 30% of oligodendrocytes, which suggests that early oligodendrocyte injury may be common to all forms of MS. If early oligodendrocyte injury is a prerequisite to MS, then what is the basis of this injury? A number of possible scenarios come to mind in view of the experimental models. Clearly, viruses are high on the list because a number of viruses have been shown to induce demyelination in animals as well as in humans (see the chapters by A.J. Bieber and by A.E. Warrington and M. Rodriguez). In particular, infection with viruses of many different families results in well-demarcated areas of demyelination in association with variable axonal loss. In addition, toxins such as cuprizone or Lysolecithin (see the chapter by W.F. Blakemore and R.J.M. Franklin) also appear to cause dysfunction of oligodendrocytes and induce very focal areas of demyelination. Finally, demyelination may result from a genetic defect that affects oligodendrocyte function. In most of these known genetic disorders, the disease manifests before myelin completely forms, and therefore, these diseases are called dysmyelinating in nature. However, in adrenoleukodystrophy, the myelin begins to degenerate after it has been completely formed. This known genetic disorder of lysosomes clearly shows evidence of inflammation as well as areas of demarcated demyelination. Therefore, it is possible that a genetic abnormality is the initial driving event in the oligodendrocytes that predisposes to long-term demyelination.

Clearly, we may not be able to identify the very early event that initiates MS, since it may occur decades before clinical presentation. However, by understanding the effector molecules initiating the demyelination process, we may be able to intervene in the disease therapeutically. What has become clear in the last few years is that one of the most important effector cells in the MS lesion is the CD8$^+$ T cell. In contrast to previous thought, which has focused primarily on the role of CD4$^+$ T cells in EAE, CD8$^+$ T cells are usually cytotoxic in nature. While some have been shown to perform a regulatory function in the immune system, many of these cells are cytotoxic in nature and recognize class I MHC antigens on the surface of cells. It was once thought that class I MHC antigens were not expressed in the central nervous system (CNS); however, recent evidence suggests that class I antigens are expressed in many of the cell types including oligodendrocytes, astrocytes, microglia, axons, and neurons. In experimental models of demyelination, class I antigens are expressed very early after the induction of virus infection. It is well known that viruses can cause the elevation of class I MHC in the CNS. It is likely that the mediators of the generation of class I MHC in the CNS are the interferons. If CD8$^+$ T cells play a major role in the disease process, then what do they recognize? It is clear that CD8$^+$ T cells recognize peptides that have been processed within the cell by macrophages or microglia. These are usually eight to ten amino acids in length. They can encompass parts of the host cell as well as exogenous factors such as viruses. It is possible that many antigens are presented in the context of class I MHC in the MS lesion to be recognized by CD8[+] T cells. It is interesting to note that experiments in the models of MS induced by viruses indicate a clear immuno-dominance of peptides recognized by CD8[+] T cells. In some experimental models, up to 60% or 70% of the CD8[+] T cells are directed against one specific immuno-dominant peptide. This provides a very interesting target for preventing the demyelinating process by immunotherapy. Unfortunately, it is difficult to isolate CD8[+] T cells from MS brain or CSF and even more difficult to culture these cells to a significant number to allow for identification of the peptides recognized by these cells.

The other aspect of immune response critical to demyelination is immunoglobu-lin. Immunoglobulins are the hallmark of the clinical assays used to diagnose MS. MS patients are known to have oligoclonal IgG and IgM bands in the CSF. These oligoclonal bands are directed against a relatively small number of antigens. Efforts have been made to identify the antigens recognized by these antibodies. In experi-mental models and viral diseases of humans demonstrating oligoclonal bands, the oligoclonal bands are directed against the infectious agent. It is possible that the same process may be occurring in the MS plaque. Therefore, continuing efforts to identify the antibodies' target are extremely important. The other possibility is that these antibodies are part of a natural immune response important in the reparative process in MS (see the chapter by A.E. Warrington and M. Rodriguez). If this is the case, then these antibodies are reparative in nature and may be part of the natural immune response that promotes remyelinating activity.

What has also become apparent is that remyelination is a common event in the MS plaques. Efforts to enhance remyelination in MS have not yet been attempted clinically. Some investigators believe that the progenitor cells within the MS plaque are depleted; therefore, it would be necessary to transplant either stem cells or puri-fied populations of oligodendrocytes into the MS plaques for remyelination to take place (see the chapter by W.F. Blakemore). Other investigators believe that the pro-genitor cells are present in MS plaque; therefore, approaches to trigger remyelina-tion by these cells are potential mechanisms of treatment (see the chapter by A.E. Warrington and M. Rodriguez). Most recently, studies have recognized natural autoantibodies directed against oligodendrocytes, and these demonstrate remarka-ble remyelination when used as treatment in experimental models of demyelina-tion. These natural autoantibodies have been cloned and sequenced and appear to have genetic sequences very close to the host germline sequences. These antibod-ies, therefore, are called natural autoantibodies, since they are directed against host-cell proteins and are present as part of the normal repertoire. Work with a human recombinant IgM antibody, isolated from a human designated 22, is nearing the late phase of completion of animal experiments and may soon be ready for application in human trials. This would be the first attempt to enhance remyelina-tion in the MS lesion and a completely different approach to the present MS treat-ments. In this case, the therapies would target the cells that make the myelin sheath (the oligodendrocytes), in contrast to all other known MS treatments, which target immune cells.

There may be other approaches to interfere with the demyelinating process. One area that has received very little attention is the study of proteases (see the chapter by I.A. Scarisbrick). Multiple proteases have been demonstrated in the CNS and have been associated with MS lesions. One specific protease identified at the Mayo Clinic (kallikrein 6) is particularly associated with active demyelination within the MS plaque. Kallikreins are a group of proteases of which the best-known member is prostate-specific antigen (PSA). PSA has become the most important marker of malignancy in clinical practice. Other proteases (and likely kallikreins) may also become specific markers of other disease processes. If these proteases are associated directly with a demyelinating event, then it would be reasonable to design protease inhibitors to target a specific population of enzymes, which could be beneficial in the MS lesion.

Axonal degeneration in MS has been an area of extensive investigation in the last few years (see the chapter by C.L. Howe on axonal pathology). It was once thought that axons were relatively preserved in MS lesions. However, loss of axons has been demonstrated in both acute and chronic plaques, since 20%-30% of axons may be lost within the lesion. Clinical deficits, especially long-term disability, best correlate with the degree of axonal loss. Therefore, understanding the mechanisms of axonal pathology in MS is important. It is possible that demyelination in itself results in axonal pathology. This is supported by the concept that oligodendrocytes provide nutritive factors to axons. Without these factors, axons would then degenerate. The other possibility is that an active immune-mediated mechanism destroys axons. Here again, CD8$^+$ T cells are the most likely culprit. Data both from experimental animals and human disease demonstrate a close association between the number of CD8$^+$ T cells and the degree of axonal pathology. In experimental animals, deletion of the CD8$^+$ T cells, either by genetic knockouts or with antibody treatment directed to these cells, results in improved function with preservation of axons. In addition, a large number of neuroprotective strategies may be applicable to the MS lesion. Traditionally, these strategies have been considered important in diseases such as stroke, where there is ischemia or anoxia. Recent evidence indicates that some of the same factors upregulated in ischemia may also be upregulated in the MS lesion (see the chapter by C.F. Lucchinetti). This suggests that similar neuroprotective factors may be utilized for treatment in MS.

The area of genetics has received wide attention in the last 20 years. MS traditionally is not considered a genetic disease, although there is an increase in concordance in identical twins in MS compared to fraternal twins. However, this concordance is only between 20% and 25%. While this indicates a genetic component, clearly environmental factors account for most of the variance. In an effort to understand the important genetic factors in MS, many large genome studies have been performed (see the chapter by J.P. McElroy and J. Oksenberg). To date, the only genetic factor consistently demonstrated to be associated with MS is HLA, specifically the DR2 haplotype associated with CD4$^+$ T cells; this has been consistently observed in most subsets of MS patients. This genetic factor, however, only explains a very small percentage of the genetic variance of MS. Clearly, other genes also play a role. Unfortunately, large genome studies have failed to identify these genes, and it is possible that the difficulty has been in grouping all MS patients together. If the neuropathological observations hold true, there may be specific subtypes of MS. It may be necessary to perform genetic studies segregating the various subtypes of MS to see if associations are stronger. The pathological substrates (see the chapter by C.F. Lucchinetti) are very distinct in that they either target the myelin sheaths or the oligodendrocytes. It would be reasonable to assume that different genetic factors play a role in each of these various subtypes.

In addition, genetics may also play a role in the degree of spontaneous remyelination occurring in MS (see the chapter by A.J. Bieber). Some genetic strains in experimental models spontaneously remyelinate following a demyelinating incident, but others do not. Mating studies between these strains have shown the remyelinating components to be dominant, such that remyelination is expressed as a dominant trait. Similar events may occur in MS lesions. Some patients spontaneously remyelinate following MS attacks and recover completely following acute events. In contrast, other patients develop an acute attack from which they never fully recover; these patients are less likely to exhibit full remyelination. No genetic studies in MS thus far have compared patients who remyelinate (recover completely from MS attack) to those who do not remyelinate (fail to recover from acute attacks). Genetic studies of the experimental models may provide unique insights on how to study the genetics of MS.

To develop successful treatments for remyelination, we will need specific surrogates of remyelination to follow in clinical trials. The most obvious surrogate for studying remyelination is magnetic resonance imaging (MRI) (see the chapter by B.J. Erickson and the chapter by I. Pirko and A.J. Johnson). Preliminary data in experimental animals suggest an association between remyelination and decreased size of T1 and T2 lesions. In addition, magnetic transfer may be a reliable measure and surrogate marker for remyelination. These observations will require detailed study in experimental animals before they can be applied to clinical trials in MS. However, given that treatment approaches for remyelination may soon reach the clinical arena, it becomes essential to develop MRI technologies to distinguish between remyelinated and non-remyelinated lesions.

Further studies in the epidemiology of MS may help determine the pathogenesis of the disease or may give a link to treatment. This has been the case in the investigation of the link between uric acid and demyelination (see the chapter by S. Spitsin and H. Koprowski). Epidemiological studies have shown that patients with high uric acid are less likely to develop MS, whereas MS tends to be associated with lower levels of uric acid. Whether this observation can be converted into a clinical treatment paradigm remains to be determined. Similarly, the statin drugs commonly used for the treatment of lipid metabolism disorders are gaining significant interest for the treatment of MS. These statin drugs may have an effect on the immune system that may be beneficial in MS. Some experimental studies using these statin drugs are in process, while others are under consideration. Of concern is the statin drugs' effect on lipid metabolism, since myelin itself is a lipid membrane. It is unknown whether statins in themselves are detrimental from the standpoint of oligodendrocyte function. It will be important to determine whether the use of statin drugs is associated with different clinical outcomes in MS. The issue is complex because there may be both beneficial and harmful effects of statins. Statins may be beneficial in downregulating the immune system; however, statins may also be harmful to lipid membranes causing injury to the oligodendrocyte (see the chapter by M.S. Weber and S.S. Zamvil).

Similarly, based on the observation that MS improves during pregnancy, there is growing interest in using hormone therapy in MS (see the chapter by E.A. Shuster). Again, hormones such as estrogen and progesterone may positively affect the immune system while potentially harming myelin/oligodendrocyte biology.

Finally, we hope that the reader will appreciate the diversity of approaches needed to understand the pathogenesis of this most disabling disease. Only by discarding the paradigm that the inflammatory response is the causative factor of MS will we make significant headway in the treatment of this disease. Clearly, inflammatory response influences pathogenesis; however, whether it is the primary contributor to the demyelinating disease process or whether it is primarily a response to an exogenous factor and therefore, playing a reparative role, still remains undetermined. The work of the talented investigators contributing to the various chapters of this book provides great hope for our patients with MS. These investigators are dedicated to finding a cure and ultimately eliminating this disease completely from the textbook of neurological diseases. One cannot help but draw analogies to human poliomyelitis. During polio outbreaks, hundreds of patients were hospitalized and required respiratory support with the use of iron lungs. The dedicated efforts of investigators, scientists, epidemiologists, virologists, immunologists and clinicians identified a single causative agent that induced poliomyelitis. Development of a vaccine for polio has led to the near disappearance of poliomyelitis in most parts of the world. We work toward a similar scenario in our lifetime with MS.

I wish to acknowledge the editorial support of Lea Dacy at Mayo Clinic College of Medicine and the production support of Anne Clauss at Springer.

Moses Rodriguez, MD

# Contents

# Contributors

A. J. Bieber
Department of Neurology, Mayo Clinic College of Medicine, 200 First Street SW,
Rochester, MN 55905, USA, bieber.allan@mayo.edu

W. F. Blakemore
Department of Veterinary Medicine and Cambridge Centre for Brain Repair,
University of Cambridge, Madingley Road, Cambridge CB3 OES, UK,
wfb1000@cam.ac.uk

B. J. Erickson
Department of Radiology, Mayo Clinic College of Medicine, 200 First Street SW,
Rochester, MN 55905, USA, BJE@mayo.edu

R. J. M. Franklin
Department of Veterinary Medicine and Cambridge Centre for Brain Repair,
University of Cambridge, Madingley Road, Cambridge CB3 OES, UK
rjf1000@cam.ac.uk

C. L. Howe
Departments of Neuroscience and Neurology, Translational Immunovirology and
Biodefense Program, Molecular Neuroscience Program, Mayo Clinic College of
Medicine, 200 First Street SW, Rochester, MN 55905, USA,
howe.charles@mayo.edu

A. J. Johnson
Department of Neurology, Waddell Center for Multiple Sclerosis, University of
Cincinnati, 231 Albert Sabin Way, ML 0525, Cincinnati, OH 45267-0525, USA

H. Koprowski
Thomas Jefferson University, 1020 Locust St, JAH Room M85, Philadelphia,
PA 19107, USA, hilary.koprowski@jefferson.edu

C. Lucchinetti
Department of Neurology, Mayo Clinic College of Medicine, 200 First Street SW,
Rochester, MN 55905, USA, clucchinetti@mayo.edu

J. P. McElroy
Department of Neurology, School of Medicine, University of California
at San Francisco, San Francisco, CA 94143, USA

J. R. Oksenberg
Department of Neurology, School of Medicine, University of California
at San Francisco, San Francisco, CA 94143, USA, Jorge.Oksenberg@ucsf.edu

I. Pirko
Department of Neurology, Waddell Center for Multiple Sclerosis,
University of Cincinnati, 231 Albert Sabin Way, ML 0525,
Cincinnati, OH 45267-0525, USA, Istvan.Pirko@uc.edu

S. J. Pittock
Department of Neurology, Mayo Clinic, College of Medicine, 200 First Street SW,
Rochester, MN 55905, USA, pittock.sean@mayo.edu

M. Rodriguez
Departments of Neurology and Immunology, Mayo Clinic, College of Medicine,
200 First Street SW, Rochester, MN 55905, USA, rodriguez.moses@mayo.edu

I. A. Scarisbrick
Departments of Physical Medicine and Rehabilitation, Neurology, Physiology
and Biomedical Engineering, Mayo College of Medicine, 200 First Street SW,
Rochester, MN 55905, USA, Scarisbrick.Isobel@Mayo.edu

E. A. Shuster
Department of Neurology, Mayo Clinic College of Medicine, Jacksoviville,
FL 32220, USA, shuster.elizabeth@mayo.edu

S. Spitsin
Thomas Jefferson University, 1020 Locust St, JAH Room M85, Philadelphia,
PA 19107, USA

A. E. Warrington
Department of Neurology, Mayo Clinic College of Medicine,
Rochester, MN 55905, USA, Warrington.arthur@mayo.edu

M. S. Weber
Department of Neurology, University of California, San Francisco, 513 Parnassus
Avenue, S-268, San Francisco, CA 94143-0435, USA

B. G. Weinshenker
Department of Neurology, Mayo Clinic College of Medicine, 200 First Street SW,
Rochester, MN 55901, USA, weinb@mayo.edu

D. M. Wingerchuk
Department of Neurology, Mayo Clinic College of Medicine, Scottsdale,
AZ, USA

S. S. Zamvil
Department of Neurology, University of California, San Francisco,
513 Parnassus Avenue, S-268, San Francisco, CA 94143-0435, USA,
zamvil@ucsf.neuroimmunol.org

# Benign Multiple Sclerosis: A Distinct Clinical Entity with Therapeutic Implications

S.J. Pittock(✉) and M. Rodriguez

**Abstract**   This chapter describes the natural history of multiple sclerosis and, in particular, reviews the controversy regarding the entity of benign multiple sclerosis. Based on the Olmsted County population prevalence cohort study performed at the Mayo Clinic, MS patients with EDSS scores of 2 or lower followed for a period of 5–10 years have a very small risk of developing disability over the next 10–20 years. Based on these findings, this chapter reviews the indications, efficacy, mode of action, and side effect profiles of the currently approved and available disease-modifying agents for the treatment of multiple sclerosis. The efficacy of these agents is discussed based on the concepts of evidence-based medicine and the natural history of the disease. We review the arguments for and against treating all patients with MS. The authors propose an individualized approach to the use of these agents in the MS population.

S.J. Pittock

Department of Neurology, Department of Laboratory Medicine and Pathology, Mayo Clinic College of Medicine, 200 First Street SW, Rochester, MN 55905, USA
e-mail: pittock.sean@mayo.edu

M. Rodriguez (ed.), *Advances in Multiple Sclerosis and Experimental*
*Demyelinating Diseases. Current Topics in Microbiology and Immunology 318.*
© Springer-Verlag Berlin Heidelberg 2008

# 1 Introduction

The past decade has witnessed significant advances in the understanding of the pathophysiology of MS and in the development of novel disease-modifying agents (DMA). The use of DMA in the treatment of patients with MS has drastically increased not only in the United States but throughout the rest of the world. Currently, in the United States, most patients given a diagnosis of relapsing-remitting MS are commenced on a DMA. Controversy still exists regarding how early DMA should be commenced and whether all patients with relapsing-remitting MS should in fact be treated [21, 54]. To answer these questions, it is important to know the natural history of the disease.

The public associates a diagnosis of MS with the need for a wheelchair and certain disability. This misinformation may motivate many patients with a recent diagnosis of MS or a clinically isolated syndrome to initiate long-term DMA. In order for the patient and physician to make the best therapeutic decision for the patient, both parties must study DMA efficacy, the side effects, mode of administration, and costs, and review the natural history of the disease.

In this chapter, we will describe the natural history of MS and review the controversies regarding the entity of benign MS. We will review the indications, efficacy, mode of action and side effect profiles of the currently available FDA approved DMA. We will discuss the importance of evidence-based medicine and natural history studies in treatment decision making. We will review the arguments for and against treating all patients. We will discuss a possible change from the blockbuster to a more individualized patient care approach.

# 2 Natural History of Multiple Sclerosis: Disability Progression

Upon receiving a diagnosis of MS, patients are generally most concerned with their long-term prognosis. Long-term follow-up studies of MS natural history cohorts from many different regions including Lyon, France [10, 11], Gothenburg Sweden [14, 58], Olmsted County, Minnesota, USA [50, 51, 57], London, Ontario, [67, 69] and British Columbia [65] Canada provide useful information on the accumulation of disability in MS. Most of these natural history studies define the course of the disease over a long period of time in an untreated population.

These studies have relied heavily on the use of the expanded disability status scale score (EDSS) as an outcome measure [35]. The EDSS, a measure of impairment, ranges from a level of zero (no disability) to ten (death). Three cutoff scores used consistently throughout natural history studies include EDSS 3 (or 4 in some), moderate dysfunction including monoparesis or mild hemiparesis; EDSS 6, which indicates a need for unilateral assistance (need for a care); and EDSS 8 (or 7 in some), in which the patient is restricted to a wheelchair but retains effective use of arms. Time from onset (or diagnosis) of MS to the assignment of one of these disability scores has been estimated in many studies and provides information regarding the rate of accumulation of physical disability.

**Table 1** Median time from onset of MS to selected EDSS levels of disability

|                                          | EDSS 3 | EDSS 6 | EDSS 8 |
| ---------------------------------------- | ------ | ------ | ------ |
| Lyon, France [8]                         | 6 [a]  |        | 18 [b] |
| Lyon, France [10]                        | 8.4 [a]| 20.1   | 29.9 [b]|
| Gothenburg, Sweden [58]                  | –      | 18     | –      |
| London, Ontario, Middlesex County [67]   | 9      | 16     | 33     |
| Olmsted County [50]                      | 23     | 28     | 52     |
| British Columbia [65]                    | –      | 28     | –      |
| Turkey [29]                              | 11     | 18     | –      |

[a] denotes median time from onset on EDSS 4;
[b] denotes median time from onset to EDSS 7

The median time from onset of MS to EDSS 3 or 4 (mild disability) reported in studies is the most variable ranging from 6 to 23 years. (Table 1) EDSS 6 is a more reliable and robust measure, and thus median times from onset of MS to EDSS 6 (need for a cane) are more consistent between studies varying from 16 to 28 years. There is a significant difference in median time from onset to EDSS 6 in the1980s compared with 2000 population-based study in Lyon, France (18 years and 30 years, respectively). This difference may be related to the fact that the 1980 cohort was exclusively hospital-based [8, 10, 11]. In addition, these results relate to all types of MS patients (relapsing-remitting and progressive).

MS type, whether relapsing or progressive, has a significant impact on disability outcome. In the Olmsted County 2000 study, the estimated median time from MS onset to EDSS 6 for patients remaining relapsing-remitting MS was 51 years. This compares with 17.9 years for secondary progressive and 6.3 years for primary progressive MS [50]. In the Lyon, France study, 1,562 patients had a relapsing course at onset and had median time from onset to EDSS 4, 6, and 7 of 11, 23, and 33 years, respectively, compared with 0, 7, and 13 years, respectively for 282 patients with a progressive course [10, 11]. This and other recent studies have reported that progression of MS was slower than had been previously reported [65] and that many patients with MS, especially those that remain relapsing-remitting, may have a more favorable outcome than previously assumed.

## 3 Benign MS: A Fallacy or a Distinct Clinical Entity?

A significant subgroup of MS patients (approximately 30%) have little disease progression and minimal or no disability after many years of disease [9]. Controversy exists regarding the definition of benign MS, which is both complicated by the limitations of measurement tools and differences in data interpretation. Though the natural history is favorable for patients considered benign after a certain disease duration, not all will remain well as time continues [24, 52, 59]. Clearly, however, the longer the duration of MS together with a low level of disability, the more likely it becomes that a patient will remain stable and not progress [52]. This is currently the best clinical predictor of long-term outcome and has been recognized for at least the past 30 years.

Charcot suggested the concept that some patients with MS may have a mild course in 1872 when he wrote "it is not rare to encounter complete remission, which is hoped to be definitive" [6]. McAlpine reported that 62 (26%) of 241 hospital-based patients followed for at least 15 years (mean disease duration of 18.2 years) were ambulatory and could walk for greater than 500 m without assistance and were "without restriction of activity for normal employment and domestic purpose but not necessarily symptom free "[44]. Multiple long-term follow-up studies of a large natural history cohort have reported a similar and strikingly consistent frequency of benign disease[9].

In the Lyon cohort of 1,844 patients, 26% of all MS patients studied had EDSS less than 4 after 20 years disease duration [10, 11]. There is currently no consensus agreement on the definition of benign MS. Before the introduction of the EDSS, various definitions existed. For example, McAlpine described it as "working away from or at home and could walk at least half a mile without a rest or support" [43], whereas Bauer defined benign course as "the ability to work after 20 years" [4]. Even after the introduction of the EDSS [35], which permitted the definition of benign course by a certain score after a specific disease duration, there still has been a lack of consensus. Definitions of benign MS have varied in terms of the disability score (0–4) and the duration of disease (5–15 years) [56]. Most consider benign MS as an EDSS ≤ 3.0 after disease duration of10 years or more. Others have suggested using a progression index (EDSS score/disease duration) [61]. An international survey by the National MS Society in the United States arrived at a consensus definition of disease in which the patient remains fully functional in all neurological systems 15 years after onset [42]. More recently, smaller studies suggested that a better definition of benign MS should be an EDSS ≤ 2 ≥ 10 years [52]. With these multiple varying definitions, it is difficult to compare results from one study with another and even more problematic to estimate the actual frequency of benign MS.

## 4  Does Benign MS Stay Benign with Increasing Disease Duration?

Another important issue is whether patients with an initial diagnosis of benign MS actually remain benign with the passage of time. In other words, how benign is benign [49]? For example, in the French cohort of 1,844 patients, 35% of patients had not reached an EDSS 4 at 15 years, 26% had not reached EDSS 4 at 20 years, and 13% had not reached EDSS 4 at 30 years. These results suggest that the likelihood of remaining benign decreases with the duration of the disease [10, 11].

Recent natural history studies have tried to address this issue. In the 2001 Olmsted County MS study, the authors investigated the level of disability and the duration of disease as predictors of subsequent EDSS a decade later [52]. All patients from the 1991 Olmsted County MS prevalence cohort who were then considered to have benign MS (EDSS ≤ 4 for ≥ 10 years) were followed up in 2001 (or ≥ 20 years disease duration). To patients with minimal disability (EDSS ≤ 2 for ≥ 10 years) in 1991, the authors asked how they were doing after an additional decade had passed. Of 28 relapsing-remitting MS patients with EDSS ≤ 2 for ≥ 10 years in 1991, 93% continued to have a low disability (EDSS ≤ 3) after an additional decade (Fig. 1a). No patient in this group developed secondary progressive MS. Most patients (all but two) continued to be employed. All described their quality of life as satisfactory or better.

For 21 patients with moderate disability (EDSS 2.5–4, for ≥ 10 years) in 1991, 43% continued to have mild to moderate disability after an additional decade, but 57% did develop significant disability (Fig. 1b). Of 21 patients, 14 (67%) had a

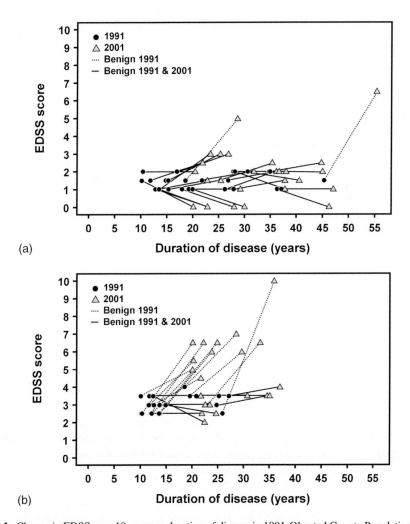

(a)

(b)

**Fig. 1** Change in EDSS over 10 years vs duration of disease in 1991-Olmsted County Population Based MS study 2001. **a** How are patients with minimal disability (EDSS ≤ 2 for ≥ 10 years) doing a further decade later? **b** How are patients with moderate disability (EDSS 2.5–4 for ≥ 10 years) doing a further decade later?

worsened EDSS, 12 (57%) progressed to EDSS >4, and eight (38%) required unilateral or bilateral assistance to walk and had developed secondary progressive MS. The authors suggested that a better definition of benign MS was an EDSS ≤ 2 for ≥ 10 years, since the chances of these patients developing significant disability in the future was less than 10%.

A recent but similar study of a large British Columbia MS cohort ($n=2,204$), reported 20-year follow-up EDSS in 169 out of 200 patients who had EDSS ≤ 3 after 10 years [59]. For patients with EDSS ≤ 2 for 10 years, 68% continued as benign at 20 years. For those with EDSS ≤ 3 for 10 years, only 52% continued to be benign, 21.3% required the use of a cane, and 23% had developed secondary progressive disease. The only variable associated with disease progression at 20 years was the 10-year EDSS score. The slight differences in likelihood of patients with EDSS ≤ 2 after 10 or more years remaining benign after 20 years or more (93% vs 68%), may be a result of differing methodologies. The Olmsted County study, though a much smaller study, was population-based with 100% ascertainment. More than half the patients, when evaluated at the first time point in 1991, had MS for more than 20 years and thus MS for more than 30 years at the 10-year follow-up point in 2001. Sayao et al.'s exclusion of patients with onset of symptoms prior to 1978 in their study (patients that accounted for 50% of the Olmsted County benign cohort) may account for some of the difference. Considering both studies, the chances of a patient with a benign course (EDSS ≤ 2 after 10 years or more) of remaining ambulatory without significant disability is between 68% and 93%. Furthermore, both studies found that the best clinical predictor of long-term outcome is how well a patient fares over the initial 10-year period, although both the above studies used ≥ 10 years from onset as the cutoff for defining a likelihood of a benign course. Further analysis of the Olmsted County data suggests the 5-year cutoff, as previously reported by Kurtzke and colleagues, as a duration of disease at which prediction of outcome was more reliable [34].

## 5  Other Clinical Predictors of MS Outcome

There have been many different variables reported in large natural history studies associated with disability outcome [9]. Most studies report that a younger age of onset, female gender, and optic neuritis as a first attack were indicators of a better prognosis [10, 11, 14, 29, 58, 67, 68]. On the other hand, cerebellar, brainstem, or motor presentations are typically associated with a worse outcome [69]. Many studies, however, have not replicated these findings, and some have even reported the opposite [3, 36, 37, 39, 40, 46].

Since one of the two most proven benefits of DMAs is the reduction in relapse rate, an important issue is whether a higher incidence of attacks early in the disease process impacts the clinical course and long-term disability in natural history studies. Unfortunately, this again is controversial. Longitudinal studies from Lyon, France, and London, Ontario, as well as a small study from

Turkey, reported a statistically significant association between numbers of relapses during the early years of MS and subsequent development of disability [8, 10, 29, 67]. However, the effect was weak. Others have not found any association between numbers of attacks in the early years of MS and disability outcome [19, 34, 48]. Whether the frequency of early attacks in MS has long-term implications remains controversial. If it does, however, natural history studies suggest that its effect is weak. This raises concern, since one of the arguments for initiating early immunomodulatory medications in patients with MS is that prevention or reduction in the frequency of early attacks may have some long-term protective benefit in terms of disability.

Despite a statistically significant *p*-value in many large natural history studies, the strength of association of all of these variables with disability outcome is weak and likely of little practical predictive value in an individual patient. Furthermore, combining clinical imaging or laboratory variables to perform multivariate analysis has been unhelpful, and combinations of predictors have not been shown to improve predictive power as many of these variables are interdependent [9].

A recent 2006 systematic review of clinical and demographic predictors of long-term disability in patients with relapsing-remitting MS reported that the most robust predictors were sphincter symptoms at onset and early disease outcomes. Incomplete recovery from the first attack and a shorter time to second attack seemed to predict a worse prognosis. Furthermore, the review found that a higher early relapse frequency was not always associated with poor prognosis [38].

# 6  Neuroimaging Studies in Benign MS

Recent magnetic transfer imaging studies reveal evidence of milder underlying brain pathology. This supports the argument that benign MS does truly exist and may be differentiated from other forms of the illness. De Stefano and colleagues carried out conventional MRI and magnetization transfer imaging in 50 patients with benign MS (EDSS< 3, disease duration >15 years) and compared their findings with 50 MS patients with early (EDSS 3, disease duration < 3 years) relapsing-remitting disease [13]. They found lesional and nonlesional magnetic transfer imaging values to be significantly less pronounced in benign MS than in the cohort of relapsing-remitting patients at their earliest disease stage. This suggests that brain tissue damage is milder in benign MS.

In a study of benign MS, secondary progressive MS, and healthy controls, spinal cord area and transverse decimeter at C5 on MRI were inversely correlated with the degree of disability; this likely reflects preservation of neural tissue in benign MS [16]. Other studies have failed to show a good correlation between amount of white matter lesions on T2-weighted MR and disability [15, 31, 53, 62]. The rate of development of new gadolinium-enhancing lesions is, however, less than in the relapsing-remitting patients [63]. Similar numbers of brain lesions have been reported for both benign and secondary progressive MS despite significant in disability in the latter [16, 17, 28, 33]. Figure 2 demonstrates the variability of MRI findings in benign MS (EDSS ≤ for > 20 years) for six patients.

Small sample size, differing definitions of clinical course, and lack of an ideal control group may explain the conflicting results reported in the literature [5, 12, 15, 16, 18, 25, 45, 64, 66]. Though differences in magnetization transfer imaging have

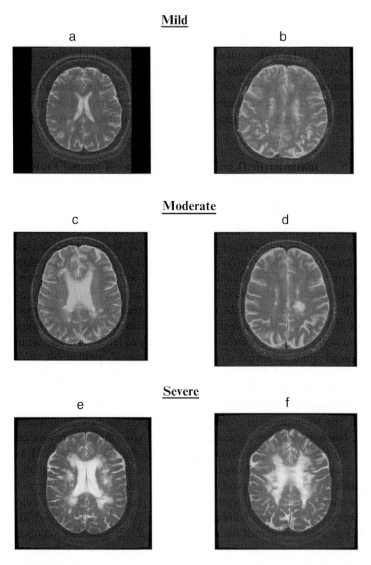

**Fig. 2A–F** Variability in MRI appearance of six patients with so-called benign MS (EDSS 3, duration >20 years). All are axial T2-weighted MRI images at or slightly above the level of the lateral ventricles

been shown between those with benign MS and those with early relapsing-remitting MS, future studies need to address whether MT measures are predictive of clinical and pathological evolution of MS.

In summary, regardless of the definition, significant numbers of patients (probably between 20% and 30%) continue to have a favorable course with low levels of disability despite a long duration of disease. A diagnosis of benign MS does not entirely guarantee a continued favorable course, but the odds are in the patient's favor. With this in mind, we need to consider the currently available immunomodulatory medications.

# 7 The Currently FDA-Approved Disease-Modifying Agents: Efficacy, Mode of Action, and Side Effects

Over the past 15 years, multiple large randomized clinical trials have shown DMA to reduce both relapse rate and the development of new MRI lesions. There are currently several licensed and FDA-approved DMA (all parenteral) for use in MS. These agents include (a) three beta interferon preparations (Avonex, Betaseron, and Rebif), (b) glatiramer acetate (Copaxone), (c) mitoxantrone (Novantrone), and (d) the monoclonal antibody natalizumab (Tysabri). The Executive Committee of the Medical Advisory Board of the National MS Society has adopted the following recommendations: "consideration of treatment as soon as possible following the definite diagnosis of MS with active disease (i.e. recent relapses and or new lesions on MRI) and may also be considered for some patients with a first attack who are at high risk in developing MS (known as clinically isolated syndrome)." The Therapeutics and Technology Assessment Committee of the American Academy of Neurology and the MS Council of Clinical Practice guidelines also suggest that it is appropriate to consider treatment with approved therapy in these patients. Furthermore, the treat all approach has been a growing trend in the United States, and this has been supported by many leaders in the field. The presentation of data to the reader can result in a significant problem when reviewing DMA efficacy in the literature. Most studies present efficacy data in terms of relative risk reduction, which overinflates benefit, especially if the control event rate is small. Here we will discuss numbers needed to treat (NNT).

## 7.1 Beta Interferon Therapies (Avonex, Betaseron, and Rebif)

### 7.1.1 Efficacy

The IFNβ drugs have been shown to reduce both relapse rate (by approximately 30%) and the accrual of new lesions on brain MRI in patients with relapsing-remitting disease [1]. For patients with a clinically isolated syndrome (CIS), seven to nine patients needed to be treated for 2 years to prevent one patient developing clinically definite MS. The Champions group compared immediate vs delayed interferon therapy in CIS and reported that 33 patients need to be treated for 5 years to prevent a single patient developing an EDSS of 2.5 [32]. Similarly, for RRMS, 6–13 patients require treatment for approximately 2 years to increase by one the number of patients free of relapse, and 8–13 patients must be treated for 2 years to prevent one patient developing an increase in EDSS [20]. The NNT mentioned above may be underestimated, since randomized control trials contain an enriched sample of patients who differ from patients seen in a population-based sample. Current data suggest that IFNβ-1a, 44 mcg subcutaneously three times per week, provides the most favorable benefit-to-risk ratio of the available DMA [20].

The role of IFNβ in secondary progressive MS is unclear. A European study reported a modest benefit [2], but subsequent North American trials [7, 22, 41, 60] did not confirm this finding.

### 7.1.2   Mode of Action

A variety of action mechanisms have been reported, including inhibition of T-cell co-stimulation and/or activation processes, modulation of anti-inflammatory and pro-inflammatory cytokines, inhibition of interferon gamma-induced class-II expression, inhibition of antigen presentation, and reduction in aberrant T-cell migration. IFNβs are administered either by subcutaneous injection (Betaseron and Rebif) or by intramuscular injection (Avonex).

### 7.1.3   Adverse Effects

Injection site reactions usually subside within weeks. Management includes icing and rotation of site, topical application of anesthetics or corticosteroid, improved injection technique, and warming the medication or using autoinjectors. Flu-like symptoms are common; dose titration, nonsteroidal anti-inflammatory drugs (NSAIDS) or acetaminophen may be helpful, though symptoms usually resolve by 3 months [70]. Symptoms occur within a few hours of each injection and last 12–24 h. Injections should be administered at night. Hematologic and hepatic function abnormalities may occur; therefore, complete blood count and liver function test monitoring is recommended at baseline, 1 week, 1 month, 3 months and then every 3–6 months thereafter. Treatment-related depression may occur, and patients and their caregivers should report any mood changes. Women may experience menstrual disorders. Women of child-bearing age should practice contraception, and women planning to become pregnant should discontinue IFNβ at least 3 months prior to discontinuation of contraception to avoid the reported risks of spontaneous abortion, still birth, and lower mean birth weight. Neutralizing antibodies (NAb) occur in up to 45% of patients on IFNβ therapy and reduce biological activity. If high titers of antibodies are identified, discontinuation of IFNβ in favor of one of the other DMAs may be appropriate [30].

## 7.2   Glatiramer Acetate (Copaxone)

### 7.2.1   Efficacy

Glatiramer acetate (GA), approved for use in relapsing-remitting MS, has mild benefits in the short term. It reduces the relapse rate and disease activity on MRI and may have some long-term disability benefit, although data are difficult to interpret because of high patient attrition in the controlled clinical trials [27, 47]. For relapsing-remitting disease, 14 patients need to be treated for 2 years to increase by one the number of patients free of relapse [20, 26].

### 7.2.2   Mode of Action

GA is administered subcutaneously daily and has multiple mechanisms of action that influence T-cell activation/proliferation, dendritic cell co-stimulation processes, antigen presentation, neurotrophic factors, cytokines, interferon gamma secretion, and regulatory TH2/3 cells [47].

### 7.2.3   Adverse Effects

GA is generally well tolerated. Injection site reaction is common and managed as for IFN reactions [70]. Lipoatrophy occurs in up to 46% of patients on long-term therapy. There is no treatment, but injection into an area of lipoatrophy should be avoided.

Lymphadenopathy (up to 30% of patients in clinical trials) is usually limited to inguinal nodes but may be generalized. Injection site rotation and/or discontinuation of injections may be beneficial. Benign systemic reaction (chest tightness, anxiety, palpitations, or dyspnea) occur in less than 15% of patients within a few minutes after injection and last 30 s to 30 min. Long-term treatment with GA does *not* result in hematologic or liver enzyme abnormalities. Binding antibodies to GA may develop within 3–4 months after initiation of therapy but do not interfere with efficacy.

## 7.3   Mitoxantrone (Novantrone)

Mitoxantrone, an anthracenedione agent, reduces relapse rate as well as numbers of T2 and gadolinium-enhancing lesions on MRI in patients with relapsing-remitting MS or early secondary progressive MS (with active inflammatory disease and evidence of substantial disease worsening over short periods of time) [23, 47]. There is no proven benefit for patients with relapse independent progression. The drug is generally used in patients with aggressive relapsing-remitting or secondary progressive disease. For patients with progressive disease, The NNT for 2 years to prevent one patient from worsening by 1 EDSS point was 11.

### 7.3.1 Mode of Action

Mitoxantrone reduces T- and B-cell immunity by inhibition of both DNA and RNA synthesis.

### 7.3.2 Adverse Effects

Patients may notice a temporary blue discoloration of the urine and sclerae. Leukopenia and neutropenia occur commonly. CBC should be monitored closely, and if the white blood cell count drops to less than $3,000/\mu l$ or if neutrophils are less than 1,500/l, mitoxantrone should be held. Liver function tests (LFTs) should also be monitored, and therapy held if LFTs increase by more than 2.5 beyond the upper limits [70].

Cardiomyopathy is dose-dependent and may be as great as 6% in patients receiving $140$ mg/m$^2$ or less [47]. Prior to each infusion, patients should have an echocardiogram to evaluate their ejection fraction. Delayed effects of mitoxantrone on cardiac function have been reported. Antiemetic premedication (with ondansetron) may alleviate nausea during and for several days after infusion. Alopecia, amenorrhea, and infertility may also occur. Mitoxantrone is teratogenic. Leukemia occurs in approximately 1% of patients and generally responds to treatment.

## 7.4 Natalizumab (Tysabri)

Natalizumab, a recombinant humanized IgG-4 kappa monoclonal antibody, appears to have significantly greater efficacy than any of the other DMAs. It reduces the rate of clinical relapse by 68% and reduced sustained disability progression at 2 years by 42%. The NNT to render one patient relapse-free after 2 years of therapy is between 2 and 4. Unfortunately, despite its greater efficacy in terms of relapse rate and MRI lesion load reduction, natalizumab (approved for use in 2004) was withdrawn from the market in 2005 due to the development of progressive multifocal leukoencephalopathy (PML) in two patients. Natalizumab has recently become available again but only under a restricted distribution program called the TOUCH (Tysabri Outreach: Unified Commitment to Health) Prescribing Program.

### 7.4.1 Mode of Action

Natalizumab inhibits the molecular interaction of alpha 4, beta 1 integrin with the vascular cell adhesion molecule (VCAM)-1 on activated vascular endothelium, thus preventing leukocyte transmigration across the blood–brain barrier. Natalizumab is administered by monthly infusions.

### 7.4.2 Adverse Effects

Two cases of PML have been reported in 1,859 MS patients treated with natalizumab. The risk of for PML in patients treated with natalizumab is roughly 1 in 1,000 patients [71]. Readers should refer to the TOUCH Prescribing Program issued by Biogen Idec and Elan for guidelines. Hypersensitivity reactions occur in 1%–4% of patients within 2 h of infusion and should be treated by stopping the infusion. Acetaminophen, antihistamines, corticosteroids, and fluids should be used as necessary. Natalizumab may increase the risk for infection; concurrent use of antineoplastic immunosuppressant or immunomodulation medications is not recommended. Approximately 6% of patients present with antinatalizumab antibodies, and the result is a reduction in efficacy and an increase in infusion-related side effects [55].

## 8  Should All MS Patients Be Treated with Disease-Modifying Therapies?

### 8.1  Clinical Implications of Benign MS

The default position regarding the use of DMA in the USA currently seems to be to treat. This, however, remains controversial [21, 54]. The decision to treat a patient with a DMA should be based upon a shared patient/physician therapeutic decision-making model. This model incorporates knowledge of the natural history of the disease, evidence-based medicine, and the patient's personal preference. Evidence-based medicine statistics inform us of the magnitude of benefit of the currently available DMA. As has been discussed above, DMA reduces relapse rate and MRI lesion accrual and has modest benefits in terms of short-term disability. However, the long-term benefits remain unproven [47]. The benefit of treating secondary progressive MS is unclear, and no benefit has been found in primary progressive MS. Patients may be overwhelmed by the data and unwilling to initiate an injectable treatment. They may have significant anxiety regarding the use of subcutaneous or intramuscular injections, although treatments generally are well tolerated and safe. MS often has a favorable natural history. The blockbuster treatment approach of MS may need to become more individualized as evidence-based medicine may not support the treat all approach.

Most natural history studies and clinical trials have been conducted using EDSS as the outcome measure. MS has effects on every aspect of the patient's life. The EDSS, albeit a good measure of MS impairment, does not measure quality of life, symptomatic complaints, employment status, or effects on activities of daily living. Though patients may do well over a long period of time in terms of EDSS measurements, they may not be doing so well in these other areas. Studies investigating these other important nonambulatory outcomes in patients deemed benign are ongoing. Furthermore, it is still unclear whether DMA benefits these outcomes over a period of many years.

One approach might be to consider initiation of DMA in patients who have active disease, either clinically (relapses) or radiographically (new or enhancing lesions) [49]. However, other patients may be appropriate candidates for a watchful waiting approach. These include patients with a greater chance of a benign course such as those with a low EDSS score at 5 years with infrequent attacks and little accumulation of MRI lesion. Likewise, patients with established progressive disease without clinical or radiologic markers of active disease might not require DMA treatment. Finally, patients with an indeterminate prognosis of clinically isolated syndrome or early relapsing-remitting MS with infrequent mild attacks lacking evidence of disease activity on MRI and a favorable prognostic profile may also benefit from postponed treatment. Patients who fully recover from their attacks may also be candidates for delayed therapy. These patients are more likely to have a remyelinating phenotype that may be altered by the drugs.

The watchful waiting approach does not imply never treat [54]. Patients in watchful waiting mode should undergo yearly neurological examination and MRI of the head. If the clinical course changes or if the MRI shows accumulation of new or enhancing lesions, the caregiver and patient should consider DMA. Some patients will request early treatment regardless of their clinical course or MRI findings, and their wishes should be respected within the shared decision-making model.

# References

1. The IFBN multiple sclerosis study group (1993) Interferon beta-1b is effective in relapsing-remitting multiple sclerosis. I. Clinical results of a multicenter, randomized, double-blind, placebo-controlled trial. Neurology 43:655–661
2. European study group in interferon beta-1b in secondary progressive MS (1998) placebo-controlled multicentre randomised trail of interferon beta-1b in treatment of secondary progressive multiple sclerosis. Lancet 352:1491–1497
3. Amato M, Ponziani G (2000) A prospective study on the prognosis of multiple sclerosis. Neurol Sci 21:831–838
4. Bauer H, Firnhaber W, Winkler W (1965) Prognostic criteria in multiple sclerosis. Ann N Y Acad Sci 122:542–551
5. Brass S, Narayanan S, Antel J, Lapierre Y, Collins L, Arnold D (2004) Axonal damage in multiple sclerosis patients with high versus low expanded disability status scale score. Can J Neurol Sci 31:225–228
6. Charcot J (1872) Leçons sur les maladies du système nerveux faites à La Salpetière. In: Delahaye A, Lecrosnier E (eds) Progres Medicale, Paris
7. Cohen J, Cutter G, Fischer J, Goodman A, Heidenreich F, Kooijmans M, Sandrock A, Rudick R, Simon J, Simonian N, Tsao E, Whitaker J, IMPACT Investigators. (2002) Benefit of interferon beta-1a on MSFC progression in secondary progressive MS. Neurology 59:679–686
8. Confavreux C, Aimard D, Devic M (1980) Course and prognosis of multiple sclerosis assessed by the computerised data processing of 349 patients. Brain 103:281–300
9. Confavreux C, Compston A (2005) The natural history of multiple sclerosis. In: Compston A, Confavreaux C, Lassmann H, McDonald I, Miller D, Noseworthy J et al., (eds) Mcalpine's multiple sclerosis, 4th edn. Churchill Livingston, Philadelphia, pp 183–272

10. Confavreux C, Vukusic S, Adeleine P (2003) Early clinical predictors and progression of irreversible disability in multiple sclerosis: An amnesic process. Brain 126:770–782
11. Confavreux C, Vukusic S, Moreau T, Adeleine P (2000) Relapses and progression of disability in multiple sclerosis. N Engl J Med 343:1430–1438
12. Davie C, Silver N, Barker G, Tofts P, Thompson AJ, McDonald W, Miller D (1999) Does the extent of axonal loss and demyelination from chronic lesions in multiple sclerosis correlate with the clinical subgroup? J Neurol Neurosurg Psychiatry 67:710–715
13. De Stefano N, Battaglini M, Stromillo ML, Zipoli V, Bartolozzi ML, Guidi L, Siracusa G, Portaccio E, Giorgio A, Sorbi S, Federico A, Amato MP (2006) Brain damage as detected by magnetization transfer imaging is less pronounced in benign than in early relapsing multiple sclerosis. Brain 129:2008–2016
14. Eriksson M, Andersen O, Runmarker B (2003) Long-term follow-up of patients with clinically isolated syndromes, relapsing-remitting and secondary progressive multiple sclerosis. Mult Scler 9:260–274
15. Falini A, Calabrese G, Filippi M, Origgi D, Lipari S, Colombo B, Comi G, Scotti G (1998) Benign versus secondary-progressive multiple sclerosis: The potential role of proton MR spectroscopy in defining the nature of disability. ANJR Am J Neuroradiol 19:223–229
16. Filippi M, Campi A, Mammi S, Martinelli V, Locatelli T, Scotti G, Amadio S, Canal N, Comi G (1995) Brain magnetic resonance imaging and multimodal evoked potentials in benign and secondary progressive multiple sclerosis. J Neurol Neurosurg Psychiatry 58:31–37
17. Filippi M, Campi A, Mammi S, Sacares P, MacManus D, Thompson A, Tofts P, McDonald W, Miller D (1994) Benign and secondary progressive multiple sclerosis: A preliminary quantitative MRI study. J Neurol 241:246–251
18. Filippi M, Inglese M, Rovaris M, Sormani M, Horsfield M, Iannucci P, Colombo B, Comi G (2000) Magnetization transfer imaging to monitor the evolution of MS: A 1-year follow-up study. Neurology 55:940–946
19. Fog T, Linnemann F (1970) The course of multiple sclerosis in 73 cases with computer-designed curves. Acta Neurol Scand 46:1–175
20. Francis G (2004) Importance of benefit-to-risk assessment for disease-modifying drugs used to treat MS. J Neurol 251:V42–V49
21. Frohman E, Havrdova E, Lublin F, Barkhof F, Achiron A, Sharief M, Stuve O, Racke M, Steinman L, Weiner H, Olek M, Zivadinov R, Corboy J, Raine C, Cutter G, Richert J, Filippi M (2006) Most patients with multiple sclerosis or a clinically isolated demyelinating syndrome should be treated at the time of diagnosis. Arch Neurol 63:614–619
22. Goodkin D, Hertsgaard D (2000) Seasonal variation of multiple sclerosis exacerbations in North Dakota. Arch Neurol 46:1015–1018
23. Hartung H, Gonsette R, Konig N, Kwiecinski H, Guseo A, Morrissey S, Krapf H, Zwingers T (2002) Mitoxantrone in progressive multiple sclerosis: A placebo-controlled, double-blind, randomised, multicentre trial. Lancet 360(9350):2018–2025
24. Hawkins S, McDonnella G (1999) Benign multiple sclerosis? Clinical course, long term follow up, and assessment of prognostic factors. J Neurol Neurosurg Psychiatry 67:148–152
25. Horsfield M, Lai M, Webb S, Barker G, Tofts P, Turner R, Rudge P, Miller D (1996) Apparent diffusion coefficients in benign and secondary progressive multiple sclerosis by nuclear magnetic resonance. Magn Reson Med 36:393–400
26. Johnson K, Brooks B, Cohen J, Ford C, Goldstein J, Lisak R, Myers L, Panitch H, Rose J, Schiffer R, Vollmer T, Weiner L, Wolinsky J (1995) Copolymer 1 reduces relapse rate and improves disability in relapsing-remitting multiple sclerosis: Results of a phase III multicenter, double-blind, placebo-controlled trial. Neurology 45:1268–1276
27. Johnson K, Brooks B, Ford C, Goodman A, Guarnaccia J, Lisak R, Myers L, Panitch H, Pruitt A, Rose J, Kachuck N, Wolinsky J (2000) Sustained clinical benefits of glatiramer acetate in relapsing multiple sclerosis patients observed for 6 years. Copolymer 1 multiple sclerosis study group. Mult Scler 6:255–266
28. Kantarci O, De Andrade M, Weinshenker B (2002) Identifying disease modifying genes in multiple sclerosis. J Neuroimmunol 123:144–159

29. Kantarci O, Siva A, Eraksoy M, Karabudak R, Sutlas N, Agaoglu J, Turan F, Ozmenoglu M, Togrul E, Demirkiran M (1998) Survival and predictors of disability in Turkish MS patients. Turkish Multiple Sclerosis Study Group (TUMSSG). Neurology 51:765–772
30. Kappos L, Clanet M, Sandberg-Wollheim M, Radue E, Hartung H, Hohlfeld R, Xu J, Bennett D, Sandrock A, Goelz S (2005) Neutralizing antibodies and efficacy of interferon beta-1a: A 4-year controlled study. Neurology 65:40–47
31. Kermode AG, Tofts PS, Thompson AJ, MacManus DG, Rudge P, Kendall BE, Kingsley DP, Moseley IF, du Boulay EP, McDonald WI (1990) Heterogeneity of blood–brain barrier changes in multiple sclerosis: An MRI study with gadolinium-DTPA enhancement. Neurology 40:229–235
32. Kinkel R (2006) Im interferon β-1a delays definite multiple sclerosis 5 years after a first demyelinating event. Neurology 66:678–684
33. Koopman R, Li D, Grochowsky E, Cutler P, Paty D (1989) Benign versus chronic progressive multiple sclerosis: Magnetic resonance imaging features. Ann Neurol 25:74–81
34. Kurtzke J (1977) Geography in multiple sclerosis. J Neurol 215:1–26
35. Kurtzke J (1983) Rating neurologic impairment in multiple sclerosis: An expanded disability status scale (EDSS). Neurology 33:1444–1452
36. Kurtzke J, Beebe G, Nagler B, Auth T, Kurland L, Nefzger M (1968) Studies on natural history of multiple sclerosis. 4: Clinical features of the onset bout. Acta Neurol Scand 44:467–499
37. Kurtzke J, Beebe G, Nagler B, Nefzger M, Auth T, Kurland L (1970) Studies on the natural history of multiple sclerosis 5: Long-term survival in young men. Arch Neurol 22:215–225
38. Langer-Gould A, Popat R, Huang S, Cobb K, Fontoura P, Gould M (2006) Clinical and demographic predictors of long-term disability in patients with relapsing-remitting multiple sclerosis. Arch Neurol 63:1686–1691
39. Leibowitz U, Alter M (1970) Clinical factors associated with increased disability in multiple sclerosis. Acta Neurol Scand 46:53–70
40. Leibowitz U, Alter M (1973) Multiple sclerosis: Clues to its cause. Amsterdam: North Holland
41. Li D, Zhao G, Paty D, University of British Columbia MS/MRI Analysis Research Group, SPECTRIMS Study Group (2001) Randomized controlled trial of interferon-beta-1a in secondary progressive MS: MRI results. Neurology 56:1505–1513
42. Lublin F, Reingold S (1996) The national multiple sclerosis society USA advisory committee on clinical trails of new agents in multiple sclerosis. Defining the clinical course of multiple sclerosis: Results of an international survey. Neurology 46:907–911
43. McAlpine D (1964) The benign form of multiple sclerosis: Results of a long-term study. BMJ 2:1029–1032
44. McAlpine D, Compston N (1952) Some aspects of the natural history of disseminated sclerosis. Q J Med 21:135–167
45. Minneboo A, Uitdehaag B, Ader H, Barkhof F, Polman C, Castelijns J (2005) Patterns of enhancing lesion evolution in multiple sclerosis are uniform within patients. Neurology 65:56–61
46. Myhr K, Riise T, Vedeler C, Nortvedt MW, Gronning R, Midgard R, Nyland HI (2001) Disability and prognosis in multiple sclerosis: demographic and clinical variables important for the ability to walk and awarding of disability pension. Mult Scler 7:59–65
47. Noseworthy J, Miller D, Compston A (2005) Disease-modifying treatments in multiple sclerosis. Churchill Livingston, London, pp 729–802
48. Patzold U, Pocklington P (1982) Course of multiple sclerosis: Results of a prospective study carried out of 102 MS patients from 1976–1980. Acta Neurol Scand 65:248–266
49. Pittock S (2007) Does benign MS today imply benign MS tomorrow? Implications for treatment. Neurology 68:480–481
50. Pittock S, Mayr W, McClelland R, Jorgensen N, Weigand S, Noseworthy J, Rodriguez M (2004) Disability profile of MS did not change over 10 years in a population-based prevalence cohort. Neurology 62:601–606

51. Pittock S, Mayr W, McClelland R, Jorgensen N, Weigand S, Noseworthy J, Weinshenker B, Rodriguez M (2004) Change in MS-related disability in a population-based cohort: A 10-year follow-up study. Neurology 62:51–59
52. Pittock S, McClelland R, Mayr W, Jorgensen N, Weinshenker B, Noseworthy J, Rodriguez M (2004) Clinical implications of benign multiple sclerosis: A 20-year population-based follow-up study. Ann Neurol 56:303–306
53. Pittock S, Noseworthy J, Rodriguez M (2007) MRI findings in benign multiple sclerosis are variable. J Neurol 254:539–541
54. Pittock S, Weinshenker B, Noseworthy J, Lucchinetti C, Keegan M, Wingerchuk D, Carter J, Shuster E, Rodriguez M (2006) Not every patient with multiple sclerosis should be treated at time of diagnosis. Arch Neurol 63:611–614
55. Polman C, O'Connor P, Havrdova E, Hutchinson M, Kappos L, Miller D, Phillips J, Lublin F, Giovannoni G, Wajgt A, Toal M, Lynn F, Panzara M, Sandrock A (2006) A randomized, placebo-controlled trial of natalizumab for relapsing multiple sclerosis. N Engl J Med 354:899–910
56. Ramsaransing G, De Keyser J (2006) Benign course in multiple sclerosis: A review. Acta Neurol Scand 113:359–369
57. Rodriguez M, Siva A, Cross S, Stolp-Smith K, O'Brien P, Kurland L (1994) Impairment, disability, and handicap in multiple sclerosis: A population-based study in Olmsted county, Minnesota. Neurology 44:28–33
58. Runmarker B, Andersen O (1993) Prognostic factors in multiple sclerosis incidence cohort with twenty-five years of follow-up. Brain 116:117–134
59. Sayao A, Devonshire V, Tremlett H (2007) Longitudinal follow-up of 'benign' multiple sclerosis at 20 years. Neurology 68:480–481
60. SPECTRIMS Study Group HR (2001) Randomized controlled trial of interferon-beta-1a in secondary progressive ms: Clinical results. Neurology 56:1496–1504
61. Thompson A (1999) Benign multiple sclerosis. J Neurol Neurosurg Psychiatry 67:138
62. Thompson A, Kermode A, MacManus D, Kendall BE, Kingsley DP, Moseley IF, McDonald WI (1990) Patterns of disease activity in multiple sclerosis: Clinical and magnetic resonance imaging study. BMJ 300:631–634
63. Thompson AJ, Miller D, Youl B, MacManus D, Moore S, Kingsley D, Kendall B, Feinstein A, Mcdonald WI (1992) Serial gadolinium-enhanced MRI in relapsing/remitting multiple sclerosis of varying disease duration. Neurology 42:60–62
64. Traboulsee A, Dehmeshki J, Peters K, Griffin C, Brex P, Silver N, Ciccarelli O, Chard D, Barker G, Thompson A, Miller D (2003) Disability in multiple sclerosis is related to normal appearing brain tissue MTR histogram abnormalities. Mult Scler 9:566–573
65. Tremlett H, Paty D, Devonshire V (2005) Disability progression in multiple sclerosis is slower than previously reported. Neurology 66:172–177
66. van Waesberghe J, Walderveen M, Castelijns J, Scheltens P, Nijeholt G, Polman C, Barkof F (1998) Patterns of lesion development in multiple sclerosis: Longitudinal observations with t1-weighted spin-echo and magnetization transfer MR. AJNR Am J Neuroradiol 19:675–683
67. Weinshenker B, Bass B, Rice G (1989a) The natural history of multiple sclerosis: A geographically based study. 1. Clinical course and disability. Brain 112:133–146
68. Weinshenker B, Bass B, Rice G, Noseworthy J, Carriere W, Baskerville J, Ebers G (1989b) The natural history of multiple sclerosis: A geographically based study. 2. Predictive value of the early clinical course. Brain 112:133–146
69. Weinshenker B, Rice G, Noseworthy J, Carriere W, Baskerville J, Ebers G (1991) The natural history of multiple sclerosis: A geographically based study. 3. Multivariate analysis of predictive factors and models of outcome. Brain 114:1045–1056
70. Wingerchuk D (2006) Multiple sclerosis disease-modifying therapies: Adverse effect surveillance and management. Expert Rev Neurotherapeutics 6:333–346
71. Yousry T, Major E, Ryschkewitsch C, Fahle G, Fischer S, Hou J, Curfman B, Miszkiel K, Mueller-Lenke N, Sanchez E, Barkhof F, Radue E, Jager H, Clifford D (2006) Evaluation of patients treated with natalizumab for progressive multifocal leukoencephalopathy. N Engl J Med 354:924–933

# Pathological Heterogeneity of Idiopathic Central Nervous System Inflammatory Demyelinating Disorders

## C. Lucchinetti

**Abstract**  The last decade has seen a resurgence of interest in MS neuropathology. This resurgence was partly fueled by the development of new molecular and histochemical tools to examine the MS lesion microscopically, as well as technological advances in neuroimaging, which permit a dynamic assessment of lesion formation and disease progression. The heterogeneous pathology of MS in relation to stage of lesion activity, phase of disease, and clinical course is discussed. Pathological studies reveal that the immune factors associated with multiple different effector mechanisms contribute to the inflammation, demyelination, and tissue injury observed in MS lesions. While many agree that pathological heterogeneity exists in white matter demyelinated lesions, it is uncertain whether these observations are patient-dependent and reflect pathogenic heterogeneity or, alternatively,

C. Lucchinetti
Mayo Clinic College of Medicine, 200 First St. SW, Rochester, MN 55905, USA
e-mail: clucchinetti@mayo.edu

M. Rodriguez (ed.), *Advances in Multiple Sclerosis and Experimental*
*Demyelinating Diseases. Current Topics in Microbiology and Immunology 318.*
© Springer-Verlag Berlin Heidelberg 2008

are stage-dependent with multiple mechanisms occurring sequentially within a given patient. Evidence supporting both concepts is presented. Remyelination is present in MS lesions; however, the factors contributing to the extent of repair and oligodendrocyte survival differ depending on the disease phase. A variable and patient-dependent extent of remyelination is observed in chronic MS cases and will likely need to be considered when designing future clinical trials aimed to promote CNS repair. MS is one member of a spectrum of CNS idiopathic inflammatory demyelinating disorders that share the basic pathological hallmark of CNS inflammatory demyelination. Advances based on recent systematic clinicopathologic-serologic correlative approaches have led to novel insights with respect to the classification of these disorders, as well as a better understanding of the underlying pathogenic mechanisms.

# 1 Introduction

Multiple sclerosis (MS) is an inherently heterogeneous disorder with respect to its clinical, radiographic, and genetic features. Its basic pathology consists of multifocal central nervous system (CNS) lesions characterized by inflammation, demyelination, astrogliosis, variable remyelination preservation, and relative axonal preservation. MS represents only one member of a family of CNS idiopathic inflammatory demyelinating disorders (IIDDs), all similarly characterized by focal demyelination, and includes acute disseminated encephalomyelitis (ADEM), acute MS (Marburg variant), Balo's concentric sclerosis (BCS), and neuromyelitis optica (NMO).

Largely due to similarities with experimental autoimmune encephalomyelitis (EAE), the role of CD4+ T cells has been emphasized in MS pathogenesis. However, accumulating in vitro and in vivo studies challenge the traditional view that MS is purely a CD4+ T cell-mediated autoimmune disease and suggest that the events involved in MS immunopathogenesis may be more complex than previously recognized. Furthermore, the advent of more sophisticated histological and molecular tools to study MS pathology has contributed to evolving concepts regarding disease initiation and progression. Although all MS lesions are characterized by destruction of myelin sheaths, they display a significant degree of pathological heterogeneity with respect to the topography of the lesions, the severity and character of the inflammatory response, the extent of remyelination and the degree and pattern of oligodendrocyte and axonal injury. It is debatable whether these observations reflect patient-dependent pathogenic heterogeneity or, alternatively, are stage-dependent with multiple mechanisms contributing to the observed pathological heterogeneity. This chapter will focus on the concept of MS pathological heterogeneity with respect to white matter lesions, the fate of the oligodendrocyte and extent of repair, and it will elaborate upon the heterogeneous clinicopathological spectrum of the CNS idiopathic inflammatory demyelinating disorders.

## 2    Heterogeneity of Multiple Sclerosis White Matter Lesions

MS pathology varies with respect to the demyelinating stage of the lesion as well as with disease duration. MS neuropathological studies are largely skewed toward the analysis of either very early lesions derived from fulminant autopsy cases, brain biopsies when the diagnosis was still in question, or very late chronic lesions from patients who died with longstanding disease. This essentially provides snapshots from which investigators attempt to draw dynamic conclusions regarding disease evolution and progression. However, pathological information is limited regarding the preclinical phase of the disease and the transition phase, when patients convert from relapsing to progressive disease.

### 2.1    Stages of Lesions

A variety of criteria have been used to stage the activity of MS lesions including the extent and activation state of lymphocytes and macrophages, the presence of MHC class II antigens, and the presence of adhesion molecules or cytokines. However, these approaches do not reliably distinguish inflammatory from demyelinating activity, and it is not uncommon to find inflammatory MS lesions with no signs of active demyelination.

Pathological studies investigating demyelinating mechanisms must therefore rely on a precise definition of demyelinating activity. At a minimum, the presence of luxol-fast blue (LFB+) myelin degradation products within the macrophage cytoplasm is a reliable indicator of ongoing demyelination [54]. A more rigorous approach to demyelination staging in MS lesions has been proposed based on the structural profile and chemical composition of myelin degradation products within macrophages in correlation to the expression of macrophage differentiation markers (Fig. 1) [18]. The time sequence of myelin degradation in macrophages is based on the evaluation of EAE lesions [55] as well as recent in vitro studies analyzing the sequential breakdown of myelin by human monocytes [37]. Whenever myelin sheaths are destroyed, macrophages or microglia cells take up the remnants. Minor myelin proteins, such as myelin oligodendrocyte glycoprotein (MOG) or myelin-associated glycoprotein (MAG), rapidly degrade within macrophages 1 to 2 days after phagocytosis. In contrast, major myelin proteins, such as myelin basic protein (MBP) and proteolipid protein (PLP), may persist in macrophages for 6–10 days. In later stages, the macrophages contain sudanophilic and periodic acid Schiff (PAS)-positive granular lipids that may persist in the lesion up to several months. Macrophages expressing distinct markers of macrophage activation and differentiation (myeloid related protein [MRP14], a member of the S100 family of calcium-binding proteins, and 27E10) infiltrate early active demyelinating MS lesions. Their cytoplasms contain myelin degradation products immunoreactive for both MOG and MAG. These minor myelin proteins disappear within late active MS lesions; however, myelin

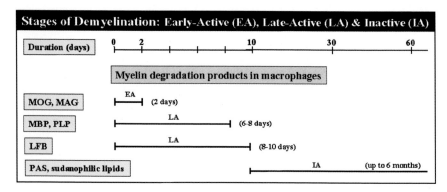

**Fig. 1** Staging of demyelinating activity. MS lesions can be classified into early active (EA), late active (LA), and inactive (IA) stages based on the type of myelin degradation products present in the macrophage cytoplasm

debris is still immunoreactive for MBP and PLP. Macrophages within inactive, completely demyelinated areas no longer contain either minor or major myelin proteins; however, PAS+ debris may still be present. Early remyelinating lesions are characterized by clusters of short, thin, irregularly organized myelin sheaths with greater MAG or CNPase reactivity relative to MOG or PLP, and PAS+ macrophages may be present. Evidence for areas of early remyelination occurring concurrently with active demyelination can also be observed.

This staging classification scheme provides a dynamic topographical framework for analyzing lesion evolution. In any MS brain, a variety of lesions at different stages of demyelinating activity may be present. Furthermore, a single MS lesion may have multiple areas of differing demyelinating activity. However, it is important to acknowledge that this staging approach may fail to capture events in lesion evolution preceding myelin degradation. Using these stringent criteria, the incidence of actively demyelinating lesions in MS brains is quite low, especially in brain bank material largely consisting of longstanding chronic MS cases.

## 2.2 MS Plaque Types

Based on the topographical distribution of the macrophages and their immunoreactivity for minor and major myelin protein degradation products, several active MS plaque types can be distinguished (Fig. 2). The acute active plaque is characterized by the synchronous destruction of myelin, with all the macrophages containing early and late myelin degradation products distributed evenly throughout the lesion. The chronic active plaque consists of numerous macrophages clustered at the radially expanding plaque edge immunoreactive for both minor and major myelin degradation products, which diminish in number toward the inactive plaque center. The

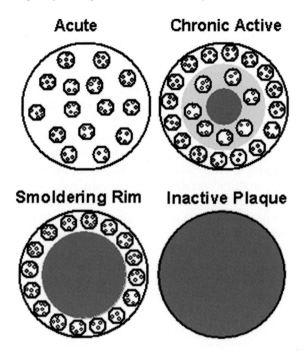

**Fig. 2** MS plaque types. The acute active plaque is characterized by the presence of macrophages containing early (*red*) and late (*green*) myelin degradation products, distributed throughout the extent of the lesion. The chronic active plaque shows the accumulation of numerous macrophages, containing both early (*red*) and late (*green*) myelin degradation products, clustered at the advancing plaque edge, and diminishing in number toward the inactive plaque center (*blue*). The smoldering rim is defined by the presence of very few macrophages restricted to the plaque edge containing early and late myelin degradation products, whereas the inactive plaque contains no early or late myelin degradation products within the macrophages

smoldering active plaque has an inactive lesion center surrounded by a rim of microglia and few activated macrophages immunoreactive for myelin degradation products, but in the majority, myelin digestion is already completed [82]. Inflammation is typically less prominent in the smoldering active plaque compared to the acute or chronic plaque. The chronic inactive MS plaque area appears sharply circumscribed; it is relatively hypocellular with marked myelin loss, prominent fibrillary astrocytosis, variably reduced axonal density, and loss of mature oligodendrocytes. There is no evidence of ongoing myelin breakdown. Inflammatory cells may still be present.

Acute active and chronic active plaques most likely represent the pathologic substrate of acute neurological dysfunction due to a combination of inflammation, edema, conduction-blocking demyelination, and variable axonal damage. They are mainly found in early-phase MS patients or in secondary progressive (SPMS) patients with ongoing clinical relapses. With increased disease duration and progression, as in SPMS and primary progressive MS, inactive plaques predominate, and acute and chronic active plaques are uncommon. Occasionally, smoldering plaques appear, and these may contribute to disease progression in SPMS [82].

Destructive plaques are characterized by demyelination associated with a pronounced destruction of other tissue elements including axons, oligodendrocytes and astrocytes. These lesions are often necrotic and cystic, resulting in encephalomalacia associated with prominent gray and white matter atrophy [109]. Destructive plaques are a hallmark of Marburg's acute MS, typically characterized by a rapidly progressive course leading to death within 1 year of onset [67]. Destructive plaques are also frequently found in patients with neuromyelitis optica (NMO), an inflammatory, typically relapsing demyelinating disorder affecting the optic nerves and spinal cord [64].

Shadow plaques are sharply demarcated plaques in a typical MS distribution, with only a moderate reduction of axonal density and a uniform presence of nerve fibers with disproportionately thin myelin sheaths. Shadow plaques typically contain few macrophages and are associated with pronounced fibrillary gliosis. Immunocytochemical and ultrastructural data suggest shadow plaques represent complete remyelination of previously demyelinated plaques [53, 79] and are characterized by reduced staining of myelin (myelin pallor) due to a decreased ratio between myelin thickness and axonal diameter. However, reduced myelin density may also present within active plaques or in areas of secondary Wallerian degeneration. Areas of active demyelination, however, are clearly defined by macrophages containing myelin degradation products, whereas areas of Wallerian degeneration have ill-defined borders and preserved nerve fibers in the lesions and show a broad range of thick to thin myelin sheaths. Shadow plaques may become targets of new demyelinating attacks [81].

## 2.3   Inflammation and Immune Effector Heterogeneity in MS

### 2.3.1   T and B Lymphocytes

The inflammatory infiltrate in active MS lesions largely consists of activated mononuclear cells, including macrophages, activated microglia, and lymphocytes. Most infiltrating lymphocytes are T cells [100], predominantly MHC class I-restricted, $CD8^+$ T lymphocytes [15] showing preferential clonal expansion [4]. The $CD8^+$ T cell repertoire appears more antigen-driven than the MHC II-restricted $CD4^+$ T cells [30], and a close apposition of activated cytotoxic T cells with degenerating oligodendrocytes and axons has been described in some acute MS lesions [71], suggesting a possible role for MHC I $CD8^+$-dependent tissue damage in MS. This hypothesis is further strengthened by recent pathologic evidence demonstrating upregulation of MHC class I expression on microglia, endothelial cells, neurons, axons, astrocytes, and oligodendrocytes within active MS lesions, suggesting these cells may become targets of an MHC class I-restricted immune response [43]. Adoptive transfer of $CD8^+$ T cells also induces EAE. This results in brain lesions with pronounced demyelination that more closely resembles MS pathology [44, 98], and disease induction is not dependent on $CD4^+$ T cells [30].

Recent studies implicate B cells and autoantibodies in MS pathogenesis. B cells, plasma cells, myelin antibodies, and immunoglobulin transcripts have all been identified in MS lesions [27, 60, 70, 83]. Molecular studies of B cells and plasma cells within MS CNS tissue and CSF suggest T cell-mediated antigen-driven clonal expansion [25, 72]. Furthermore, the H chain variable (V) regions of immunoglobulin (Ig) expressed in MS plaques and CSF reveals a limited repertoire. The VH sequences are oligoclonal, extensively mutated and derived in part from clonally expanded B cell populations, all features suggestive of antigenic stimulation [7, 75, 76, 84, 93, 105]. Pathologic studies have described the co-deposition of immunoglobulin (Ig) and activated terminal lytic complement complex in active MS lesions [62, 97]. These findings, coupled with the presence in CSF of membrane attack complex-enriched membrane vesicles, also indicate a potential role for complement-mediated injury in MS [38].

Although MS patients have presented with elevated antibody titers to a number of self and foreign antigens [5, 68, 73, 99], none have proven pathogenic [25]. MOG has received much attention as a possible autoantigen; however, its role in MS pathogenesis remains uncertain. Demyelination is often limited in T cell models of EAE; however, the presence of autoantibodies directed against MOG extensively amplifies the extent of demyelination [58]. Serum MOG antibodies have been described in MS patients [11]; however, they are also present in patients with noninflammatory neurological diseases and in normal controls. Although an increased risk of progression to clinically definite MS in patients with serum MOG antibodies has been reported [11], a recent study failed to confirm this association [51].

Structures suggestive of lymphoid B cell follicles have appeared in the meninges of patients in the late progressive disease phase, suggesting that ectopic lymphoid follicle formation maintains humoral autoimmunity and contributes to disease severity and progression in chronic MS [89]. Clonally expanded populations of Ig variable gene-mutated B cells appear in the CNS of MS patients, supporting the occurrence of a germinal center-like reaction [23]. Furthermore, the CSF of MS patients is enriched with centroblasts and B cells with a memory phenotype compared to peripheral blood. In the same individuals, antibody-secreting cells are detected in the CSF and appear to correlate with CNS inflammation. These B cell subsets are the output of a germinal center reaction thought to occur in the CNS. Recent findings suggest that the inflamed brain becomes a favorable niche for B cell survival and proliferation and, under some circumstances, sustains the formation of ectopic lymphoid structures. B cells might therefore expand and mature inside the CNS, giving rise to antibody-secreting cells, which could play an effector role in disease pathogenesis [22].

### 2.3.2 Macrophages/Microglia

Hematogenous macrophages and activated CNS microglia are important antigen-presenting and myelin-phagocytizing cells involved in active demyelination [88] and significantly outnumber lymphocytes within active MS lesions. However, macrophages exert both beneficial and detrimental effects on lesion evolution [16, 88] and are subclassified into two phenotypes. The M1 phenotype produces pro-inflammatory mediators and reactive oxygen species (ROS) [42, 65] and is predominantly involved in Th1 cell responses. The M2 phenotype, on the other hand, produces anti-inflammatory mediators and is associated with Th2 responses, tissue scavenging, tissue remodeling, and repair and resolution of inflammation [66]. Additionally, M2-induced signals inhibit M1-induced chemokines [65, 66]. Active MS lesions contain numerous foamy macrophages, reflecting ingestion and accumulation of myelin lipids. A recent MS immunocytochemical in vitro study suggested that the foamy macrophages found at the MS plaque edge is mainly involved in myelin phagocytosis, whereas those located in the plaque center demonstrate an M2 phenotype and may, therefore, contribute to the resolution of inflammation, limit further lesion development, and promote tissue repair [16]. Macrophages may also contribute to lesion repair and neuroprotection by promoting the clearance of cell debris [88] as well as by the secretion of neurotrophic factors and cytokines [48, 49, 95].

### 2.3.3   Excitotoxicity, Nitric Oxide, and Histotoxic Hypoxia

Glutamate is the most abundant excitatory neurotransmitter in the CNS. It is secreted in large amounts by macrophages. An excess of glutamate causes excitotoxicity, which can lead to neuronal and oligodendrocyte damage and degeneration during CNS inflammation. Prolonged activation of neurons by glutamate may be damaging via production of nitric oxide (NO), reactive oxygen species (ROS), arachidonic acid, phospholipase A2, and proteases such as calpain-causing calcium influx [69]. Impaired glutamate clearance and degradation by astrocytes and oligodendrocytes and inhibited clearance by pro-inflammatory cytokines may all contribute to excess extracellular glutamate [41]. Glutamate receptors in the CNS of MS patients reportedly had altered expression, and the presence of a specific glutamate receptor correlated with the presence of axonal damage [34]. In MS, macrophages and microglia were immunoreactive for the glutamate-producing enzyme glutaminase, which co-localized with dystrophic axons [104].

Nitric oxide (NO) is a signal transducer involved in glutamate-induced excitation, is expressed by activated microglia, astrocytes, and macrophages during inflammation in the CNS [14], and is induced by several different cytokines including IFN-γ, TNF-α, and IL-1β [28]. NO directly affects CNS inflammation via induction of encephalitogenic T cell apoptosis and contributes to demyelination, oligodendrocyte destruction, and axonal injury [92]. Although not detected in the normal human CNS, iNOS is abundantly expressed by astrocytes in plaque areas in MS autopsies [36] and was demonstrated in a biopsy taken 33 days after onset of disseminated symptoms in a patient with fulminant MS [13]. Inducible NOS labeling decreases as lesions age and become less active [26, 59]. Oligodendrocytes and axons are highly vulnerable to NO. NO induces a functional and reversible conduction block in demyelinated axons [85]; however, repetitively stimulated axons ultimately degenerate upon exposure to NO [91]. NO impairs mitochondrial electron transport and, therefore, oxidative phosphorylation [17]. Exposing CNS white matter to NO also causes ATP depletion and irreversible injury [32]. These observations suggest that irreversible axonal damage by NO results from the combined effect of direct toxicity and energy failure.

When inflammatory mediators, such as reactive oxygen and nitrogen species, are excessively liberated, they contribute to mitochondrial dysfunction and a state of histotoxic hypoxia [2]. Hypoxic brain damage leads to the destruction of glial cells and neurons in the lesions. If the hypoxia is incomplete, a cascade of events occurs to increase the resistance of the tissue to subsequent hypoxic damage and thus limit structural damage from the insult. This is referred to as hypoxic preconditioning [90]. One master switch in the induction of hypoxic preconditioning is the expression of hypoxia-inducible factors (HIFs) $\alpha$ and $\beta$ [90]. They act as transcription factors to induce gene expression of downstream molecules involved in neuroprotection, vasomotor control, angiogenesis, cell growth, and energy metabolism [2]. These proteins render the tissue resistant to further hypoxia-induced injury.

Sublethal hypoxia at the border of a stroke lesion also induces the expression of stress proteins, especially hsp70, a molecular chaperone that re-natures damaged proteins and protects the tissue against further insult [21, 103]. The expression of these survival proteins is not restricted to hypoxic or ischemic lesions. HIF expression can be induced or increased by pro- or anti-inflammatory cytokines, and protein denaturation in injured tissue induces HSP expression [2, 90]. All these proteins are expressed at the border between active inflammatory lesions and the adjacent normal tissue. While hsp70 is found at the edges of all inflammatory lesions in the CNS, the expression of HIF-1$\alpha$ is restricted to lesions following hypoxia-like tissue injury [1]. In a systematic study in over 80 cases of inflammatory and degenerative CNS white matter diseases and 20 controls, HIF-1$\alpha$ expression was significantly associated ($p<0.0000001$) with a subset of MS lesions, various viral encephalitides, metabolic encephalopathy, and acute stroke lesions characterized by a preferential loss of MAG, and a distal oligodendrogliopathy with apoptotic oligodendrocyte cell death. Similar patterns of tissue injury and HIF-1$\alpha$ expression between these viral, demyelinating, and ischemic disorders suggest a shared pathogenesis related to energy failure and histotoxic hypoxia.

## 2.4 Evidence for Immunopathogenic Heterogeneity in Multiple Sclerosis

Pathological studies suggest that the immune factors associated with multiple different effector mechanisms contribute to the inflammation, demyelination, and tissue injury observed in MS lesions. Binding T cells to myelin epitopes leads to macrophage activation and secondary myelin destruction. T cells and microglia/macrophages release a variety of toxic mediators including cytokines, proteases, reactive oxygen, and nitrogen species or excitotoxins, which result in direct tissue damage. Antibodies mediate tissue damage via complement activation or interaction with activated macrophages. Cytotoxic T cells directly attack oligodendrocytes and axons. However, it is unclear whether a dominant immune effector pathway of active MS lesion formation operates with a given patient or, alternatively, whether multiple immune effector pathways occurring either in parallel or sequentially within a given patient produce the active white matter lesion.

Analyzing large samples of human brain biopsies and autopsies during early disease revealed patterns of demyelination that were homogenous in multiple active lesions of the same patient but differed between patients [62]. Active demyelinating lesions were classified into four patterns based on plaque geography, myelin protein expression, pattern of oligodendrocyte pathology, and presence of immune complex deposition (Fig. 3). Only T cells and macrophages dominated the

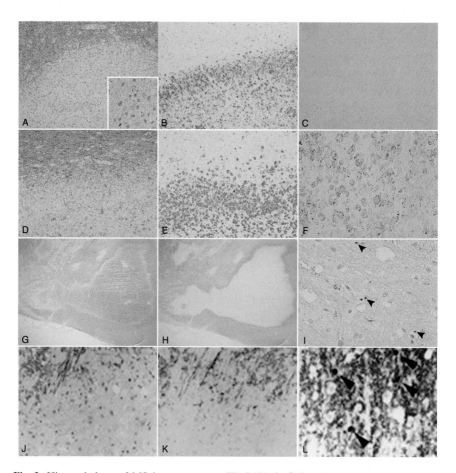

**Fig. 3** Histopathology of MS immunopattern (IP) I–IV. **A–C** IP I. **A** A perivenous confluent active demyelinating lesion. Macrophages contain myelin debris within their cytoplasm (*inset*). **B** Macrophages accumulate in a sharp rim at the lesion border. **C** Complement deposition is absent.

active lesions in Pattern I, whereas Pattern II lesions were additionally characterized by Ig deposition and products of complement activation at sites of active myelin breakdown, suggesting the involvement of pathogenic antibodies. Pattern III lesions had pronounced oligodendrocyte apoptosis associated with a preferential loss of MAG and CNPase, in a pattern of tissue injury closely resembling acute white matter infarcts [1]. These lesions appear to be driven by an exaggerated production of oxygen and nitric oxide radicals resulting in mitochondrial dysfunction and subsequent histotoxic hypoxia. Pattern IV lesions had extensive oligodendrocyte degeneration in the periplaque white matter adjacent to the active lesion, suggesting an increased susceptibility of the target tissue for immune-mediated injury. Although these four MS immunopathological patterns share similarities with existing animal models, the reason for this complex pathology is unknown. Different inciting factors may result in immunopathological heterogeneity; however, pathological heterogeneity may also result from different genetic factors influencing immune-mediated inflammation, as well as glial, axonal, and neuronal survival.

Regardless, these observations suggest fundamental differences in the pathogenic mechanisms leading to focal demyelination in MS between different patient subgroups and may, in part, account for the variable treatment response often observed among MS patients. However, applying these findings to MS patients requires technologies that allow the stratification of MS pathologic subtypes without dependence on brain biopsies. Studies to identify immunopathological, specific clinical, and paraclinical surrogate markers are ongoing. To date, pattern IV has been seen exclusively in three patients with PPMS; however, Patterns I, II, and III do not correlate with a specific clinical course (RR, SP, PP), or early disability [78]. Longer clinical follow-up, however, is needed to determine whether immunopathological patterns differentially impact long-term clinical course and disability. Despite the apparent lack of correlation between immunopathological patterns and prototypic MS clinical course in early MS, a striking correlation has been reported between therapeutic response to plasma exchange (PLEX) administered for steroid-unresponsive fulminant MS attacks and immunopathological pattern. Only Pattern II MS patients with active lesions characterized by antibody and complement deposition responded to PLEX, in contrast to no response in either pattern I or III patients [47].

---

**Fig. 3** (continued)   **D–F** IP II. **D** A perivenous confluent active demyelinating lesion. Clustering of oligodendrocytes and labeling of delicate oligodendrocyte processes is suggestive of concurrent ongoing remyelination. **E** Macrophages accumulate in a sharp rim at the lesion border. **F** Macrophages contain complement-positive myelin debris within their cytoplasm. **G–I** IP III. **G** MOG overexpression within active MS lesion compared to adjacent NAWM. **H** A striking loss of MAG is demonstrated within the lesion corresponding to the region of MOG overexpression. **I** Condensed oligodendrocyte nuclei suggestive of apoptosis (*arrowheads*). Note residual MAG immunoreactivity in the oligodendrocyte process at *upper left corner*. **J–L** IP IV. **J, K** Distribution of myelin antigens MO (**J**) and MAG (**K**) is similar in the lesions. **L** DNA fragmentation of oligodendrocytes is seen in the periplaque white matter [double staining of in situ tailing (DNA fragmentation) and CNPase (myelin and oligodendrocytes)]. (Reprinted with permission from Lucchinetti et al 2000)

How long these patterns persist in disease course is unknown, since the mechanisms of MS lesion formation in chronic active, late-phase plaques are not well understood. Slowly expanding rims of active demyelination with microglial activation and limited inflammation have been described [82]; however, whether the immunopathologic heterogeneity seen in early active MS lesions persists in these later phases is uncertain. Perhaps a common mechanism underlies disease progression among all patients once the active demyelinating phase subsides. Ongoing studies address the impact of these different pathological subtypes on long-term clinical and radiographic progression.

## 2.5   *Immunopathologic Heterogeneity May Be Stage-Dependent*

There have been recent challenges to both the primary role for inflammation in MS pathogenesis and the concept of interindividual heterogeneity of MS lesions [10]. Based on extensive oligodendrocyte apoptosis in the absence of inflammation in a pediatric MS patient who died 9 months after disease onset (and 17 h after presentation with acute pulmonary edema) as well as 12 other cases reportedly demonstrating similar pathological findings, the authors proposed that a primary oligodendrocyte injury preceding inflammation and active myelin breakdown represents the initial lesion in all RRMS patients. This study questions whether inflammation is a prerequisite in MS pathogenesis. However, lymphocyte subsets were not examined, and the index patient was treated with high-dose corticosteroids prior to death, which may have dampened the inflammatory response.

This study also reported the coexistence of different tissue injury patterns within the same patient [10]. The authors described the presence of oligodendrocyte apoptosis in the absence of overt inflammation in some areas as well as complement activation with evidence of remyelination in others, which was interpreted as evidence of an overlap of features typically associated with both Patterns III and II, respectively, within a single patient, thus challenging the hypothesis of MS immunopathogenic interindividual heterogeneity. The authors suggest that these Pattern III-like apoptotic lesions are prephagocytic and represent an early stage in the formation of most, if not all, lesions in RRMS (starter lesion) [9]. They further propose that these apoptotic lesions evolve directly into demyelinated lesions or, once remyelinated, become the targets of additional demyelinating episodes. However, in this study, the definition of complement activation, as well as the immunopathological classification of the lesions, partially differed from that described in the original publication [62]. Whether methodological differences explain the divergent results or whether, in some patients, different mechanisms of tissue injury occur side by side is not yet resolved. However, in our studies based on a large sample of cases, including serial biopsies and autopsies as well as detailed follow-up studies with MRI, such an overlap has not been observed [61]. Furthermore, the presence of probable hypoxia related to the patient's known perimortem pulmonary edema may result in an identical pattern of myelin and oligodendrocyte pathology [1, 2].

## 3   Remyelination in MS

Remyelination is present both in early [63] and chronic MS lesions [77] (Fig. 5). Early in the disease, remyelination may be extensive; however, the extent of oligodendrocyte loss in these early MS lesions is highly variable with two distinct patterns of oligodendrocyte pathology described [63]. The first pattern is characterized by oligodendrocyte survival or progenitor recruitment, and the second is characterized by extensive oligodendrocyte destruction. The pattern remains uniform among multiple active MS plaques examined from a single patient, arguing against this variability simply reflecting varying severity of a single inciting event but rather suggesting that myelin and mature oligodendrocytes and/or their progenitors are differentially affected among MS patients. The extent of remyelination in early MS lesions apparently depends on the availability of oligodendrocytes or their progenitor cells. Furthermore, evidence for early remyelination is found in actively demyelinating lesions, suggesting both destructive and reparative capabilities in the inflammatory microenvironment (Fig. 4). Mononuclear immune cells, such as T cells, release anti-inflammatory cytokines, such as IL-4 and IL-10, and neurotrophic factors, such as brain-derived neurotrophic factor (BDNF) [48]. Recent histopathological studies have produced clear

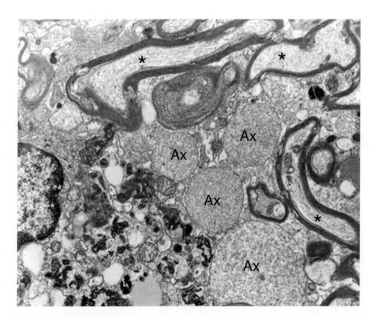

**Fig. 4** Remyelination and demyelination in MS. Electron microscopy of an early MS lesion reveals active demyelination occurring simultaneously with remyelination. A macrophage-containing myelin debris is in proximity of a field of both denuded, completely demyelinated axons (*Ax*), as well as thinly remyelinated axons (*). (Provided courtesy of Moses Rodriguez, Mayo Clinic, Rochester, MN, USA)

evidence that immune cells within MS lesions produce BDNF [95]. These findings support a potentially important role for inflammation in lesion repair. In addition, the induction of inflammation can transform a non-remyelinating experimental situation into a remyelinating one [29]. It is therefore possible that the complete blockage of all inflammatory responses in the MS lesion is counterproductive.

The factors influencing the extent of remyelination may differ with disease chronicity. The density of mature oligodendrocytes within chronic MS plaques is low [107]. When remyelination is present, it is either restricted to the plaque edge or may extend throughout the lesion and form a completely remyelinated shadow plaque. A radiologic–pathologic correlative study reported that more than 40% of MS lesions showed signs of remyelination [8]. However, a recent study indicates significant interindividual heterogeneity in the extent of remyelination present in chronic MS cases [77]. In up to 20% of the cases, the plaques analyzed in the forebrain were completely remyelinated shadow plaques; in other cases, the extent of remyelination was sparse. This diverse capacity to form shadow plaques does not correlate with clinical subtype, age at disease onset, or gender. In fact, shadow plaques are not restricted to patients with early and relapsing MS but are particularly prominent in patients with long-standing chronic disease who died at an advanced age.

It is not clear why remyelination is extensive in some patients yet is limited in others. Lesions located in the subcortical or deep white matter have a higher remyelination potential than those present in the periventricular white matter [77]. Axonal health and density are also key factors impacting the extent of remyelination. It is also plausible, though not yet proven, that genetic factors contribute to the variable extent of remyelination observed among chronic MS patients. Recent studies on Theiler's murine encephalomyelitis (TMEV) MS model demonstrate that hereditary factors contribute to the remyelinating capacity following inflammatory demyelination. Crossing mice strains that lack spontaneous remyelination with strains that demonstrate extensive remyelination, leads to an inherited, dominant reparative phenotype [12]. Although the variable and patient-dependent aspects of remyelination observed in MS need to be considered in the design of future clinical trials aimed to promote CNS repair, investigators still lack magnetic resonance tools that reliably distinguish demyelinated from remyelinated lesions.

# 4 The Clinicopathologic Spectrum of CNS Idiopathic Inflammatory Demyelinating Disorders

Relapsing-remitting and progressive (primary or secondary) MS represents the most common CNS idiopathic inflammatory demyelinating disorder (IIDD); however, there is a broad clinicopathologic spectrum of IIDDs that share the basic pathological hallmark of CNS inflammatory demyelination (Fig. 5). These disorders vary in their clinical course, regional distribution and specific pathological features and include the fulminant demyelinating disorders (e.g., acute disseminated encephalomyelitis [ADEM], the Marburg variant of acute MS, tumefactive MS, and

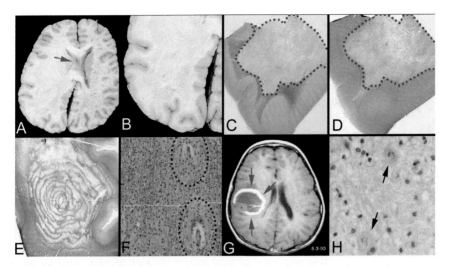

**Fig. 5** Spectrum of CNS idiopathic inflammatory demyelinating disorders. **A, B** Macroscopy of Marburg's type MS. Large confluent lesions lead to mass effect and herniation. **C, D** Microscopy of the lesion shown in **A** and **B** with extensive demyelination (LFB-PAS) and axonal loss (Bielschowsky's silver impregnation). E. Balo's concentric sclerosis showing the characteristic alternating bands of demyelination and preserved myelin. **F** ADEM lesions are characterized by perivascular inflammation and only minimal, mainly perivenular demyelination (*circles*). **G** Tumefactive lesion with severe edema and mass effect. **H** Hypertrophic astrocyte (Creutzfeld-Peters cell) in an acute demyelinating lesion

Balo's concentric sclerosis) as well as the recurrent demyelinating disorders with a restricted topographical distribution (e.g., NMO). Although the clinical and pathological characteristics of these disorders are diverse, the presence in some cases of transitional forms suggests a spectrum of inflammatory demyelinating disorders that share a pathogenic relationship. A.B. Baker acknowledged this broad spectrum and stated, "In all probability, what is generally known as multiple sclerosis is not a single disease but a group of diseases with certain clinical similarities. From the standpoint of clinical research, the present state of affairs is not satisfactory. In order to conduct clinical research in MS, it is imperative that very rigid criteria for diagnosing this disease be developed [6]." Advances based on recent systematic clinicopathologic–serologic correlative approaches have led to novel insights with respect to the classification of these disorders as well as a better understanding of the underlying pathogenic mechanisms.

## 4.1 Acute Disseminated Encephalomyelitis

ADEM is clinically defined as an acute or subacute monophasic, multifocal, steroid-responsive CNS syndrome occurring after infection or vaccination and is often considered in the differential diagnosis when a patient presents with a first attack of IIDD of the CNS. However, most first attacks of IIDD, especially in adults, are harbingers of MS and, accordingly, indicate a significant risk of future relapse and disability. A hallmark of ADEM is its monophasic course, which imparts a more favorable prognosis largely because of a tendency not to recur. Early and accurate distinction between ADEM and other IIDDs, especially MS and neuromyelitis optica (NMO), is important for prognostication and treatment, especially for patients presenting with fulminant or progressive disease. Still, there is considerable overlap in the epidemiologic, clinical, CSF and imaging features of ADEM and MS. This often makes it difficult to distinguish reliably between the two following a single demyelinating event. However, important pathological differences exist between ADEM and MS.

In ADEM, the postmortem brain is edematous, and yellow or grayish perivascular halos corresponding to microscopic inflammatory infiltrates surrounding vessels may be visualized. ADEM lesions are microscopic and diffusely involve the brain and spinal cord. In contrast, in rare cases of fatal MS, the brain may also be edematous, but circumscribed demyelinated plaques are easily visible and sometimes massive, particularly in cases of Marburg acute MS [40, 67, 80, 102] .

Histopathologically, ADEM is characterized by a prominent perivenular pattern of predominantly macrophage infiltration associated with the hallmark of restricted perivenular "sleeves of demyelination" [40, 74]. These areas of inflammation and demyelination are limited to an approximately 1- or 2-mm margin around the vessel or extend less than the diameter of the vessel (Fig. 5F). Although these perivenular lesions may coalesce and appear confluent in places, their perivenular pattern remains evident, and the lesions do not become globoid or ellipsoid as in MS [74]. Confluent sheets of inflammation and demyelination are not characteristic of ADEM but rather are the pathological hallmarks of the MS lesion. ADEM lesions are typically of the similar histological age, in keeping with a monophasic process [101]. Though diffuse, certain areas may have a regional predominance. Microscopic lesions predominantly affect white matter, but gray matter may also be involved as well as the brainstem (especially ventral pons), cerebellum, optic nerves, deep gray matter, and spinal cord. A mild lymphocytic meningeal infiltrate and subpial layer of microglial cells are also characteristic. Acute hemorrhagic leukoencephalitis (AHLE) is a very rare condition pathologically similar to ADEM with the additional evidence of petechial hemorrhages and venular necrosis. AHLE is considered to be a severe form of ADEM with a high mortality rate.

## 4.2   Marburg Variant of Acute MS

Otto Marburg recognized acute MS as a subtype of the disease in 1906 [67]. Clinically, this entity is characterized by rapid progression and an exceptionally severe course, which typically ends in death within 1 year of presentation. The course is generally monophasic and relentlessly progressive, with death usually secondary to brainstem involvement. Although for most patients, this is the presenting episode of demyelination, there are a several recorded cases of well-documented MS that subsequently progressed to a fulminant terminal stage.

Pathologically, the lesions are more destructive than typical MS or ADEM lesions and are characterized by massive macrophage infiltration, acute axonal injury, and necrosis (Fig. 5A–D). Multiple small lesions may be disseminated throughout the brain and spinal cord and may result in large confluent white matter plaques. In some cases, there is widespread diffuse demyelination throughout the white matter. Despite the destructive nature of these lesions, remyelination is often observed.

One study suggests that this acute form of MS is associated with immature myelin basic protein (MBP) [108]. An autopsy study on a single case of Marburg's disease documented pronounced posttranslational changes that converted mature MBP to an extensively citrullinated and poorly phosphorylated immature form. These changes were thought to render myelin more susceptible to breakdown. More recent neuropathological studies suggest that these fulminant destructive lesions are often associated with deposition of immunoglobulins (mainly IgG) and pronounced complement activation at sites of active myelin destruction [33, 97]. These observations suggest an important role for demyelinating antibodies.

## 4.3   Tumefactive MS

MS occasionally presents as a mass lesion indistinguishable clinically and radiographically from a brain tumor. These patients often present with cerebral symptoms of headache, aphasia, disturbance in consciousness, or seizures. Neuroimaging often reveals unifocal or multifocal enhancing lesions with associated mass effect and brain edema (Fig. 5G, H). These patients pose considerable diagnostic difficulty and often require brain biopsy to confirm a diagnosis. Even the biopsy specimen may resemble a brain tumor given the hypercellular nature of these lesions, which are often associated with bizarre astrocyte morphology (nuclear inclusions and mitoses). However, the presence of large numbers of infiltrating macrophages in the setting of myelin loss and relative axonal preservation ultimately confirms the diagnosis of inflammatory demyelinating disease. It is difficult to classify these tumefactive lesions within the spectrum of IIDDs. Although some cases behave like the acute Marburg variant of MS or have features suggestive of Balo's concentric sclerosis, there are other examples in which the course is monophasic and self-limited. Some tumefactive MS patients develop typical MS, whereas others have recurring tumor-like lesions.

## 4.4   Balo Concentric Sclerosis

Considered a variant of inflammatory demyelinating disease closely related to MS, Balo concentric sclerosis (BCS) is characterized pathologically by large demyelinating lesions with a peculiar pattern of alternating layers of preserved and destroyed myelin, mimicking the rings of a tree trunk (Fig. 5E). Clinically, BCS resembles Marburg MS with similar acute fulminant onset followed by rapid progression to major disability and death within months [24, 52, 67]. Of interest, one of the cases in Marburg's original series (Case no. 3) contained extensive concentric lesions [67]. There are reports of less fulminant disease [50, 86], and smaller concentric rims of demyelination have been observed in lesions from some MS patients with a more classical acute or chronic disease course. T2-weighted MR images may reveal a distinct pattern of hypointense/isointense and hyperintense rings corresponding to bands of preserved and destroyed myelin and permit *ante mortem* diagnosis [20, 31, 35, 39, 46, 50, 94].

A recent report described MAG loss and hypoxia-like tissue injury in Balo concentric sclerosis lesions in a pattern similar to other Pattern III MS lesions [96]. This study analyzed 12 autopsied cases with Balo-type concentric lesions and reported that all actively demyelinating concentric lesions followed a pattern of demyelination, suggesting hypoxia-like tissue injury. Active lesions were associated with high expression of iNOS in macrophages and microglia. Proteins involved in tissue preconditioning, such as *hsp*70, HIF-1α, and D-110, were upregulated at the edge of actively demyelinating Balo lesions, as well as in the outermost myelinated layers of the concentric lesion. Due to their neuroprotective effects, the rim of periplaque tissue expressing these proteins may be resistant to further hypoxia-like injury in an expanding lesion and therefore remain as a rim of preserved myelin. Hypoxic preconditioning may therefore explain the concentric pattern of demyelination found in Balo's concentric sclerosis [96].

## 4.5   Neuromyelitis Optica

Neuromyelitis optica (NMO; Devic disease) is an idiopathic inflammatory CNS demyelinating disease characterized by monophasic or relapsing attacks of optic neuritis and myelitis that, unlike classical MS, tends to spare the brain in early stages. Debate continues as to whether NMO is an MS variant or a separate disease. Most experts now regard NMO as a relapsing demyelinating disease distinguished from classical MS by clinical, neuroimaging, laboratory, and pathological criteria [106]. Pathologically, NMO lesions demonstrate extensive demyelination across multiple spinal cord levels, associated with necrosis and cavitation, as well as acute axonal damage in both gray and white matter. Active NMO lesions are characterized by Ig and complement deposition in a characteristic rim and rosette vasculocentric pattern, quite distinct from the pattern of immune complex deposition observed in a subset of active MS lesions (Fig. 6) [64].

The recent discovery of a specific serum autoantibody biomarker, NMO-IgG, which distinguishes NMO from MS, provides further evidence that NMO and MS may be distinct pathogenic entities [57]. NMO-IgG binds at or near the blood–brain barrier (BBB) and outlines CNS microvessels, pia, subpial, and the Virchow-Robin spaces. The staining pattern of patients' serum IgG binding to mouse spinal cord is

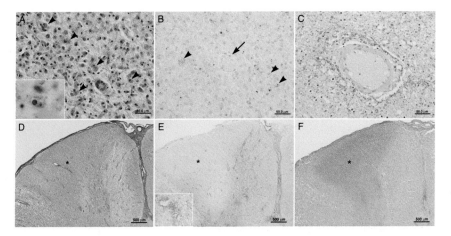

**Fig. 6** AQP4 Immunoreactivity (IR) in acute pattern II MS (**A–C**) and NMO (**D–F**) lesions. **A** Numerous macrophages containing myelin debris are dispersed throughout the active lesion (*arrowheads* and *inset*; LFB/PAS). **B** C9neo antigen is present within macrophages (*arrowheads*), but absent around blood vessels (*arrow*). **C** Higher magnification reveals AQP4 IR is prominent in a rosette pattern surrounding a penetrating blood vessel in the lesion. **D** In NMO, there is extensive demyelination involving both gray and white matter (LFB/PAS); (*) indicates preserved myelin in the PPWM. **E** C9neo is deposited in a vasculocentric rim and rosette pattern (*inset*) within the active lesions, but not in the PPWM (*). **F** The lesions lack AQP4, which is retained in the PPWM (*) and gray matter. **A, D** LFB/PAS; **B, E** C9neo IHC; **C, F** AQP4 IHC

remarkably similar to the vasculocentric pathologic pattern of immunoglobulin and complement deposition seen in NMO lesions. Sensitivity and specificity for this autoantibody are 73% (95% Cl, 60%–86%) and 91% (95% Cl, 79%–100%) for NMO in North American patients and 58% (95% Cl, 30%–86%) and 100% for optic-spinal multiple sclerosis in Japanese patients [57]. Clinical correlations of NMO-IgG seropositivity have extended the NMO spectrum to include cases of Asian optic-spinal MS, recurrent myelitis associated with longitudinally extensive spinal cord lesions, recurrent isolated optic neuritis, and either optic neuritis or myelitis occurring in the context of systemic autoimmune diseases.

NMO-IgG binds selectively to the mercurial-insensitive water channel protein aquaporin-4 (AQP4), which is concentrated in astrocytic foot processes at the BBB [56]. AQP4 is the predominant water channel in the brain and is also expressed to a limited extent in stomach, kidney, lung, skeletal muscle and inner ear [3]. AQP4 has an important role in brain water homeostasis and, consistent with its location in the CNS, is involved in the development, function, and integrity of the interface between the brain and blood and brain and cerebrospinal fluid [45]. In contrast to MS lesions, which exhibit stage-dependent loss of AQP4, all NMO lesions demonstrate a striking loss of AQP4, regardless of the stage of demyelinating activity, extent of tissue necrosis, or site of CNS involvement [87]. These data strongly suggest a pathogenic role for a complement-activating AQP4-specific autoantibody as the initiator of the NMO lesion and further distinguish NMO from MS. A direct antibody-mediated injury against this astrocytic protein would be expected to disrupt essential homeostatic functions, including regulation of water flux, ions, and neurotransmitter levels, ultimately resulting in irreversible tissue damage. The divergent immunopathogenic concepts for NMO and MS have important therapeutic consequences.

# Conclusions

The pathological hallmarks of the basic MS lesion, namely focal demyelination, inflammation, gliosis, and relative axonal preservation, were described over 160 years ago [19]. However, the last decade has seen closer examination of the MS lesion with newer, more sophisticated immunological and molecular tools. Although the cause of the disease remains elusive, recent studies have yielded novel pathogenic insights into the multiple potential effector mechanisms involved in lesion formation, the possible factors contributing to remyelination, and the spectrum of the CNS idiopathic inflammatory demyelinating disorders. The dominant effector mechanisms involved in the formation of the MS lesion may be heterogeneous and differ between patients. The extent of remyelination varies between patients and is independent of disease course. In addition, major advances have been made in understanding the pathogenic basis of the unique pathology associated with both Balo's concentric sclerosis and neuromyelitis optica. A better understanding of the diverse immune effector mechanisms and targets involved in the pathogenesis of MS and other CNS inflammatory demyelinating disorders will lead to more effective therapeutic strategies, better tailored for the specific patient, as well as the specific inflammatory demyelinating disorder.

# References

1. Aboul-Enein F, Lassmann H (2005) Mitochondrial damage and histiotoxic hypoxia: a pathway of tissue injury in inflammatory brain disease. Acta Neuropathol 109:49–55
2. Aboul-Enein F, Rauschka H, Kornek B, Stadelmann C, Stefferl A, Bruck W, Lucchinetti C, Schmidbauer M, Jellinger K et al (2003) Preferential loss of myelin-associated glycoprotein reflects hypoxia-like white matter damage in stroke and inflammatory brain diseases. J Neuropathol Exp Neurol 62:25–33
3. Amiry-Moghaddam M, Otsuka T, Hurn PD, Traystman RJ, Haug FM, Froehner SC, Adams ME, Neely JD, Agre P, Ottersen OP, Bhardwaj A (2003) An alpha-syntrophin-dependent pool of AQP4 in astroglial end-feet confers bidirectional water flow between blood and brain. Proc Natl Acad Sci U St A 100:2106–2111
4. Babbe H, Roers A, Waisman A, Lassmann H, Goebels N, Hohlfeld R, Friese M, Schroder R, Deckert M, Schmidt S, Ravid R, Rajewsky K (2000) Clonal expansion of CD8(+) T cells dominate the T cell infiltrate in active multiple sclerosis lesions as shown by micromanipulation and single cell polymerase chain reaction. J Exp Med 192:393–404

5. Baig S, Olsson O, Olsson T, Love A, Jeansson S, Link H (1989) Cells producing antibody to measles and herpes simplex virus in cerebrospinal fluid and blood of patients with multiple sclerosis and controls. Clin Exp Immunol 78:390–395
6. Baker AB (1968) Problems in the classification of multiple sclerosis. In: Alter M, Kurtzke JF (eds) The epidemiology of multiple sclerosis. Charles C. Thomas, Springfield, IL, pp 14–25.
7. Baranzini SE, Jeong MC, Butunoi C et al (1999) B cell repertoire diversity and clonal expansion in multiple sclerosis brain lesions. J Immunol 163:5133–5144
8. Barkhof F, Bruck W, De Groot C, Bergers E, Hulshof S, Geurts J, Polman CH, van der Valk P (2003) Remyelinated lesions in multiple sclerosis: magnetic resonance image appearance. Arch. Neurol. 60:1073–1081
9. Barnett MH, Prineas JW (2004) Pathological heterogeneity in multiple sclerosis: a reflection of lesion stage? Ann Neurol 56:309
10. Barnett MH, Prineas JW (2004) Relapsing and remitting multiple sclerosis: pathology of the newly forming lesion. Annals of Neurology 55:458–468
11. Berger T, Rubner P, Schautzer F, Egg R, Ulmer H, Mayringer I, Dilitz E, Deisenhammer F, Reindl M (2003) Antimyelin antibodies as a predictor of clinically definite multiple sclerosis after a first demyelinating event. N Engl J Med 349:139–145
12. Bieber AJ, Ure DR, Rodriguez M (2005) Genetically dominant spinal cord repair in a murine model of chronic progressive multiple sclerosis. J Neuropathol Exp Neurol 64:46–57
13. Bitsch A, Bruhn H, Vougioukas V, Stringaris A, Lassmann H, Frahm J, Bruck W (1999) Inflammatory CNS demyelination: histopathologic correlation with in vivo quantitative proton MR spectroscopy. AJNR Am J Neuroradiol 20:1619–1627
14. Bo L, Dawson T, Wesselingh S et al (1994) Induction of nitric oxide synthase in demyelinating regions of multiple sclerosis brains. Ann Neurol 36:778–786
15. Booss J, Esiri MM, Tourtellotte WW, Mason DY (1983) Immunohistological analysis of T lymphocyte subsets in the central nervous system in chronic progressive multiple sclerosis. J Neurol Sci 62:219–232
16. Boven LA, Van Meurs M, Van Zwam M, Wierenga-Wolf A, Hintzen RQ, Boot RG et al (2006) Myelin-laden macrophages are anti-inflammatory consistent with foam cells in multiple sclerosis. Brain 129:517–526
17. Brown GC, Borutaite V (2002) Nitric oxide inhibition of mitochondrial respiration and its role in cell death. Free Radic Biol Med 33:1440–1450
18. Bruck W, Porada P, Poser S, Rieckmann P, Hanefeld F, Kretchmar HA, et al (1995) Monocyte-macrophage differentiation in early multiple sclerosis lesions. Ann Neurol 38:788–796
19. Charcot JM (1868) Histologie de la sclérose en plaques. Gaz Hop Civils Militaires 140, 141, 143:554–555, 557–558, 566
20. Chen C, Ro L, Chang C, Ho Y, Lu C (1996) Serial MRI studies in pathologically verified Balo's concentric sclerosis. J Comput Assist Tomogr 20:732–735
21. Christians ES, Yan LJ, Benjamin IJ (202) Heat shock factor 1 and heat shock proteins: critical partners in protection against acute cell injury. Crit Care Med 30:S43–S50
22. Corcione A, Aloisi F, Serafini B, Capello E, Mancardi GL, Pistoia V, Uccelli A (2005) B-cell differentiation in the CNS of patients with multiple sclerosis. Autoimmun Rev 4:594–654
23. Corcione A, Casazza S, Ferretti E, Giunti G, Zappia E, Pistorio A, Gambini C, Mancardi GL, Uccelli A, Pistoia V (2004) Recapitulation of B cell differentiation in the central nervous system of patients with multiple sclerosis. Proc Natl Acad Sci USA 10:11064–11069
24. Courville C (1970) Concentric sclerosis. In: Bruyn PV (ed) Handbook of Clinical Neurology. Elsevier, Amsterdam, pp 437–451.
25. Cross A, Trotter J, Lyons J (2001) B cells and antibodies in CNS demyelinating disease. J Neuroimmunol 112:1–14
26. De Groot C, Ruuls S, Theeuwes J, Dijkstra C, van der Valk P (1997) Immunocytochemical characterization of the expression of inducible and constitutive isoforms of nitric oxide synthase in demyelinating multiple sclerosis lesions. J Neuropathol Exp Neurol 56:10–20

27. Esiri MM (1977) Immunoglobulin-containing cells in multiple sclerosis plaques. Lancet 2:478
28. Forstermann U, Kleinert H (1995) Nitric oxide synthase: expression and expressional control of the three isoforms. Naunyn-Schmiedebergs Arch Pharmacol 352:351–364
29. Franklin RJ (2002) Why does remyelination fail in multiple sclerosis? Nat Rev Neurosci 3:705–714
30. Friese M, Fugger L (2005) Autoreactive CD8+ T cells in multiple sclerosis: a new target for therapy? Brain 128:1747–1763
31. Garbern J, Spence A, Alvord E (1986) Balo's concentric demyelination diagnosed premortem. Neurology 36:1610–1614
32. Garthwaite G, Goodwin DA, Batchelor AM et al (2002) Nitric oxide toxicity in CNS white matter: an in vitro study using rat optic nerve. Neuroscience 109:145–155
33. Genain CP, Cannella B, Hauser SL, Raine CS (1999) Identification of autoantibodies associated with myelin damage in multiple sclerosis. Nat Med 5:170–175
34. Geurts JJ, Wolswijk G, Bo L, van der Valk P, Polman CH, Troost D, Aronica E (2003) Altered expression patterns of group I and II metabotropic glutamate receptors in multiple sclerosis. Brain 126:1755–1766
35. Gharagozloo A, Poe L, Collins G (1994) Antemortem diagnosis of Balo concentric sclerosis: correlative MR imaging and pathologic features. Radiology 191:817–819
36. Giovannoni G, Heales S, Land J, Thompson E (1998) The potential role of nitric oxide in multiple sclerosis. Multiple Sclerosis 4:212–216
37. Goes vd A, Boorsma W, Hoekstra K, Montagne L, De Groot CJ, Dijkstra CD (2005) Determination of the sequential degradation of myelin proteins by macropahges. J Neuroimm 161:12–20
38. Hafler DA, Slavik JM, Anderson DE, O'Connor KC, De Jager P, Baecher-Allan C (2005) Multiple sclerosis. Immunol Rev 204:208–231
39. Hanemann C, Kleinschmidt A, Reifenberger G, Freud H, Seitz R (1993) Balo concentric sclerosis followed by MRI and positron emission tomography. Neuroradiology 35:578–580
40. Hart M, Earle K (1975) Haemorrhagic and perivenous encephalitis: a clinical-pathological review of 38 cases. J Neurol Neurosurg Psychiatry 38:585–591
41. Hendricks JJ, Teunissen CE, de Vries HE, Dijkstra CD (2005) Macrophages and neurodegeneration. Brain Res Reviews 48:185–195
42. Hill KE, Zollinger LV, Watt HE, Carlson NG, Rose JW (2004) Inducible nitric oxide synthase in chronic active multiple sclerosis plaques: distribution, cellular expression, and association with myelin damage. J Neuroimmunol 151:171–179
43. Hoftberger R, Aboul-Enein F, Brueck W, Lucchinetti CF, Rodriguez M, Schmidbauer M, Jellinger K et al (2004) Expression of major histocompatibility complex class I molecules on the different cell types in multiple sclerosis lesions. Brain Pathol 14:43–50
44. Huseby ES, Liggitt D, Brabb T, Schnabel B, Öhlén C, Goverman J (2001) A pathogenic role for myelin-specific CD8+ T cells in a model for multiple sclerosis. J Exp Med 194:669–676
45. Jung J, Bhat R, Preston G, Guggino W, Baraban J, Agre P (1994) Molecular characterization of an aquaporin cDNA from brain: candidate osmoreceptor and regulator of water balance. Proc Natl Acad Sci USA 91:13052–13056
46. Karaarslan E, Altintas A, Senol U, Yeni N, Dincer A, Bayindir C, KIaraagac N, Siva A (2001) Balo's concentric sclerosis: clinical and radiologic features of five cases. AJNR Am J Neuroradiol 22:1362–1367
47. Keegan M, Konig F, McClelland R, Bruck W, Morales Y, Bitsch A, Panitch H, Lassmann H, Weinshenker B, Rodriguez M, Parisi J, Lucchinetti CF (2005) Relation between humoral pathological changes in multiple sclerosis and response to therapeutic plasma exchange. Lancet 366:579–582
48. Kerschensteiner M, Gallmeier E, Behrens L, Klinkert WEF, Kolbeck R, Hoppe E, Oropeza-Wekerle RL, Bartke I, Stadelmann C, Lassmann H, Wekerle H, Hohlfeld R (1999) Activated human T cells, B cells and monocytes produce brain-derived neurotrophic factor (BDNF) in vitro and in brain lesions: a neuroprotective role for inflammation? J Exp Med 189:865–870

49. Kerschensteiner M, Stadelmann C, Dechang G, Wekerle H, Hohlfeld R (2003) Neurotrophic cross-talk between the nervous and immune systems: implications for neurological diseases. Ann Neurol 53:292–304
50. Korte J, Born E, Vos L, Breuer T, Wondergem J (1994) Balo concentric sclerosis: MR diagnosis. AJNR Am J Neuroradiol 15:1284–1285
51. Kuhle J, Pohl, Mehling M, Edan G, Freedman M, Hartung HP, Polman C, Miller D, Montalban X, Barkhof F, Bauer L, Dahms S, Lindberg R, Kappos L, Sandbrink R (2007) Lack of association between antimyelin antibodies and progression to multiple sclerosis. N Engl J Med 356:371–378
52. Kuroiwa Y (1982) Clinical and epidemiological aspects of multiple sclerosis in Japan. Jpn J Med 21:135–140
53. Lassmann H (1983) Comparative neuropathology of chronic experimental allergic encephalomyelitis and multiple sclerosis. Springer Schriftenr Neurol 25:1–135
54. Lassmann H, Raine C, Antel J, Prineas J (1998) Immunopathology of multiple sclerosis: Report on an international meeting held at the Institute of Neurology of the University of Vienna. J Neuroimmunol 86:213–217
55. Lassmann H, Wisniewski HM (1979) Chronic relapsing experimental allergic encephalomyelitis: morphological sequence of myelin degradation. Brain Res 169:357–368
56. Lennon VA, Kryzer TJ, Pittock SJ, Verkman AS, Hinson SR (2005) IgG marker of opticspinal MS binds to the aquaporin-4 water channel. J Exp Med 202:473–477
57. Lennon VA, Wingerchuk DM, Kryzer TJ, Pittock SJ, Lucchinetti CF, Fujihara K, Nakashima I, Weinshenker BG (2004) A serum autoantibody marker of neuromyelitis optica: Distinction from multiple sclerosis. Lancet 364:2106–2112
58. Linington C, Bradl M, Lassmann H, Brunner C, Vass K (1988) Augmentation of demyelination in rat acute allergic encephalomyelitis by circulating mouse monoclonal antibodies directed against a myelin/oligodendrocyte glycoprotein. Am J Pathol 130:443–454
59. Liu J, Zhao M, Brosnan C, Lee S (2001) Expression of inducible nitric oxide synthase and nitrotyrosine in multiple sclerosis lesions. Am J Pathol 158:2057–2066
60. Lock C, Hermans G, Pedotti R et al (2002) Gene-microarray analysis of multiple sclerosis lesions yields new targets validated in autoimmune encephalomyelitis. Nat Med 8:500–508
61. Lucchinetti CF, Bruck W, Lassmann H (2004) Evidence for pathogenic heterogeneity in multiple sclerosis. Ann Neurol 56:308
62. Lucchinetti CF, Bruck W, Parisi J, Scheithauer B, Rodriguez M, Lassmann H (2000) Heterogeneity of multiple sclerosis lesions: implications for the pathogenesis of demyelination. Ann Neurol 47:707–717
63. Lucchinetti CF, Brueck W, Rodriguez M, Parisi J, Scheithauer B, Lassmann H (1999) A quantitative study on the fate of the oligodendrocyte in multiple sclerosis lesions: a study of 113 cases. Brain 122:2279–2295
64. Lucchinetti CF, Mandler RN, McGavern D, Bruck W, Gleich G, Ransohoff RM, Trebst C, Weinshenker B, Wingerchuk D, Parisi JE, Lassmann H (2002) A role for humoral mechanisms in the pathogenesis of Devic's neuromyelitis optica. Brain 125:1450–1461
65. Mantovani A, Sica A, Locati M (2005) Macrophage polarization comes of age. Immunity 23:344–346
66. Mantovani A, Sica A, Sozzani S, Allavena P, Vecchi A, Locati M (2004) The chemokine system in diverse forms of macrophage activation and polarization. Trends Immunol 25:677–686
67. Marburg O (1906) Die sogenannte "akute Multiple Sklerose". J Psychiatr Neurol 27:211–212
68. Martino G, Olsson T, Fredrikson S, Hojeberg B, Kostulas V, Grimaldi LM, Link H (1991) Cells producing antibodies specific for myelin basic protein region 70–89 are predominant in cerebrospinal fluid from patients with multiple sclerosis. Eur J Immunol 21:2971–2976
69. Matute C, Alberdi E, Domercq M, Perez-Cerda F, Perez-Samartin A, Sanchez-Gomez MV (2001) The link between excitotoxic oligodendroglial death and demyelinating diseases. Trends Neurosci 24:224–230

70. Mehta PD, Frisch S, Thormar H et al (1981) Bound antibody in multiple sclerosis brains. J Neurol Sci 49:91–98
71. Neumann H, Medana IM, Bauer J, Lassmann H (2002) Cytotoxic T lymphocytes in autoimmune and degenerative CNS diseases. Trends Neurosci 25:313–319
72. O'Connor KC B-OA, Hafler DA (2001) The neuroimmunology of multiple sclerosis: possible roles of T and B lymphocytes in immunopathogenesis. J Clin Immunol 21:81–92
73. Olsson T, Zhi WW, Hojeberg B, Kostulas V, Jiang YP, Anderson G, Ekre HP, Link H (1990) Autoreactive T lymphocytes in multiple sclerosis determined by antigen-induced secretion of interferon-gamma. J Clin Invest 86:981–985
74. Oppenheimer DR (1976) Demyelinating diseases. In: Blackwood W, Corsellis JAN (eds) Greenfield's neuropathology. Edward Arnold, London pp 470–499
75. Owens GP, Kraus H, Burgoon MP et al (1998) Restricted use of VH4 germline segments in an acute multiple sclerosis brain. Ann Neurol 43:236–243
76. Owens GP, Ritchie AM, Burgoon MP et al (2003) Single-cell repertoire analysis demonstrates that clonal expansion is a prominent feature of the B cell response in multiple sclerosis cerebrospinal flu. J Immunol 171:2725–2733
77. Patrikios P, Stadelmann C, Kutzelnigg A, Rauschka H, Schmidbauer M, Laursen H, Sorensen.P, Brück W, Lucchinetti CF, Lassmann H (2006) Remyelination is extensive in a subset of multiple sclerosis patients. Brain 129:3165–3172
78. Pittock SJ, McClelland RL, Achenbach SJ, Konig F, Bitsch A, Bruck W, Lassmann H, Parisi J, Lucchinetti CF (2005) Clinical course, pathologic correlations and outcome of biopsy proven inflammatory demyelinating disease. J Neurol Neurosurg Psychiatry 767:1693–1697
79. Prineas J (1985) The neuropathology of multiple sclerosis. In: Vinken P, Bruyn G, Klawans H (eds) Handbook of clinical neurology. Elsevier Science, New York pp 213–257
80. Prineas J, McDonald WI, Franklin JM (2002) Demyelinating diseases. In: Graham LP (ed) Greenfield's neuropathology. Edward Arnold, London pp 471–550.
81. Prineas JW, Barnard RO, Revesz T, Kwon EE, Sharer L, Cho ES (1993) Multiple sclerosis. Pathology of recurrent lesions. Brain 116:681–693
82. Prineas JW, Kwon EE, Cho ES, Sharer LR, Barnett MH, Oleszak EL, Hoffman B, Morgan BP (2001) Immunopathology of secondary-progressive multiple sclerosis. Ann Neurol 50:646–657
83. Prineas JW, Wright RG (1978) Macrophages, lymphocytes, and plasma cells in the perivascular compartment in chronic multiple sclerosis. Lab Invest 38:409–421
84. Qin Y, Duquette P, Zhang Y et al (1998) Clonal expansion and somatic hypermutation of V (H) genes of B cells from cerebrospinal fluid in multiple sclerosis. J Clin Invest 102:1045–1050
85. Redford EJ, Kapoor R, Smith KJ (1997) Nitric oxide donors reversibly block axonal conduction: demyelinated axons are especially susceptible. Brain 120:2149–2157
86. Revel M, Valiente E, Gray F, Beges C, Degos J, Brugieres P (1993) Concentric MR patterns in multiple sclerosis. Report of two cases. J Neuroradiol 20:252–257
87. Roemer SF, Parisi JE, Lennon VA, Benarroch EE, Lassmann H, Bruck W, Mandler RN, Weinshenker BG, Pittock SJ, Wingerchuk DM, Lucchinetti CF (2007) Pattern specific loss of aquaporin 4 immunoreactivity distinguishes neuromyelitis optica from multiple sclerosis. Brain 130:1174–1205
88. Schwartz M, Butovsky O, Bruck W et al (2006) Microglial phenotype: is the commitment reversible? Trends Neurosci 29:68–74
89. Serafini B, Rosicarelli B, Magliozzi R et al (2004) Detection of ectopic B-cell follicles with germinal centers in the meninges of patients with secondary progressive multiple sclerosis. Brain Pathol 14:164–174
90. Sharp FR, Bernaudin M (2004) HIF1 and oxygen sensing in the brain. Nat Rev Neurosci 5:437–448
91. Smith KJ, Kapoor R, Hall SM, Davies M (2001) Electrically active axons degenerate when exposed to nitric oxide. Ann Neurol 49:470–476

92. Smith KJ, Lassmann H (2002) The role of nitric oxide in multiple sclerosis. Lancet Neurol 1:232–241
93. Smith-Jensen T, Burgoon MP, Anthony J et al (2000) Comparison of immunoglobulin G heavy-chain sequences in MS and SSPE brains reveals an antigen-driven response. Neurology 54:1227–1232
94. Spiegel M, Kruger H, Hofmann E, Kappos L (1989) MRI study of Balo's concentric sclerosis before and after immunosuppressant therapy. J Neurol 236:487–488
95. Stadelmann C, Kerschensteiner M, Misgeld T et al (2002) BDNF and gp145trkB in multiple sclerosis brain lesions: neuroprotective interactions between immune cells and neuronal cells. Brain 125:75–85
96. Stadelmann C, Ludwin SK, Tabira T, Guseo A, Lucchinetti C, Brück W, Lassmann H (2005) Hypoxic preconditioning explains concentric lesions in Balo's type of multiple sclerosis. Brain 128:979–987
97. Storch MK, Piddlesden S, Haltia M, Livanainen M, Morgan P, Lassmann H (1998) Multiple sclerosis: in situ evidence for antibody- and complement-mediated demyelination. Ann Neurol 43:465–471
98. Sun D, Whitaker JN, Huang Z, Liu D, Coleclough C, Wekerle H, Raine CS (2001) Myelin antigen-specific CD8+ T cells are encephalitogenic and produce severe disease in C57BL/6 mice. J Immunol 166:7579–7587
99. Sun J, Link H, Olsson T et al (1991) T and B cell responses to myelin-oligodendrocyte glycoprotein in multiple sclerosis. J Immunol 146:1490–1495
100. Traugott U (1983) Multiple sclerosis: relevance of class I and class II MHC-expressing cells to lesion development. J Neuroimmunol 16:283–302
101. Turnbull HM, McIntosh J (1926) Encephalomyelitis following vaccination. Br J Exp Pathol 7:181–222
102. Van Bogaert L (1950) Post-infectious encephalomyelitis and multiple sclerosis; the significance of perivenous encephalomyelitis. J Neuropathol Exp Neurol 9:219–249
103. Vass K, Welch WJ, Nowak TS (1988) Localization of 70-kDa stress protein induction in gerbil brain after ischemia. Acta Neuropathol 77:128–135
104. Werner P Pitt D, Raine CS (2001) Multiple sclerosis: altered glutamate homeostasis in lesions correlates with oligodendrocyte and axonal damage. Ann Neurol 50:169–180
105. Williamson RA, Burgoon MP, Owens GP et al (2001) Anti-DNA antibodies are a major component of the intrathecal B cell response in multiple sclerosis. Proc Natl Acad Sci USA 98:1793–1798
106. Wingerchuk D, Pittock S, Lennon V, Lucchinetti C, Weinshenker B (2005) Neuromyelitis optica diagnostic criteria revisited: validation and incorporation of the NMO-IgG serum autoantibody. Neurology 64:A38
107. Wolswijk G (1998) Chronic stage multiple sclerosis lesions contain a relatively quiescent population of oligodendrocyte precursor cells. J Neurosci 18:601–609
108. Wood DD, Bilbao JM, O'Connors P, Moscarello MA (1996) Acute multiple sclerosis (Marburg type) is associated with developmentally immature myelin basic protein. Ann Neurol 40:18–24
109. Youl BD, Kermode AG, Thompson AJ, Revesz T, Scaravilli F, Barnard RO, Kirkham FJ, Kendall BE, Kingsley D, Moseley IF (1991) Destructive lesions in demyelinating disease. J Neurol Neurosurg Psychiatry 54:288–292

# Multiple Sclerosis Genetics

**J.P. McElroy and J.R. Oksenberg(✉)**

**Abstract** Multiple sclerosis (MS) clusters with the so-called complex genetic diseases, a group of common disorders characterized by modest disease risk heritability and multifaceted gene–environment interactions. The major histocompatibility complex (MHC) is the only genomic region consistently associated with MS, and susceptible MHC haplotypes have been identified. Although the MHC does not account for all genetic contribution to MS, the other genetic contributors have been elusive. Microarray gene-expression studies, which also have not identified a major MS locus, have, however, been promising in elucidating some of the possible pathways involved in the disease. Yet, microarray studies thus far have been unable to separate the genetic causes of MS from the expression consequences of MS. The use of new methodologies and technologies to refine the phenotype, such as brain spectroscopy, PET and functional magnetic resonance imaging combined with novel computational tools and a better understanding of the human genome architecture, may help resolve the genetic causes of MS.

J.R. Oksenberg
Department of Neurology, School of Medicine, University of California at San Francisco, San Francisco, CA 94143, USA
e-mail: Jorge.Oksenberg@ucsf.edu

M. Rodriguez (ed.), *Advances in Multiple Sclerosis and Experimental Demyelinating Diseases. Current Topics in Microbiology and Immunology 318.*
© Springer-Verlag Berlin Heidelberg 2008

# 1 Introduction

Although the etiology of multiple sclerosis (MS) is unknown, it is widely accepted to be caused by a complex interaction between environmental factors and genetics (Table 1). Possible environmental influences on MS susceptibility are geography, pathogen or chemical exposure, exposure to sunlight, month of birth, and nutrition. Evidence supporting genetic influence on MS susceptibility comes from familial aggregation and ethnic group susceptibility data. Heterogeneity has been observed in terms of whether the inflammatory infiltrate is associated with the deposition of antibody and activation of complement, and whether the target of the pathology is the myelin sheath or the oligodendrocyte [76]. A key but unresolved question is whether a single genetic mechanism of tissue damage is operative in MS, or whether fundamentally distinct pathologies are present in different genetic backgrounds.

Cases of MS often cluster in families. The risk of MS increases with relatedness to an MS-affected individual, although inheritance of MS does not follow simple mendelian inheritance patterns [108]. Monozygotic twins have a concordance rate of approximately 25%–30%, whereas dizygotic twins and full sibs have a concordance of about 2%–5% [107, 86]. While the greater concordance of monozygotic twins as compared to dizygotic twins indicates a strong genetic component, a monozygotic twin concordance rate of 30% is also consistent with strong environmental and/or epigenetic risk factors. To separate the shared family environment from the genetic risk of sib concordance, Sadovnick et al. [109] studied half-sib individuals who did or did not reside in the same household. They found that half-sibs raised together did not have a higher concordance than half-sibs raised apart, which indicates a lack of environmental influence within families on the risk of developing MS. Ebers et al. [37] studied MS patients who were adopted as children or who had first-degree adopted relatives. Adoption into a family with a first-degree relative who developed MS did not increase the risk of the adoptee developing MS. Also, no first-degree family members developed MS after adopting an individual who developed MS. These results also point to a lack of intra-family environmental

**Table 1** Model of genetic contributions in MS

1. Difficult to identify nonheritable (environmental factors)
2. Unknown genetic parameters and mode of inheritance
3. Multiple genes of moderate and cumulative effect dictate susceptibility and influence disease course
4. Etiologic heterogeneity. Identical genes, different phenotype
5. Genetic heterogeneity. Different genes, identical phenotype
6. Allelic heterogeneity. Identical genes, different alleles, identical phenotype
7. Postgenomic (transcriptional) mechanisms
8. Complex gene–gene and gene–environment interactions
9. Gender effect in susceptibility

influence on the risk of developing MS and indicate that intra-family aggregation of MS is primarily a result of genetic or epigenetic factors.

Differences in prevalence of MS between different ethnic groups residing in the same locations provide evidence supporting the genetic control of MS. For instance, people of European descent living in South Africa have higher prevalence of MS than native South Africans [30]. However, reports of altered susceptibilities for individuals moving between geographic regions with different prevalence provide evidence for environmental influences on MS [8, 30, 67, 82]. In addition, symptoms of the disease vary across ethnicities. For example, optic and spinal involvement is more common in patients of Asian descent than in White patients [64]. The results of these studies emphasize the role of both genetics and environment in MS.

## 2 Major Histocompatibility Complex and Multiple Sclerosis

The only genomic region consistently shown to have a large effect on multiple sclerosis susceptibility across studies is the major histocompatibility complex (MHC; human leukocyte antigen [HLA] in humans), which spans about 3.5 Mb on chromosome *6p21.3*. The HLA contains a large array of highly polymorphic genes involved in immune response and self-recognition [78]. The major classes of the HLA genes are the class I and class II genes, located telomerically and centromerically, respectively (Fig. 1). In an immune response, the cell surface HLA proteins present fragmented antigen proteins to T cells. The highly polymorphic regions of the class I and class II HLA genes correspond to the peptide-binding grove of the protein, which indicates that the polymorphisms likely developed to battle varying pathogenic challenges throughout evolution. Because of its role in antigen recognition, including self-antigens, the HLA system has been extensively studied in autoimmunity.

The association between the HLA and MS was first reported in 1972. Since then, many linkage scans and HLA directed analyses have confirmed this association. In most populations studied, the HLA class II *DR2* haplotype (*HLA-DRB1\*1501-*

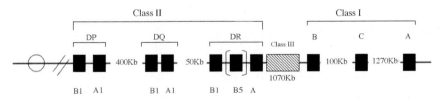

**Fig. 1** The HLA region, the genomic region most strongly associated with MS susceptibility, is divided into three classes of immune-related genes with the class II located centromerically, class I located telomerically, and class III genes between

*DQA1\*0102-DQB1\*0602*) has been associated with MS susceptibility [91], and studies have found a DR2 dose effect on MS susceptibility [13, 85, 14]. The HLA locus has been estimated to explain 15%–60% of the genetic contribution to MS susceptibility [55].

There is a clear association between MS susceptibility and the HLA region and the DR2 haplotype. However, the causative gene or genes within the HLA have not been clearly identified because of the extensive linkage disequilibrium and high gene density within the region. Some studies have attempted to distinguish the effects of *DQB1* from *DRB1* in Northern Europeans [119, 7, 18]. Taken together, however, the results were inconclusive. Using a multivariate logistic model including the effects of the *DRB1\*1501*, *DQA1\*0102*, and *DQB1\*0602*, Fernandez et al. [42] found that only the *DQB1* gene was significantly associated with MS in a Spanish population. The high level of linkage disequilibrium between *DQB1\*0602* and *DRB1\*1501* seen in people of European ancestry is not seen in people of African origin, which is more conducive to analyzing the effects of the genes separately. Oksenberg et al. [92] studied the HLA locus in African Americans for an association to MS. They found an association with *DRB1\*15* and MS that was independent of *DQB1\*0602*, and that the *DRB1\*1503* and *DRB1\*0301* alleles were also associated with MS. Another conclusion from this study, based on the haplotype data in the African American population, was that the MS-associated genes in the HLA developed prior to the divergence of human ethnic groups.

Non-*DRB1\*1501* alleles and interactions between different alleles of the *DRB1* gene may also affect MS susceptibility. Ligers et al. [71] found an association between MS susceptibility and the *DRB1* gene in *DRB1\*15*-negative Canadian families, indicating that other *DRB1* alleles may also modestly affect MS susceptibility. The *DRB1\*0301* and *DRB1\*0405* alleles were associated with MS in a Sardinian population [80]. Dyment et al. [33] studied a Canadian population of 873 families with 1,781 MS-affected individuals for the HLA *DRB1* locus. They found that, in addition to the *DRB1\*15* allele, the *DRB1\*17* allele was also associated with susceptibility and that the *DRB1\*14* and *DRB1\*01* alleles, which are both commonly in disequilibrium with *DQA1\*01* and *DQB1\*05* in Whites, were associated with MS resistance in the presence of the *DRB1\*1501* allele. An interaction was found between the *DRB1\*15* and the *DRB1\*08* alleles in association with susceptibility. Results from a population of 1,339 families of European descent with 1,571 affected individuals were recently reported by Barcellos et al. [14]. In addition to confirming the well-known association of *DRB1\*15* with MS, they identified several other interesting associations. *DRB1\*03* was also identified as a susceptibility allele. As in the Dyment et al. [33] study, the *DRB1\*14* was identified as a resistance allele, and the *DRB1\*15/DRB1\*08* allelic combination was identified as conferring high risk for MS. These studies illustrate the complexity of the genetic contribution to MS and the complexity of the HLA effect.

Some studies suggest that genes in the HLA region other than the *DRB1* and *DQB1* may also affect MS susceptibility. In Japanese MS patients with neuromyelitis optica, a subset disease of MS predominantly involving the optic nerve and spinal cord, the *HLA DPA1\*0202* [60, 133] and *HLA DPB1\*0501* alleles [133] were found to be associated with susceptibility. However, Fukazawa et al. [45] found that while the *DPB\*0501* allele was associated with MS susceptibility, it did not distinguish between opticospinal MS and nonopticospinal MS in *DPB1\*0301*-negative patients. The *DPB\*0301* allele was associated with a nonopticospinal disease course. Palacio et al. [94] and de Jong et al. [29] found associations with loci inside the class III HLA region, and others have found associations between loci telomeric to or within the class I region and MS [117, 44, 80, 70, 104]. Finally, *HLA-DRβ 5DRα* heterodimers also appear to be effective myelin antigen-presenting molecules [118], and recently published experiments using triple DRB1-DRB5-hTCR transgenics support functional epistasis between *DRB1* and *DRB5* genes [52].

To summarize, without question, the HLA region is associated with MS susceptibility. Most of the studies have shown the *HLA-DRB1\*1501-DQA1\*0102-DQB1\*0602* haplotype to increase susceptibility. The effect of the *DRB1* gene has been demonstrated separately from the *DQB1* gene and vice versa. The causal genes are still not clear, although it is possible that several or even many genes in the HLA region may have an effect on MS susceptibility.

# 3  Genetic Analyses

The majority of attempts to identify genetic polymorphisms associated with MS susceptibility have come in the form of candidate gene (hypothesis-driven) analyses or linkage and association scans (hypothesis-neutral). In the candidate gene approach, polymorphisms in genes are screened for an association with a trait of interest. Genes are chosen for the candidate gene approach based on known or hypothesized function, location in the genome, and/or function in other species. In linkage and association analyses, markers are chosen throughout the genome without prior knowledge of a hypothetical association with the trait of interest (although they are sometimes chosen based on a positional association with a trait) to test for an association with a phenotype of interest. The advantage of this approach is that the whole genome can be surveyed to identify genes that may affect a trait even in the absence of prior knowledge of function; the disadvantage is the large number of tests for which significance values need to be corrected. However, the candidate gene approach would also suffer from multiple testing if the total number of candidate genes analyzed for a trait (from multiple studies) were taken into account.

Linkage disequilibrium, which is a statistical association between two or more genetic loci, extends further in a group of related individuals than in a group of unrelated individuals. This is because many of the genomic regions in members of the same family are identical by descent (IBD), i.e., inherited as large segments of DNA from a recent common ancestor. Because the goal of the candidate gene approach is to identify an association between a specific gene and a trait, a population with lower linkage disequilibrium, such as a group of unrelated individuals, is ideal. Studying a population with limited linkage disequilibrium increases the likelihood that observed associations between a gene and a trait are due to the effects of the gene being scrutinized, instead of another linked gene. Since a linkage analysis is typically an exploratory experiment to identify trait-associated regions of the genome, populations with higher linkage disequilibrium, such as families, are ideal for identifying the trait-associated genomic regions that may not be close to the markers under analysis. With the high number of polymorphisms across the genome now available for genotyping on some predesigned arrays (>500,000), the need for extended regions of disequilibrium is minimized. Therefore, a whole genome association scan can be performed in a population of unrelated individuals while still maintaining reasonable power to detect trait-associated regions.

## 3.1   Linkage Analyses and Association Scans

The first genome scans to identify genomic regions associated with MS were reported in 1996. The three studies utilized sib-pair data structures and microsatellite markers. Haines et al. [54] analyzed 443 markers in 52 American families with multiple MS-affected individuals. They identified 19 genomic regions of suggestive association with MS including the HLA region. The analysis concluded that there was no single locus with a large effect on MS susceptibility. A genome scan in a UK population of 129 families was reported by Sawcer et al. [114]. Using 311 markers, 19 suggestive genomic regions were identified with two regions reaching significance:6p21 (HLA) and 17q22. Ebers et al. [36] studied 257 markers in a population of Canadian families with 100 sib-pairs. Five loci were suggestively associated with MS. Surprisingly, the HLA showed no linkage, but a marker near the HLA region did show a significant correlation with MS. Taken together, the results from the three pivotal studies supported a role for the HLA in MS and showed that other loci additively affecting MS susceptibility probably have small overall effects on the disease. The following year, Kuokkanen et al. [66] reported an analysis of 328 markers in 16 Finnish families with MS-affected individuals, followed by analysis of additional markers in the ten most interesting regions in 21 families (which included the 16 families from the first stage of the analysis). They found several regions, including the HLA locus, which were mildly associated with MS in the first stage of the study and suggestive significance at the *17q22-q24* region in the second stage of the study. Although no genomic regions showed striking associations with MS across the four studies, there were some overlapping regions between the studies. These included *1p36-p33, 2p23-21, 3p14-p13, 3q22-24, 4q31-qter, 5p14-p12, 5q12-q13, 6p21, 6q22-27, 7q11-q22, 17q22-24, 18p11,* and *19q12-13* [90].

Following these studies, many other MS linkage or association studies were conducted either as whole genome scans or as follow-up studies to investigate specific genomic regions of interest. These studies utilized many different ethnic and/or national populations (Table 2). The most comprehensive was conducted by the International MS Genetics Consortium [113], which included 2,692 individuals from 730 multiplex families of Northern European descent genotyped for 4,506

**Table 2** Summary of linkage/association scans in MS. The only region of the genome consistently having a large effect on MS susceptibility has been the MHC. However, the regions 17q22–24 and 19p13 have been found to be associated with MS susceptibility in several studies

| Population | N | Genomic regions/markers of interest | References |
|---|---|---|---|
| African Americans | 605 A/1043 C[2] | 1 cent. | Reich et al. [101] |
| Australians | 54 sib-pairs | 2p13, 4q26–28, 6q26, Xp11 | Ban et al. [10] |
| | 217 A/187 C | 12q15, 16p13, 18p11, 19q13, 11q12, 11q23, 14q21 | Ban et al. [9] |
| Belgians | 204 A/198 C; 131 trios | HLA Class I and II, 5q14, 8q, 20p13 | Goris et al. [51] |
| Canadians | 219 and 333 sib-pairs | HLA Class II DRB1, 17q22 | Dyment et al. [35] |
| | 552 and 333 sib-pairs | 6p21, 2q27, 5p15, 18p11, 9q21, 1p31, 17q | Dyment et al. [34] |
| Chinese and White Americans | 152 A/139 C | HLA class II, 19q13.2 | Barcellos et al. [15] |
| Finnish | 27, 125, and 135 families | Negative: 19q13.2–13.3 | Reunanen et al. [102] |
| | 22 families | 17q22–24 | Saarela et al. [106] |
| | 195 A/205 C | 1q43, 2p16, 4p15, 4q34, 6p21 | Laaksonen et al. [68] |
| French | 200 A/200 C; 200 trios | TNFα, D6S265, D7S1824, D12S1064, D14S1426, D14S605, D21S2051 | Alizadeh et al. [6] |
| French and White Americans | 245 families | 1q, 6p, 9q, 16p, 3q, 5q, 18p, 1p, 22q, 2q, 6q, 13q, 16q | Kenealy et al. [63] |
| | 188 families | 1p34, 3p14, 19q13 | Pericak-Vance et al. [96] |
| Germans | 198 A/ 198 C | 87 markers across the genome including 6p21 | Goedde et al. [48] |
| | 234 A/ 209 C; 68 trios | 2p24, 2q33, 6p21, 6p25, 11q23, 12q13, 15q24, 17p13, 19q13, Xq13 | Weber et al. [127] |
| Hungarians | 88 A/128 C | 33 markers across the genome | Rajda et al. [98] |
| Icelandics | 200 A/ 200 C | 3q25, 6p21.3, 19q13 | Jonasdottir et al. [62] |
| Northern European Descendants | 730 families | 5q33, 6p21, 17q23, 19p13 | Sawcer et al. [113] |
| Northern Irish | 200 A/ 200 C | 22 markers across the genome including 6p21 and 19q13 | Heggarty et al. [57] |
| | 200 A/ 200 C; 215 A/290 C | 1p13, 2p13, 2q14, 3p23, 7q21, 13q14, 15q13, 17p13, 18q21, 20p12 | Abdeen et al. [1] |
| Northern Irish and Sardinian | 368 A/174 C; 217 trios | 7q21–22 | Vandenbroeck et al. [124] |
| Polish | 200 A/200C; 129 trios | HLA, 2p16, 3p13, 7p22, 15q26 | Bielecki et al. [16] |
| Portuguese | 200 A/ 200 C | 6p21.3, 6q14.1, 7q34 | Martins Silva et al. [81] |
| | 188 A/ 188 C | 4q, 5q, 6p, 7q, 10p, 11p, 11q | Santos et al. [110] |

(continued)

**Table 2** (continued)

| Population | N | Genomic regions/markers of interest | References |
|---|---|---|---|
| Sardinians and Italians | 69 families | 2p11, 3q21.1, 7p15.2, 22q13.1 | D'Alfonso et al. [28] |
| | 254 families | 19q13.13 | D'Alfonso et al. [27] |
| | 40 families | None | Broadley et al. [20] |
| | 49 families | 1q31, 10q23, 11p15 | Coraddu et al. [25] |
| | 229 A/264 C; 235 trios | 2q36, 6p21, 6p25, 7p12, 16p12 | Coraddu et al. [24] |
| | 224 A/231 C; 185 trios | 2p21–22 | Liguori et al. [72] |
| Scandinavians | 106 sib-pairs; 106 A/100 C | 5p, 6p21 | Oturai et al. [93] |
| | 115 families | 17q | Larsen et al. [69] |
| | 136 sib-pairs | 17 regions across the genome including 6p21 and 17q25 | Akesson et al. [5] |
| | 199 A/200 C; 201 A/200 C | 1p33, 3q13, 6p21, 6q14, 7p22, 9p21, Xq22 | Harbo et al. [56] |
| Spanish | 200 A/200 C | 15 regions across the genome including 6p21, 17q21–24, and 19q13 | Goertsches et al. [49] |
| Swedish | 46 and 28 families; 190 A 148 C | 12q23, 7ptr-15 | Xu et al. [131] |
| | 74 families | 12p13.3, 7q35 | Xu et al. [132] |
| | 54 A and 114 healthy family members | 2q23–31, 6p24–21, 6q25–27, 14q24–32, 16p13–12, 17q12–24 | Giedraitis et al. [47] |
| Turks | 197 A/199 C | 1p35, 2p25–22, 3q13, 5q22–23, 5p15, 6q14, 8q24, 9q34, 11q13, 12q24, 19q13 | Eraksoy et al. [38] |
| | 43 families | 13q, 18q23 | Eraksoy et al. [39] |
| U.K. | 129 and 98 sib-pairs | 1cen, 3p, 6p, 7p, 14q, 17q, 22q, X | Chataway et al. [22] |
| | 744 trios | 17q23 | Chataway et al. [23] |
| | 216 A/219 C; 745 trios | HLA, 1p, 1q, 2p, 4q, 17q, 19q | Sawcer et al. [115] |
| | 226 families | 1p, 6p, 10p, 11p, 14q, 17q, 19p, 20p, Xq | Hensiek et al. [58] |
| | 16 trios | HLA, 5q13.2, 10q22–23 | Yeo et al. [134] |
| | 937 trios | Negative: 17q21 inversion | Goris et al. [50] |
| White Americans | 98 families | 19q13 | Pericak-Vance et al. [97] |
| | 98 families | 6p21, 6q27, 19q13, 12q23–24, 16p137q21–22, 13q33–34 | Haines et al. [53] |
| | 361 families | 17q11 | Vyshkina and Kalman [126] |

[1] A = MS Affected
[2] C = "Healthy" Control

**Table 3** Genomic regions associated with MS from Sawcer et al. [113], the most comprehensive genome screen for MS to date

| Chromosome | MLS | Sib allele sharing (%) | s[a] |
|---|---|---|---|
| 6p21 | 11.66 | 58.5 | 1.51 |
| 17q23 | 2.45 | 53.8 | 1.18 |
| 5q33 | 2.18 | 54.0 | 1.19 |
| 20p12 | 1.83 | 54.0 | 1.09 |
| 3p26 | 1.74 | 53.4 | 1.16 |

[a] s<CHFAN> is the relative risk attributed to the locus [103]

markers, resulting in a mean information extraction of 79.3%. The study identified several regions associated with MS (Table 3). Considering all of these studies together, no genomic regions other than the HLA region were either very strongly associated with MS in multiple studies or moderately associated with MS in a majority of the studies. However, across studies, two regions of the genome do seem to stand out more than the other regions:*17q22-24* and *19q13*.

A meta-analysis combines the data from several separate studies to gain more power for identifying loci affecting a trait. Several meta-analyses have been conducted for MS using data from some of the studies mentioned above. Wise et al. [130] used a novel meta-analysis method (the Genome Search Meta-analysis method: GSMA) to analyze the data from the first four [54, 114, 36, 66] genome scan studies. Taking all four studies into account, significant associations were detected on chromosomes 6p (HLA), 19p, 5p, 17q, 2p, and 14q. Additional significant associations were identified on chromosomes 3, 4, and 7 when the Finnish data [66] were removed; however, the significance was reduced for chromosomes 2, 5, 14, and 17. The GSMA method utilized the statistical results of the four studies, but it should have been more powerful to combine the raw data of the studies for a single large analysis. The Transatlantic Multiple Sclerosis Genetics Cooperative [122] combined the raw data from the three 1996 genome scan studies for a meta-analysis. Although no genetic regions reached genome-wise significance, there were several suggestive regions:*17q11*, *6p21* (HLA), *5q11*, *17q22*, *16p13*, *3p21*, *12p13*, and *6qtel*. Another meta-analysis reported by the GAMES and the Transatlantic Multiple Sclerosis Genetics Cooperative in 2003 [46] included the raw data from nine populations [54, 36, 114, 66, 20, 25, 5, 10, 39] previously studied. A genome-wise significant association was found for chromosome *6p21* (HLA), and a suggestive association was found for chromosomes *17q21* and *22q13*. To further investigate a genomic region associated with MS in several studies, Akesson et al. [4] genotyped individuals from the studies for additional markers on chromosome 10, and did a combined analysis across the data sets. The results of the study support an MS-associated locus on chromosome *10p15*. Fernald et al. [41] conducted a meta-analysis of all published whole genome screens for MS, whole genome screens for experimental autoimmune encephalomyelitis (EAE), and large-scale expression analyses for MS and EAE. The meta-analysis of the genome screen studies revealed several interesting regions of consensus across multiple studies, including chromosomes 2q, 5p, 6p (MHC), 7p, 7q, 11q, 16q, 17q, and 18p (Fig. 2).

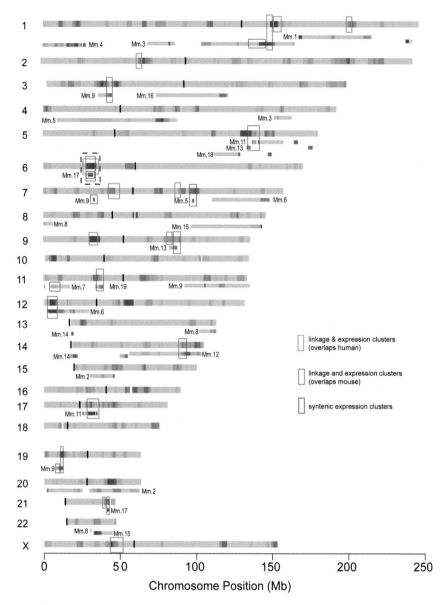

**Fig. 2** Figure from Fernald et al. [41] showing the overlap in MS- or EAE-associated genomic regions from linkage and expression studies in humans and mice. Human chromosomes are shown in their entirety and the corresponding syntenic regions of the mouse genome are indicated below each chromosome. The *intensity of red* is proportional to the value of the Z-statistic for the marker data in the 10 Mb window around each point. Consensus susceptibility regions that overlap with differentially expressed genes are indicated in *green* (human) and *blue* (mouse) *boxes*. *Red boxes* indicate syntenic regions where clusters of DEG were identified. (Reprinted from Fernald GH, Yeh RF, Hauser SL et al. 2005. Mapping gene activity in complex disorders: integration of expression and genomic scans for multiple sclerosis. J Neuroimmunol 67:157–169, with permission from Elsevier)

With the exception of the MHC region, chromosome 17q had the largest consensus across studies. A meta-analysis of 18 populations previously studied for MS susceptibility was conducted by Abdeen et al. [1], followed by a screen of the most interesting genomic region from the meta-analysis in a Northern Irish population. Ten significantly MS-associated genomic regions were identified: *1p13, 2p13, 2q14, 3p23, 7q21, 13q14, 15q13, 17p13, 18q21,* and *20p12.*

Taken together, two points are evident from the linkage/association studies and meta-analyses of these studies: the MHC is important in MS and the genetic contribution to MS is complex. The complexity of MS genetics indicates the need to use more elaborated statistical models than have currently been employed to identify new MS genes. Enough evidence exists to facilitate follow-up studies for a few regions, such as *17q22-24* and *19q13,* to identify the causative mutations resulting in the MS associations. However, attempts thus far to identify the causative mutations in these regions have not yielded definitive new MS genes. The lack of reproducibility between many of the linkage/association studies is likely a result of several factors, including insufficient power, small single-gene effects, genetic heterogeneity, phenotypic heterogeneity, genetic interactions, and false-positives. These factors are discussed in depth in relation to candidate gene studies below. The advent of whole genome association studies with dense sets of markers (>500,000) that are currently underway will facilitate more in-depth analysis of these regions without the need to design genomic region-specific studies. A screen of such type in 931 MS trio families was recently completed by an international consortium. The study yielded a large number of promising leads, which were pursued in a confirmatory dataset. A combined analysis from more than 12,000 sample identified a number of genes involved in disease susceptibility including the interleukin 2 receptor (also known as CD25) on chromosome 10p15 and the interleukin 7 receptor (CD127) on chromosome 5p13 [New Reference #1].

## 3.2   Non-MHC Candidate Genes

Many non-MHC genes have been investigated individually for an association with MS (Table 4). The majority of the genes studied are related to immune response, and many genes have been initially reported to have an association with MS. However, until now, the only non-MHC gene–MS association that has been consistently replicated across studies and populations is the interleukin 7 receptor alpha chain [New References #1, #2, #3], and the estimated effect size of this gene on MS susceptibility is small in these very recent studies. The general lack of replication is probably due to insufficient power (low numbers of individuals), small single-gene effects, genetic heterogeneity, phenotypic heterogeneity, genetic interactions, and false-positives. Low numbers and small single-gene effects jointly contribute to a lack of reproducibility. If the contribution of a gene is small, detecting its effect in a small population would require a chance-positive association between the effect and random error. This could inflate the observed effect of the gene enough to be significant in the small population. Since the associated error is a random occurrence, it would not be expected to happen by chance in another similarly small independent population. Therefore, the association is not

**Table 4** Examples of non-MHC candidate genes that have been recently associated with MS. Although the results of these studies are promising, they require replication for validation of gene effects

| Gene | Chromosomal location | Population(s) | Biological function(s) | Reference |
| --- | --- | --- | --- | --- |
| CD24 molecule (*CD24*) | 6q21 | Central Ohio case-control | Apoptosis Immune response | Zhou et al. [135] |
| Neuropeptide prepro-tachykinin-1 (*TAC1*) | 7q21–22 | Northern Irish case-control | Neurotransmission Vasodilatation Behavior | Cunningham et al. [26] |
| Interleukin 4 receptor (*IL4R*) | 16p11–12 | Single case US MS families | Immune response | Mirel et al. [84] |
| MHC class II transactivator (*Mhc2ta*) | 16p13 | Nordic case-control | Regulation of MHC class II expression | Swanberg et al. [121] |
| Nitric acid synthase (*NOS2a*) | 17q11 | Multi-case US families and African-American case-control | Neurotransmission Antimicrobial Immune response | Barcellos et al. [12] |
| Beta-chemokines or CC chemokine ligands (*CCLs*) | 17q11 | Multi-case US and Canadian families | Immune response | Vyshkina et al. [125] |
| Protein kinase C alpha (*PRKCA*) | 17q24 | Multi-case Finnish and Canadian MS families | Cell adhesion Cell transformation Cell cycle check-point | Saarela et al. [105] |
| 2′,5′- oligoad-enylate synthetase 1 (OAS1) | 12q24.1 | Spaniard case-control | Innate antivirus response | Fedetz et al. [40] |
| Angiotensin-converting enzyme (ACE) | 17q23.3 | Slovania and Croatia case-control | Renin-angiotensin system | Lovrecic et al. [75] |
| alphaB-crystal-lin gene (CRYAB) | 11q22.3-q23.1 | Denmark case-control | Molecular chaperon Myelin component | Stoevring et al. [120] |

replicated in the other populations. Note that this is an issue of power rather than false-positives, since the gene does have an effect on the trait.

Mutations in some genes may be sufficient, but not required, for an individual to develop MS. For instance, a mutation in one of several genes in the same biological pathway may be sufficient to alter the pathway and contribute to MS. This redundancy would dilute the statistical effect of any one of those genes when being studied in a population segregating susceptible alleles at all of the loci. Also, genetic stratification, which can occur when different ethnicities are present in a population, can increase the genetic heterogeneity of the disease in that population. Genetic heterogeneity can result in a lack of reproducibility when studying populations with different genetic backgrounds (ethnicity) or with different allelic frequencies at the susceptible loci. It is noteworthy that genetic heterogeneity may occur even within seemingly homogeneous populations such as Europeans [116]. In addition, phenotypic heterogeneity, which may be a reflection of genetic heterogeneity, can result in a lack of reproducible associations. While there may be some genetic overlap, populations with different disease manifestations may very well have different genetic causes, and therefore it is unclear whether individuals with these diseases should be analyzed separately.

Statistical genetic interactions, which may or may not be a result of direct biological interactions of molecules, also reduce the power of an analysis. The aforementioned redundancy of or within biological pathways would result in a statistical interaction, even if the products of the genes involved do not molecularly interact with each other to affect the disease. On the other hand, a complex protein, such as some hormones, may have several components from different genes. Combinations of specific alleles of the different genes may result in an aberrant function of the protein that individual mutations in the genes by themselves could not manufacture.

Finally, many irreproducible gene–MS associations may be false-positives. For those associations, the random error, by chance, has a configuration that results in a statistical association between the genes and MS. Although there are many reported significant gene–MS associations, there are surely more non-reported gene–MS non-associations that have been identified. As the number of genes independently tested within and between labs increases (while using significance thresholds that are not adjusted correspondingly), the probability of getting a false-positive increases [83]. Since it is not feasible to correct for all genes tested, especially when many tests are unreported, reproducibility is relied on as the standard for declaring true effects. Unfortunately, consistent reproducibility is a standard that only the HLA and the interleukin 7 receptor have achieved in MS genetic research.

# 4 Microarray Studies

Another method to identify genes associated with a trait is gene expression studies. Unlike the linkage and candidate gene analyses, in which genetic polymorphisms are analyzed for associations with a trait, gene expression studies identify genes whose RNA expression levels are associated with a trait. Microarrays survey the expression levels of many genes (from thousands to tens of thousands) throughout the genome to determine if differing expression levels are associated with differing trait values. As with the genome scans using markers, microarrays involve a large number of tests and therefore suffer from high significance thresholds required for multiple testing.

Microarray studies in MS have primarily used either brain tissue or blood [74, 2]. Each tissue has advantages. Since the primary site of damage in MS is in the brain, brain tissue gene expression may be more MS-specific than gene expression in the blood. Also, use of brain tissue is conducive to analysis of more precise phenotypic characteristics, such as lesion type or lesion region (margin vs center), and allows a comparison of normal-appearing tissue with abnormal tissue within the same individual. Brain tissue samples, however, are obtained at autopsy and therefore will also reflect many non-MS physiological events. Further, the normal-appearing tissue or other control tissue may be plagued by pathological confounding events. Alternatively, blood samples from patients are much more easily obtained and are acquired from living subjects. In addition, since MS may be autoimmune in origin, the immune cells in the periphery, prior to entering the brain, may be the proper targets for analysis.

## 4.1  Brain Microarray Studies

The first microarray analysis of MS brain tissue was conducted on a single 46-year-old male patient [128]. Acute white matter plaque tissue was contrasted with normal-appearing white matter to determine differentially expressed genes between the samples. Sixty-two differentially expressed genes (out of more than 5,000 genes surveyed) were identified, including several genes related to the brain or inflammation. In a follow-up paper, Whitney et al. [129] compared the gene expression from lesions in two MS patients and brains of EAE mice with normal-appearing white matter using a microarray consisting of 2,798 human genes. They found that the myelin basic protein gene was under expressed in the MS lesions as compared to normal white matter, indicating that the oligodendrocytes in the lesions were not properly functioning or dead. One interesting upregulated gene that was upregulated in both the MS lesions and the EAE brains was arachidonate 5-lipoxygenase. The product of this gene is involved in the formation of biologically active leukotrienes, which play a role in allergic reactions and immune response. Chabas and colleagues [21] sequenced cDNA libraries to identify RNA transcripts present in two MS brain lesion libraries but not in a healthy control brain library. The most abundant transcripts in the MS lesions not found in the healthy controls were alpha B-crystallin, prostaglandin D synthase, prostatic binding protein, ribosomal protein L17, and osteopontin. The researchers also found increased levels of osteopontin in the spinal cord of rats with EAE but not in rats protected from EAE. In a follow-up study, Hur et al. [59] also found that osteopontin exacerbated EAE and promoted the survival of activated T cells. Lock et al. [73] compared gene expression levels between brain lesion samples from four MS patients and brains of two control individuals. The inflammatory cytokines interleukin-6, interleukin-17, and interferon-γ were among the genes upregulated in the MS samples. The group also found differentially expressed genes between two extremes of MS pathology – acute inflammatory lesions and noninflammatory silent lesions. They then chose two of these differentially expressed genes, immunoglobulin Fc receptor common γ chain and granulocyte colony stimulating factor, to test their effects on EAE in mice. Immunoglobulin Fc receptor common γ chain (which was downregulated in acute/active lesions) knockout and granulocyte colony stimulating factor injection both ameliorated EAE. Mycko et al. [87] used microarray analysis to compare the margins and centers active and silent lesions in four MS patients. They found that the majority of the differentially expressed genes among the four groups (silent/margin, silent/center, active/margin, and active/center) resulted from upregulated genes in the margin of the active lesions, which is known to be the main site of lesion activity. The group also found that many of the differentially expressed genes between the margins and centers of active lesions were related to inflammation and immune response. In a later study [88], the group compared the margins and centers of chronic active and chronic inactive lesions in four MS patients. They found that more immune-related genes were expressed in the margins and centers of chronic active lesions, whereas more apoptosis-related genes were expressed in the margins and centers of the chronic inactive lesions. More recently, Dutta et al. [32] compared the gene expression of 33,000 genes between postmortem nonlesioned motor cortexes from the brains of six MS cases and six controls. They found that some genes affecting mitochondrial functions had lower expression in MS samples and that the motor neurons in MS patients had impaired mitochondrial function and decreased inhibitory innervation, which may contribute to progressive neurological disability in MS patients.

## 4.2    Microarray Studies from Blood

The first microarray study in MS using blood was reported by Ramanathan et al. [99]. They compared the peripheral blood mononuclear cell (PBMC) gene expression of 15 RRMS patients to 15 healthy controls using a 4,000-gene array. Thirty-four genes were differentially expressed, and 13 of these were immune response-related. To determine the gene expression similarities between normal immune response and autoimmune diseases, Maas et al. [77] compared the expression levels of more than 4,000 genes in PBMCs from nine healthy controls, pre- and post-flu vaccination, with individuals having four different autoimmune diseases including four individuals with MS. The results indicated that the gene expression patterns of individuals with different autoimmune diseases were similar but differed from the expression patterns of the immunized individuals. The major classes of genes that were upregulated in the autoimmune group were receptors, inflammatory mediators, signaling/second messenger molecules, and putative autoantigens, while the major downregulated classes of genes were related to apoptosis and ubiquitin/proteasome function. Bomprezzi et al. [17] compared the PBMC gene expression levels of 24 RR or SPMS samples with 21 healthy controls. Applying a novel analytical algorithm, they were able to use the expression levels to distinguish MS patients from most of the healthy controls and found that the MS patients had expression profiles indicating anti-apoptosis and autoreactive T-cell activation states. Achiron et al. [3] used a 12,000-gene array to compare the gene expression patterns in PBMCs between 26 relapsing-remitting MS patients and 18 healthy controls. Identified differentially expressed genes were also involved in T cell activation and expansion, inflammation, and anti-apoptotic mechanisms. In another study by the same group, Mandel et al. [79] compared the PBMC gene expression profiles of 13 RRMS patients, five systemic lupus erythematosus (SLE) patients, and 18 healthy controls, followed by verification of differentially expressed genes by RT-PCR and ELISA in 15 RRMS patients, eight SLE patients, and ten healthy controls. As in the Maas et al. [77] study (which also included SLE), the MS and SLE patients had a similar gene expression pattern that distinguished them from the healthy controls but also had expression profiles that distinguished the two disease groups. The genes that best distinguished individuals with disease from healthy individuals were involved in inflammation, apoptosis, and activated immune cell proliferation. MS patients were best distinguished from healthy controls by impairment of apopto-sis-related pathways. Genes encoding heat shock protein 70 were downregulated in MS patients, which was also the case in the Bomprezzi et al. [17] study. RT-PCR or ELISA verified the association between IL1B, IL8, *NR4A1*, and *CD1D* with MS. Satoh et al. [111] compared the gene expression profiles of T- and non-T-blood cells of 72 MS patients with 22 healthy controls using a microarray con-sisting of 1,258 genes. Many of the most significantly expressed genes indicated both pro- and anti-apoptotic pathways involved in MS, and some cell cycle and maintenance genes were underexpressed in MS.

Some of the microarray studies show evidence for subtypes of MS within groups of MS patients based on gene expression clustering. Van Baarsen et al. [123] used peripheral blood cell microarrays to contrast 29 RRMS patients with 25 healthy controls. Using cluster analysis of the expression data, the patients could be divided into two, approximately even groups. One of these groups of patients showed ele-vated expression of pathways known to be involved in response to viral pathogens. Satoh et al. [112] used T cell RNA with a 1,258-gene array to identify differential gene expression between 72 Japanese untreated RR and SPMS patients and 22 control subjects. Then 46 of the MS patients were treated with IFN-β for 2 years, and responders were compared to nonresponders. Between the untreated individu-als and controls, 286 genes were differentially expressed. The genes clustered the MS patients into four subgroups, and several chemokine and growth factor genes were overexpressed in the MS patients (across all subgroups) as compared to con-trols. Upregulated genes in the MS patients included *IL-12p40*, *IL-10*, *GCSF*, *PDGFRA*, *TGFβ2*, *IGF-II*, and *NR4A2*; the latest is involved in the induction of the osteopontin gene, which Chabas et al. [21] found to be overexpressed in MS patients' brain lesions and brains of EAE-susceptible mice. Although not significant, there were clear differences in the percentages of IFN-β responders between the different subgroups. This finding is important to note because it suggests the possibility of predicting IFN-β response in MS patients prior to administration of IFN-β, using the results of a gene expression study. Using the expression of 70 genes, Baranzini et al. [11] were also able to predict response to IFN-β prior to administration of the drug in 52 RRMS patients.

The results of the gene expression analyses have been promising. Interpretation of the results of post-disease onset gene expression studies, however, is not straightforward because the contributions of cause and effect are confounded. Distinguishing a differentially expressed disease-causing gene from a gene that is differentially expressed in reaction to disease is usually not possible when the expression analysis is performed after the onset of the disease. However, the studies do provide insights into the pathways involved in the disease, whether they are causative or not, and may still illuminate points of intervention for treatment. Follow-up studies of interesting genes, such as those performed by Lock et al. [73] in EAE mice, are important to help clarify the roles of the differential expressed genes in disease.

# 5   Future Directions

MS is at least partially affected by genetics. Many different strategies have been used in an effort to identify the genetic determinants of MS, including microarray studies, candidate gene studies, and linkage scans. Thus far, only one genetic region has been unambiguously identified as having a major effect on MS susceptibility: the MHC, which accounts for 15%–60% of the genetic contribution to MS susceptibility [55]. The interleukin 7 receptor has also been found to have a consistent effect, but this effect is relatively small. Efforts to identify other genomic regions conferring susceptibility have been largely unsuccessful. Some other non-MHC MS-associated loci have been identified in single studies, but the associations have not been widely replicated across studies. New experimental strategies and technologies may elucidate the genetic control of MS in the near future.

Because of the complexity of MS and the genetic and phenotypic heterogeneity involved in the disease, the use of more precise and well-defined MS traits may promote the identification of the genes involved. This strategy includes analyzing specific phenotypic characteristics that are heterogeneous in the general disease but amenable to rigorous quantitation, such as MRI abnormalities (lesion location and volume; the number of lesions). Several studies have used nonsusceptibility clinical characteristics with limited success [91]. These studies attempt to identify genes modifying the disease (age of onset, time for disease progression, severity, etc.) rather than causing the disease, and some of these phenotypes may be less genetically complex. Nevertheless, identification of these modifier genes can add pieces to the puzzle of the genetic causes of susceptibility. As this field of study progresses, it will be important to identify relevant clinical features that can be used as phenotypes for analysis.

Because of redundancy and gene–gene interactions inherent in complex molecular pathways, MS candidate gene studies should move from the single gene, reductionist strategy to a more holistic approach. Some important pathways in MS have been identified through microarray analysis, and more will likely be identified. As the knowledge of these pathways and their involvement in MS is refined, candidate gene studies should focus on the multiple genes involved in these pathways and their interactions, such as done by Brassat et al. [19]. This strategy also requires a change in the statistical methodologies currently used in many of the one-gene-at-a-time candidate gene analyses that are currently employed. The large-scale association studies (>500,000 SNPs) now underway to identify MS genes will be invaluable to test candidate genes identified in other studies, as well as to identify interactions between specific genes of interest. However, the enormous number of genotypes creates a considerable challenge to a systematically nondirected search for genetic interactions.

The efforts of the Human Genome Project to define the basic organization of the genome and its polymorphism content, together with advances in cost-efficient/genome-wide genotyping technology and analysis, have laid the groundwork for the final deconstruction of the MS genome. The potential of gene identification in complex diseases was recently highlighted by the discovery of the *Complement Factor H* gene associated with age-related macular degeneration [65]. In another example, Duerr et al. [31] demonstrated an association between variants in the *IL23R* gene and Crohn disease. In both cases, genetic discoveries led to a major leap in the understanding of disease pathogenesis. Several genome-wide association studies are underway in MS, but there are three important lessons coming from the Crohn disease and macular degeneration studies. First, replication of association findings is essential to distinguish artifacts from genuine positive results. Second, attention to phenotypic specificity reduces a primary source of heterogeneity and increases power. Third, very large sample data sets are needed to identify the full array of disease loci beyond the "low-hanging fruit." In light of the significant clinical and locus heterogeneity that is pervasive to MS as well as the modest individual gene effects, achieving adequate statistical power constitutes the most important requisite to generate definite results.

Microarray analysis is an important tool in understanding the molecular pathways involved in MS. However, microarray analysis cannot distinguish a causative gene from an MS-reactive gene when performed after disease onset. An ideal microarray analysis would compare gene expression between healthy controls and genetically susceptible individuals prior to onset of disease. A resource yet to be used for this purpose is unaffected identical twins of MS patients. Comparison of the gene expression of these individuals with that of healthy controls might elucidate the susceptible expression profiles or the expression profiles of very early (preclinical) disease states. In addition, microarray analyses have been able to separate MS patients into groups based on expression profiles. If these findings are indeed indicative of different disease types, then candidate gene and linkage studies may have more power if conducted within each of these groups, as a result of reduced disease heterogeneity.

New genetic technologies may prove vital in uncovering the genetic causes of MS. Recently, a new kind of polymorphic variation in the copy number of DNA sequence was described. Copy number variants (CNVs) are a major source of human genetic variation [89]. CNVs affect more nucleotides than single nucleotide polymorphisms (SNPs) and cover about 12% of the genome [100]. More than 3,800 CNVs have been identified in the human genome (Database of Genomic Variants: http://projects.tcag.ca/variation [Dec. 2006]). CNVs are a result of duplications or deletions of genomic regions and can affect one or more genes in that region. Studying chromosomal aberrations, such as CNVs, may be "the most rapid approach to identify candidate susceptibility loci and genes" in complex diseases [43]. CNV patterns can be identified by a technique called comparative genome hybridization (SNP-CGH [95]). SNP-CGH uses high-density SNP genotyping panels to survey the genome for these genetic aberrations. Applying this technology to new and already available data sets may prove invaluable to MS genetic research.

Another relatively new technology that has yet to be utilized in MS is genetical genomics (GG [61]). The first step of a GG experiment is microarray analysis to identify genes with transcript levels associated with a trait of interest. Then markers throughout the genome are scrutinized for an association with the expression levels of the transcripts. Genes that are important in MS because of their expression levels are identified in the GG method, as well as the regions of the genome (and eventually the genes) containing polymorphisms that regulate the gene expression. Networks of genetic control of expression and affected pathways can then be identified. The main limiting factor for a GG experiment is cost. Microarray studies typically use low numbers of individuals (~4 to ~100 individuals so far in MS) because of the per-individual cost of the experiment. These numbers of individuals are very low for detecting modest effect regulatory polymorphisms in the linkage step of the study. Ideally, the number of individuals used in a GG study would be commensurate with the numbers used in some of the larger linkage studies (>400).

Until now, studies to identify the genetic determinants of MS have had limited success. Identification of the genetic basis for MS is still very important for the development of cures or treatments. Use of the newest genetic technologies combined with the identification of better phenotypic descriptors of MS and rapidly improving understanding of the human genome architecture will certainly uncover the full array of genes contributing to MS.

# References

1. Abdeen H, Heggarty S, Hawkins SA, Hutchinson M, McDonnell GV, Graham CA (2006) Mapping candidate non-MHC susceptibility regions to multiple sclerosis. Genes Immun 7:494–502
2. Achiron A and Gurevich M (2006) Peripheral blood gene expression signature mirrors central nervous system disease: the model of multiple sclerosis. Autoimmun Rev 5(8):517–522
3. Achiron A, Gurevich M, Friedman N, Kaminski N and Mandel M (2004) Blood transcriptional signatures of multiple sclerosis: unique gene expression of disease activity. Ann Neurol 55(3):410–417
4. Akesson E, Coraddu F, Marrosu MG, Massacesi L, Hensiek A, Harbo HF, Oturai A, Trojano M, Momigliano-Richiardi P, Cocco E, Murru R, Hillert J, Compston A, Sawcer S (2003)

Refining the linkage analysis on chromosome 10 in 449 sib-pairs with multiple sclerosis.
J Neuroimmunol 143:31–38

5. Akesson E, Oturai A, Berg J, Fredrikson S, Andersen O, Harbo HF, Laaksonen M, Myhr KM,
   Nyland HI, Ryder LP, Sandberg-Wollheim M, Sorensen PS, Spurkland A, Svejgaard A,
   Holmans P, Compston A, Hillert J, Sawcer S (2002) A genome-wide screen for linkage in
   Nordic sib-pairs with multiple sclerosis. Genes Immun 3:279–285

6. Alizadeh M, Genin E, Babron MC, Birebent B, Cournu-Rebeix I, Yaouanq J, Dreano S,
   Sawcer S, Compston A, Clanet M, Edan G, Fontaine B, Clerget-Darpoux F, Semana G
   (2003) Genetic analysis of multiple sclerosis in Europeans: French data. J Neuroimmunol
   143:74–78

7. Allen M, Sandberg-Wollheim M, Sjogren K, Erlich HA, Petterson U, Gyllensten U (1994)
   Association of susceptibility to multiple sclerosis in Sweden with HLA class II DRB1 and
   DQB1 alleles. Hum Immunol 39:41–48

8. Alter M, Halpern L, Kurland LT, Bornstein B, Leibowitz U, Silberstein J (1962) Multiple sclerosis in Israel. Prevalence among immigrants and native inhabitants. Arch Neurol 7:253–263

9. Ban M, Sawcer SJ, Heard RN, Bennetts BH, Adams S, Booth D, Perich V, Setakis E,
   Compston A, Stewart GJ (2003) A genome-wide screen for linkage disequilibrium in
   Australian HLA-DRB1*1501 positive multiple sclerosis patients. J Neuroimmunol
   143:60–64

10. Ban M, Stewart GJ, Bennetts BH, Heard R, Simmons R, Maranian M, Compston A, Sawcer
    SJ (2002) A genome screen for linkage in Australian sibling-pairs with multiple sclerosis.
    Genes Immun 3:464–469

11. Baranzini SE, Mousavi P, Rio J, Caillier SJ, Stillman A, Villoslada P, Wyatt MM, Comabella
    M, Greller LD, Somogyi R, Montalban X, Oksenberg JR (2005) Transcription-based predic-
    tion of response to IFNbeta using supervised computational methods. PLoS Biol 3:e2

12. Barcellos LF, Begovich AB, Reynolds RL, Caillier SJ, Brassat D, Schmidt S, Grams SE,
    Walker K, Steiner LL, Cree BA, Stillman A, Lincoln RR, Pericak-Vance MA, Haines JL,
    Erlich HA, Hauser SL, Oksenberg JR (2004) Linkage and association with the NOS2A locus
    on chromosome 17q11 in multiple sclerosis. Ann Neurol 55:793–800

13. Barcellos LF, Oksenberg JR, Begovich AB, Martin ER, Schmidt S, Vittinghoff E, Goodin
    DS, Pelletier D, Lincoln RR, Bucher P, Swerdlin A, Pericak-Vance MA, Haines JL, Hauser
    SL (2003) HLA-DR2 dose effect on susceptibility to multiple sclerosis and influence on dis-
    ease course. Am J Hum Genet 72:710–716

14. Barcellos LF, Sawcer S, Ramsay PP, Baranzini SE, Thomson G, Briggs F, Cree BC,
    Begovich AB, Villoslada P, Montalban X, Uccelli A, Savettieri G, Lincoln RR, DeLoa C,
    Haines JL, Pericak-Vance MA, Compston A, Hauser SL, Oksenberg JR (2006) Heterogeneity
    at the HLA-DRB1 locus and risk for multiple sclerosis. Hum Mol Genet 15:2813–2824

15. Barcellos LF, Thomson G, Carrington M, Schafer J, Begovich AB, Lin P, Xu XH, Min BQ,
    Marti D, Klitz W (1997) Chromosome 19 single-locus and multilocus haplotype associations
    with multiple sclerosis. Evidence of a new susceptibility locus in Caucasian and Chinese
    patients. JAMA 278:1256–1261

16. Bielecki B, Mycko MP, Tronczynska E, Bieniek M, Sawcer S, Setakis E, Benediktsson K,
    Compston A, Selmaj KW (2003) A whole genome screen for association in Polish multiple
    sclerosis patients. J Neuroimmunol 143:107–111

17. Bomprezzi R, Ringner M, Kim S, Bittner ML, Khan J, Chen Y, Elkahloun A, Yu A,
    Bielekova B, Meltzer PS, Martin R, McFarland HF, Trent JM (2003) Gene expression profile
    in multiple sclerosis patients and healthy controls: identifying pathways relevant to disease.
    Hum Mol Genet 12:2191–2199

18. Boon M, Nolte IM, Bruinenberg M, Spijker GT, Terpstra P, Raelson J, De Keyser J,
    Zwanikken CP, Hulsbeek M, Hofstra RM, Buys CH, te Meerman GJ (2001) Mapping of a
    susceptibility gene for multiple sclerosis to the 51 kb interval between G511525 and
    D6S1666 using a new method of haplotype sharing analysis. Neurogenetics 3:221–230

19. Brassat D, Motsinger AA, Caillier SJ, Erlich HA, Walker K, Steiner LL, Cree BA, Barcellos
    LF, Pericak-Vance MA, Schmidt S, Gregory S, Hauser SL, Haines JL, Oksenberg JR, Ritchie

MD (2006) Multifactor dimensionality reduction reveals gene-gene interactions associated with multiple sclerosis susceptibility in African Americans. Genes Immun 7:310–315

20. Broadley S, Sawcer S, D'Alfonso S, Hensiek A, Coraddu F, Gray J, Roxburgh R, Clayton D, Buttinelli C, Quattrone A, Trojano M, Massacesi L, Compston A (2001) A genome screen for multiple sclerosis in Italian families. Genes Immun 2:205–210

21. Chabas D, Baranzini SE, Mitchell D, Bernard CC, Rittling SR, Denhardt DT, Sobel RA, Lock C, Karpuj M, Pedotti R, Heller R, Oksenberg JR, Steinman L (2001) The influence of the proinflammatory cytokine, osteopontin, on autoimmune demyelinating disease. Science 294:1731–1735

22. Chataway J, Feakes R, Coraddu F, Gray J, Deans J, Fraser M, Robertson N, Broadley S, Jones H, Clayton D, Goodfellow P, Sawcer S, Compston A (1998) The genetics of multiple sclerosis: principles, background and updated results of the United Kingdom systematic genome screen. Brain 121:1869–1887

23. Chataway J, Sawcer S, Feakes R, Coraddu F, Broadley S, Jones HB, Clayton D, Gray J, Goodfellow PN, Compston A (1999) A screen of candidates from peaks of linkage: evidence for the involvement of myeloperoxidase in multiple sclerosis. J Neuroimmunol 98:208–213

24. Coraddu F, Lai M, Mancosu C, Cocco E, Sawcer S, Setakis E, Compston A, Marrosu MG (2003) A genome-wide screen for linkage disequilibrium in Sardinian multiple sclerosis. J Neuroimmunol 143:120–123

25. Coraddu F, Sawcer S, D'Alfonso S, Lai M, Hensiek A, Solla E, Broadley S, Mancosu C, Pugliatti M, Marrosu MG, Compston A (2001) A genome screen for multiple sclerosis in Sardinian multiplex families. Eur J Hum Genet 9:621–626

26. Cunningham S, Patterson CC, McDonnell G, Hawkins S, Vandenbroeck K (2005) Haplotype analysis of the preprotachykinin-1 (TAC1) gene in multiple sclerosis. Genes Immun 6:265–270

27. D'Alfonso S, Nistico L, Bocchio D, Bomprezzi R, Marrosu MG, Murru MR, Lai M, Massacesi L, Ballerini C, Repice A, Salvetti M, Montesperelli C, Ristori G, Trojano M, Liguori M, Gambi D, Quattrone A, Tosi R, Momigliano-Richiardi P (2000) An attempt of identifying MS-associated loci as a follow-up of a genomic linkage study in the Italian population. J Neurovirol 6 [Suppl 2]: S18–S22

28. D'Alfonso S, Nistico L, Zavattari P, Marrosu MG, Murru R, Lai M, Massacesi L, Ballerini C, Gestri D, Salvetti M, Ristori G, Bomprezzi R, Trojano M, Liguori M, Gambi D, Quattrone A, Fruci D, Cucca F, Richiardi PM, Tosi R (1999) Linkage analysis of multiple sclerosis with candidate region markers in Sardinian and Continental Italian families. Eur J Hum Genet 7:377–385

29. de Jong BA, Huizinga TW, Zanelli E, Giphart MJ, Bollen EL, Uitdehaag BM, Polman CH, Westendorp RG (2002) Evidence for additional genetic risk indicators of relapse-onset MS within the HLA region. Neurology 59:549–555

30. Dean G (1967) Annual incidence, prevalence, and mortality of multiple sclerosis in white South-African-born and in white immigrants to South Africa. BMJ 2:724–730

31. Duerr RH, Taylor KD, Brant SR, Rioux JD, Silverberg MS, Daly MJ, Steinhart AH, Abraham C, Regueiro M, Griffiths A, Dassopoulos T, Bitton A, Yang H, Targan S, Datta LW, Kistner EO, Schumm LP, Lee AT, Gregersen PK, Barmada MM, Rotter JI, Nicolae DL, Cho JH (2006) A genome-wide association study identifies IL23R as an inflammatory bowel disease gene. Science 314:1461–1463

32. Dutta R, McDonough J, Yin X, Peterson J, Chang A, Torres T, Gudz T, Macklin WB, Lewis DA, Fox RJ, Rudick R, Mirnics K, Trapp BD (2006) Mitochondrial dysfunction as a cause of axonal degeneration in multiple sclerosis patients. Ann Neurol 59:478–489

33. Dyment DA, Herrera BM, Cader MZ, Willer CJ, Lincoln MR, Sadovnick AD, Risch N, Ebers GC (2005) Complex interactions among MHC haplotypes in multiple sclerosis: susceptibility and resistance. Hum Mol Genet 14:2019–2026

34. Dyment DA, Sadovnick AD, Willer CJ, Armstrong H, Cader ZM, Wiltshire S, Kalman B, Risch N, Ebers GC (2004) An extended genome scan in 442 Canadian multiple sclerosis-affected sibships: a report from the Canadian Collaborative Study Group. Hum Mol Genet 13:1005–1015

35. Dyment DA, Willer CJ, Scott B, Armstrong H, Ligers A, Hillert J, Paty DW, Hashimoto S, Devonshire V, Hooge J, Kastrukoff L, Oger J, Metz L, Warren S, Hader W, Power C, Auty

A, Nath A, Nelson R, Freedman M, Brunet D, Paulseth JE, Rice G, O'Connor P, Duquette P, Lapierre Y, Francis G, Bouchard JP, Murray TJ, Bhan V, Maxner C, Pryse-Phillips W, Stefanelli M, Sadovnick AD, Risch N, Ebers GC (2001) Genetic susceptibility to MS: a second stage analysis in Canadian MS families. Neurogenetics 3:145–151

36. Ebers GC, Kukay K, Bulman DE, Sadovnick AD, Rice G, Anderson C, Armstrong H, Cousin K, Bell RB, Hader W, Paty DW, Hashimoto S, Oger J, Duquette P, Warren S, Gray T, O'Connor P, Nath A, Auty A, Metz L, Francis G, Paulseth JE, Murray TJ, Pryse-Phillips W, Nelson R, Freedman M, Brunet D, Bouchard JP, Hinds D, Risch N (1996) A full genome search in multiple sclerosis. Nat Genet 13:472–476

37. Ebers GC, Sadovnick AD, Risch NJ (1995) A genetic basis for familial aggregation in multiple sclerosis. Canadian Collaborative Study Group. Nature 377:150–151

38. Eraksoy M, Hensiek A, Kurtuncu M, Akman-Demir G, Kilinc M, Gedizlioglu M, Petek-Balci B, Anlar O, Kutlu C, Saruhan-Direskeneli G, Idrisoglu HA, Setakis E, Compston A, Sawcer S (2003a) A genome screen for linkage disequilibrium in Turkish multiple sclerosis. J Neuroimmunol 143:129–132

39. Eraksoy M, Kurtuncu M, Akman-Demir G, Kilinc M, Gedizlioglu M, Mirza M, Anlar O, Kutlu C, Demirkiran M, Idrisoglu HA, Compston A, Sawcer S (2003b) A whole genome screen for linkage in Turkish multiple sclerosis. J Neuroimmunol 143:17–24

40. Fedetz M, Matesanz F, Caro-Maldonado A, Fernandez O, Tamayo JA, Guerrero M, Delgado C, Lopez-Guerrero JA, Alcina A (2006) OAS1 gene haplotype confers susceptibility to multiple sclerosis. Tissue Antigens 68:446–449

41. Fernald GH, Yeh RF, Hauser SL, Oksenberg JR, Baranzini SE (2005) Mapping gene activity in complex disorders: integration of expression and genomic scans for multiple sclerosis. J Neuroimmunol 167:157–169

42. Fernandez O, Fernandez V, Alonso A, Caballero A, Luque G, Bravo M, Leon A, Mayorga C, Leyva L, de Ramon E (2004) DQB1*0602 allele shows a strong association with multiple sclerosis in patients in Malaga, Spain. J Neurol 251:440–444

43. Feuk L, Marshall CR, Wintle RF, Scherer SW (2006) Structural variants: changing the landscape of chromosomes and design of disease studies. Hum Mol Genet 15 Spec No 1: R57–R66

44. Fogdell-Hahn A, Ligers A, Gronning M, Hillert J, Olerup O (2000) Multiple sclerosis: a modifying influence of HLA class I genes in an HLA class II associated autoimmune disease. Tissue Antigens 55:140–148

45. Fukazawa T, Kikuchi S, Miyagishi R, Miyazaki Y, Yabe I, Hamada T, Sasaki H (2006) HLA-dPB1*0501 is not uniquely associated with opticospinal multiple sclerosis in Japanese patients. Important role of DPB1*0301. Mult Scler 12:19–23

46. GAMES and Cooperative TMSG (2003) A meta-analysis of whole genome linkage screens in multiple sclerosis. J Neuroimmunol 143:39–46

47. Giedraitis V, Modin H, Callander M, Landtblom AM, Fossdal R, Stefansson K, Hillert J, Gulcher J (2003) Genome-wide TDT analysis in a localized population with a high prevalence of multiple sclerosis indicates the importance of a region on chromosome 14q. Genes Immun 4:559–563

48. Goedde R, Sawcer S, Boehringer S, Miterski B, Sindern E, Haupts M, Schimrigk S, Compston A, Epplen JT (2002) A genome screen for linkage disequilibrium in HLA-DRB1*15-positive Germans with multiple sclerosis based on 4666 microsatellite markers. Hum Genet 111:270–277

49. Goertsches R, Villoslada P, Comabella M, Montalban X, Navarro A, de la Concha EG, Arroyo R, Lopez de Munain A, Otaegui D, Palacios R, Perez-Tur J, Jonasdottir A, Benediktsson K, Fossdal R, Sawcer S, Setakis E, Compston A (2003) A genomic screen of Spanish multiple sclerosis patients reveals multiple loci associated with the disease. J Neuroimmunol 143:124–128

50. Goris A, Maranian M, Walton A, Yeo TW, Ban M, Gray J, Compston A, Sawcer S (2006) No evidence for association of a European-specific chromosome 17 inversion with multiple sclerosis. Eur J Hum Genet 14:1064

51. Goris A, Sawcer S, Vandenbroeck K, Carton H, Billiau A, Setakis E, Compston A, Dubois B (2003) New candidate loci for multiple sclerosis susceptibility revealed by a whole genome association screen in a Belgian population. J Neuroimmunol 143:65–69

52. Gregory, SG, Schmidt S, Seth P, Oksenberg JR, Hart J, Prokop A, Caillier SJ, Ban M, Goris A, Barcellos LF, Lincoln R, McCauley JL, Sawcer SJ, Compston DA, Dubois B, Hauser SL, Garcia-Blanco MA, Pericak-Vance MA, and Haines JL (2007) Interleukin 7 receptor alpha chain (IL7R) shows allelic and functional association with multiple sclerosis. Nat Genet 39:1083–1091

53. Gregersen JW, Kranc KR, Ke X, Svendsen P, Madsen LS, Thomsen AR, Cardon LR, Bell JI, Fugger L (2006) Functional epistasis on a common MHC haplotype associated with multiple sclerosis. Nature 443:574–577

54. Haines JL, Bradford Y, Garcia ME, Reed AD, Neumeister E, Pericak-Vance MA, Rimmler JB, Menold MM, Martin ER, Oksenberg JR, Barcellos LF, Lincoln R, Hauser SL (2002) Multiple susceptibility loci for multiple sclerosis. Hum Mol Genet 11:2251–2256

55. Haines JL, Ter-Minassian M, Bazyk A, Gusella JF, Kim DJ, Terwedow H, Pericak-Vance MA, Rimmler JB, Haynes CS, Roses AD, Lee A, Shaner B, Menold M, Seboun E, Fitoussi RP, Gartioux C, Reyes C, Ribierre F, Gyapay G, Weissenbach J, Hauser SL, Goodkin DE, Lincoln R, Usuku K, Oksenberg JR et al (1996) A complete genomic screen for multiple sclerosis underscores a role for the major histocompatability complex. The Multiple Sclerosis Genetics Group. Nat Genet 13:469–471

56. Haines JL, Terwedow HA, Burgess K, Pericak-Vance MA, Rimmler JB, Martin ER, Oksenberg JR, Lincoln R, Zhang DY, Banatao DR, Gatto N, Goodkin DE, Hauser SL (1998) Linkage of the MHC to familial multiple sclerosis suggests genetic heterogeneity. The Multiple Sclerosis Genetics Group. Hum Mol Genet 7:1229–1234

57. Harbo HF, Datta P, Oturai A, Ryder LP, Sawcer S, Setakis E, Akesson E, Celius EG, Modin H, Sandberg-Wollheim M, Myhr KM, Andersen O, Hillert J, Sorensen PS, Svejgaard A, Compston A, Vartdal F, Spurkland A (2003) Two genome-wide linkage disequilibrium screens in Scandinavian multiple sclerosis patients. J Neuroimmunol 143:101–106

58. Heggarty S, Sawcer S, Hawkins S, McDonnell G, Droogan A, Vandenbroeck K, Hutchinson M, Setakis E, Compston A, Graham C (2003) A genome-wide scan for association with multiple sclerosis in a N. Irish case control population. J Neuroimmunol 143:93–96

59. Hensiek AE, Roxburgh R, Smilie B, Coraddu F, Akesson E, Holmans P, Sawcer SJ, Compston DA (2003) Updated results of the United Kingdom linkage-based genome screen in multiple sclerosis. J Neuroimmunol 143:25–30

60. Hur EM, Youssef S, Haws ME, Zhang SY, Sobel RA, Steinman L (2007) Osteopontin-induced relapse and progression of autoimmune brain disease through enhanced survival of activated T cells. Nat Immunol 8:74–83

61. Ito H, Yamasaki K, Kawano Y, Horiuchi I, Yun C, Nishimura Y, Kira J (1998) HLA-DP-associated susceptibility to the optico-spinal form of multiple sclerosis in the Japanese. Tissue Antigens 52:179–182

62. Jansen RC, Nap JP (2001) Genetical genomics: the added value from segregation. Trends Genet 17:388–391

63. Jonasdottir A, Thorlacius T, Fossdal R, Jonasdottir A, Benediktsson K, Benedikz J, Jonsson HH, Sainz J, Einarsdottir H, Sigurdardottir S, Kristjansdottir G, Sawcer S, Compston A, Stefansson K, Gulcher J (2003) A whole genome association study in Icelandic multiple sclerosis patients with 4804 markers. J Neuroimmunol 143:88–92

64. Kenealy SJ, Babron MC, Bradford Y, Schnetz-Boutaud N, Haines JL, Rimmler JB, Schmidt S, Pericak-Vance MA, Barcellos LF, Lincoln RR, Oksenberg JR, Hauser SL, Clanet M, Brassat D, Edan G, Yaouanq J, Semana G, Cournu-Rebeix I, Lyon-Caen O, Fontaine B (2004) A second-generation genomic screen for multiple sclerosis. Am J Hum Genet 75:1070–1078

65. Kira J (2003) Multiple sclerosis in the Japanese population. Lancet Neurol 2(2):117–127

66. Klein RJ, Zeiss C, Chew EY, Tsai JY, Sackler RS, Haynes C, Henning AK, SanGiovanni JP, Mane SM, Mayne ST, Bracken MB, Ferris FL, Ott J, Barnstable C, Hoh J (2005) Complement factor H polymorphism in age-related macular degeneration. Science 308:385–389
67. Kuokkanen S, Gschwend M, Rioux JD, Daly MJ, Terwilliger JD, Tienari PJ, Wikstrom J, Palo J, Stein LD, Hudson TJ, Lander ES, Peltonen L (1997) Genomewide scan of multiple sclerosis in Finnish multiplex families. Am J Hum Genet 61:1379–1387
68. Kurtzke JF, Hyllested K (1987) MS epidemiology in Faroe Islands. Riv Neurol 57:77–87
69. Laaksonen M, Jonasdottir A, Fossdal R, Ruutiainen J, Sawcer S, Compston A, Benediktsson K, Thorlacius T, Gulcher J, Ilonen J (2003) A whole genome association study in Finnish multiple sclerosis patients with 3669 markers. J Neuroimmunol 143:70–73
70. Larsen F, Oturai A, Ryder LP, Madsen HO, Hillert J, Fredrikson S, Sandberg-Wollheim M, Laaksonen M, Harbo HF, Sawcer S, Fugger L, Sorensen PS, Svejgaard A (2000) Linkage analysis of a candidate region in Scandinavian sib pairs with multiple sclerosis reveals linkage to chromosome 17q. Genes Immun 1:456–459
71. Lie BA, Akselsen HE, Bowlus CL, Gruen JR, Thorsby E, Undlien DE (2002) Polymorphisms in the gene encoding thymus-specific serine protease in the extended HLA complex: a potential candidate gene for autoimmune and HLA-associated diseases. Genes Immun 3:306–312
72. Ligers A, Dyment DA, Willer CJ, Sadovnick AD, Ebers G, Risch N, Hillert J (2001) Evidence of linkage with HLA-DR in DRB1*15-negative families with multiple sclerosis. Am J Hum Genet 69:900–903
73. Liguori M, Sawcer S, Setakis E, Compston A, Giordano M, D'Alfonso S, Mellai M, Malferrari G, Trojano M, Livrea P, De Robertis F, Massacesi L, Repice A, Ballerini C, Biagioli T, Bomprezzi R, Cannoni S, Ristori G, Salvetti M, Grimaldi LM, Biunno I, Comi G, Leone M, Ferro I, Naldi P, Milanese C, Gellera C, Loredana LM, Savettieri G, Salemi G, Aridon P, Caputo D, Rosa Guerini F, Ferrante P, Momigliano-Richiardi P (2003) A whole genome screen for linkage disequilibrium in multiple sclerosis performed in a continental Italian population. J Neuroimmunol 143:97–100
74. Lock C, Hermans G, Pedotti R, Brendolan A, Schadt E, Garren H, Langer-Gould A, Strober S, Cannella B, Allard J, Klonowski P, Austin A, Lad N, Kaminski N, Galli SJ, Oksenberg JR, Raine CS, Heller R, Steinman L (2002) Gene-microarray analysis of multiple sclerosis lesions yields new targets validated in autoimmune encephalomyelitis. Nat Med 8:500–508
75. Lock CB, Heller RA (2003) Gene microarray analysis of multiple sclerosis lesions. Trends Mol Med 9:535–541
76. Lovrecic L, Ristic S, Starcevic-Cizmarevic N, Jazbec SS, Sepcic J, Kapovic M, Peterlin B (2006) Angiotensin-converting enzyme I/D gene polymorphism and risk of multiple sclerosis. Acta Neurol Scand 114:374–377
77. Lucchinetti CF, Bruck W, Parisi J, Scheithauer B, Rodriguez M, Lassmann H (2000) Heterogeneity of multiple sclerosis lesions: implications for pathogenesis of demyelination. Ann Neurol 47:707–717
78. Lundmark F, Duvefelt K, Iacobaeus E, Kockum I, Wallstrom E, Khademi M, Oturai A, Ryder LP, Saarela J, Harbo HF, Celius EG, Salter H, Olsson T, and Hillert J (2007) Variation in interleukin 7 receptor alpha chain (IL7R) influences risk of multiple sclerosis. Nat Genet 39:1108–1113
79. Maas K, Chan S, Parker J, Slater A, Moore J, Olsen N, Aune TM (2002) Cutting edge: molecular portrait of human autoimmune disease. J Immunol 169:5–9
80. Mak TW, Simard JJL (1998) Handbook of immune response genes. New York, Plenum Press
81. Mandel M, Gurevich M, Pauzner R, Kaminski N, Achiron A (2004) Autoimmunity gene expression portrait: specific signature that intersects or differentiates between multiple sclerosis and systemic lupus erythematosus. Clin Exp Immunol 138:164–170
82. Marrosu MG, Murru R, Murru MR, Costa G, Zavattari P, Whalen M, Cocco E, Mancosu C, Schirru L, Solla E, Fadda E, Melis C, Porru I, Rolesu M, Cucca F (2001) Dissection of the

HLA association with multiple sclerosis in the founder isolated population of Sardinia. Hum Mol Genet 10:2907–2916

83. Martins Silva B, Thorlacius T, Benediktsson K, Pereira C, Fossdal R, Jonsson HH, Silva A, Leite I, Cerqueira J, Costa PP, Marta M, Foltynie T, Sawcer S, Compston A, Jonasdottir A (2003) A whole genome association study in multiple sclerosis patients from north Portugal. J Neuroimmunol 143:116–119

84. Martyn CN, Gale CR (1997) The epidemiology of multiple sclerosis. Acta Neurol Scand Suppl 169:3–7

85. McElroy JP (2005) Mapping quantitative trait loci for economic traits in chickens. Genetics. PhD Thesis, Iowa State University, Ames, IA

86. Mirel DB, Barcellos LF, Wang J, Hauser SL, Oksenberg JR, Erlich HA (2004) Analysis of IL4R haplotypes in predisposition to multiple sclerosis. Genes Immun 5:138–141

87. Modin H, Olsson W, Hillert J, Masterman T (2004) Modes of action of HLA-DR susceptibility specificities in multiple sclerosis. Am J Hum Genet 74:1321–1322

88. Mumford CJ, Wood NW, Kellar-Wood H, Thorpe JW, Miller DH, Compston DA (1994) The British Isles survey of multiple sclerosis in twins. Neurology 44:11–15

89. Mycko MP, Papoian R, Boschert U, Raine CS, Selmaj KW (2003) cDNA microarray analysis in multiple sclerosis lesions: detection of genes associated with disease activity. Brain 126:1048–1457

90. Mycko MP, Papoian R, Boschert U, Raine CS, Selmaj KW (2004) Microarray gene expression profiling of chronic active and inactive lesions in multiple sclerosis. Clin Neurol Neurosurg 106:223–229

91. Nadeau JH, Lee C (2006) Genetics: copies count. Nature 439:798–799

92. Oksenberg JR, Baranzini SE, Barcellos LF, Hauser SL (2001) Multiple sclerosis: genomic rewards. J Neuroimmunol 113:171–184

93. Oksenberg JR, Barcellos LF (2005) Multiple sclerosis genetics: leaving no stone unturned. Genes Immun 6:375–387

94. Oksenberg JR, Barcellos LF, Cree BA, Baranzini SE, Bugawan TL, Khan O, Lincoln RR, Swerdlin A, Mignot E, Lin L, Goodin D, Erlich HA, Schmidt S, Thomson G, Reich DE, Pericak-Vance MA, Haines JL, Hauser SL (2004) Mapping multiple sclerosis susceptibility to the HLA-DR locus in African Americans. Am J Hum Genet 74:160–167

95. Oturai A, Larsen F, Ryder LP, Madsen HO, Hillert J, Fredrikson S, Sandberg-Wollheim M, Laaksonen M, Koch-Henriksen N, Sawcer S, Fugger L, Sorensen PS, Svejgaard A (1999) Linkage and association analysis of susceptibility regions on chromosomes 5 and 6 in 106 Scandinavian sibling pair families with multiple sclerosis. Ann Neurol 46:612–616

96. Palacio LG, Rivera D, Builes JJ, Jimenez ME, Salgar M, Anaya JM, Jimenez I, Camargo M, Arcos-Burgos M, Sanchez JL (2002) Multiple sclerosis in the tropics: genetic association to STR's loci spanning the HLA and TNF. Mult Scler 8:249–255

97. Peiffer DA, Le JM, Steemers FJ, Chang W, Jenniges T, Garcia F, Haden K, Li J, Shaw CA, Belmont J, Cheung SW, Shen RM, Barker DL and Gunderson KL (2006) High-resolution genomic profiling of chromosomal aberrations using Infinium whole-genome genotyping. Genome Res 16:1136–1148

98. Pericak-Vance MA, Rimmler JB, Haines JL, Garcia ME, Oksenberg JR, Barcellos LF, Lincoln R, Hauser SL, Cournu-Rebeix I, Azoulay-Cayla A, Lyon-Caen O, Fontaine B, Duhamel E, Coppin H, Brassat D, Roth MP, Clanet M, Alizadeh M, Yaouanq J, Quelvennec E, Semana G, Edan G, Babron MC, Genin E, Clerget-Darpoux F (2004) Investigation of seven proposed regions of linkage in multiple sclerosis: an American and French collaborative study. Neurogenetics 5:45–48

99. Pericak-Vance MA, Rimmler JB, Martin ER, Haines JL, Garcia ME, Oksenberg JR, Barcellos LF, Lincoln R, Goodkin DE, Hauser SL (2001) Linkage and association analysis of chromosome 19q13 in multiple sclerosis. Neurogenetics 3:195–201

100. Rajda C, Bencsik K, Seres E, Jonasdottir A, Foltynie T, Sawcer S, Benediktsson K, Fossdal R, Setakis E, Compston A, Vecsei L (2003) A genome-wide screen for association in Hungarian multiple sclerosis. J Neuroimmunol 143:84–87

101. Ramanathan M, Weinstock-Guttman B, Nguyen LT, Badgett D, Miller C, Patrick K, Brownscheidle C, Jacobs L (2001) In vivo gene expression revealed by cDNA arrays: the pattern in relapsing-remitting multiple sclerosis patients compared with normal subjects. J Neuroimmunol 116:213–219

102. Redon R, Ishikawa S, Fitch KR, Feuk L, Perry GH, Andrews TD, Fiegler H, Shapero MH, Carson AR, Chen W, Cho EK, Dallaire S, Freeman JL, Gonzalez JR, Gratacos M, Huang J, Kalaitzopoulos D, Komura D, MacDonald JR, Marshall CR, Mei R, Montgomery L, Nishimura K, Okamura K, Shen F, Somerville MJ, Tchinda J, Valsesia A, Woodwark C, Yang F, Zhang J, Zerjal T, Zhang J, Armengol L, Conrad DF, Estivill X, Tyler-Smith C, Carter NP, Aburatani H, Lee C, Jones KW, Scherer SW, Hurles ME (2006) Global variation in copy number in the human genome. Nature 444:444–454

103. Reich D, Patterson N, De Jager PL, McDonald GJ, Waliszewska A, Tandon A, Lincoln RR, DeLoa C, Fruhan SA, Cabre P, Bera O, Semana G, Kelly MA, Francis DA, Ardlie K, Khan O, Cree BA, Hauser SL, Oksenberg JR, Hafler DA (2005) A whole-genome admixture scan finds a candidate locus for multiple sclerosis susceptibility. Nat Genet 37:1113–1118

104. Reunanen K, Finnila S, Laaksonen M, Sumelahti ML, Wikstrom J, Pastinen T, Kuokkanen S, Saarela J, Uimari P, Ruutiainen J, Ilonen J, Peltonen L, Tienari PJ (2002) Chromosome 19q13 and multiple sclerosis susceptibility in Finland: a linkage and two-stage association study. J Neuroimmunol 126:134–142

105. Risch N (1990) Linkage strategies for genetically complex traits. I. Multilocus models. Am J Hum Genet 46:222–228

106. Rubio JP, Bahlo M, Butzkueven H, van Der Mei IA, Sale MM, Dickinson JL, Groom P, Johnson LJ, Simmons RD, Tait B, Varney M, Taylor B, Dwyer T, Williamson R, Gough NM, Kilpatrick TJ, Speed TP, Foote SJ (2002) Genetic dissection of the human leukocyte antigen region by use of haplotypes of Tasmanians with multiple sclerosis. Am J Hum Genet 70:1125–1137

107. Saarela J, Kallio SP, Chen D, Montpetit A, Jokiaho A, Choi E, Asselta R, Bronnikov D, Lincoln MR, Sadovnick AD, Tienari PJ, Koivisto K, Palotie A, Ebers GC, Hudson TJ and Peltonen L (2006) PRKCA and multiple sclerosis: association in two independent populations. PLoS Genet 2:e42

108. Saarela J, Schoenberg Fejzo M, Chen D, Finnila S, Parkkonen M, Kuokkanen S, Sobel E, Tienari PJ, Sumelahti ML, Wikstrom J, Elovaara I, Koivisto K, Pirttila T, Reunanen M, Palotie A, Peltonen L (2002) Fine mapping of a multiple sclerosis locus to 2.5 Mb on chromosome 17q22-q24. Hum Mol Genet 11:2257–2267

107. Sadovnick AD, Armstrong H, Rice GP, Bulman D, Hashimoto L, Paty DW, Hashimoto SA, Warren S, Hader W, Murray T et al (1993) A population-based study of multiple sclerosis in twins: update. Ann Neurol 33:281–285

108. Sadovnick AD, Baird PA, Ward RH (1988) Multiple sclerosis: updated risks for relatives. Am J Med Genet 29:533–541

109. Sadovnick AD, Ebers GC, Dyment DA, Risch NJ (1996) Evidence for genetic basis of multiple sclerosis. The Canadian Collaborative Study Group. Lancet 347:1728–1730

110.Santos M, Pinto-Basto J, Rio ME, Sa MJ, Valenca A, Sa A, Dinis J, Figueiredo J, Bigotte de Almeida L, Coelho I, Sawcer S, Setakis E, Compston A, Sequeiros J, Maciel P (2003) A whole genome screen for association with multiple sclerosis in Portuguese patients. J Neuroimmunol 143:112–115

111. Satoh J, Nakanishi M, Koike F, Miyake S, Yamamoto T, Kawai M, Kikuchi S, Nomura K, Yokoyama K, Ota K, Kanda T, Fukazawa T, Yamamura T (2005) Microarray analysis identifies an aberrant expression of apoptosis and DNA damage-regulatory genes in multiple sclerosis. Neurobiol Dis 18:537–550

112. Satoh J, Nakanishi M, Koike F, Onoue H, Aranami T, Yamamoto T, Kawai M, Kikuchi S, Nomura K, Yokoyama K, Ota K, Saito T, Ohta M, Miyake S, Kanda T, Fukazawa T, Yamamura T (2006) T cell gene expression profiling identifies distinct subgroups of Japanese multiple sclerosis patients. J Neuroimmunol 174:108–118

113. Sawcer S, Ban M, Maranian M, Yeo TW, Compston A, Kirby A, Daly MJ, De Jager PL, Walsh E, Lander ES, Rioux JD, Hafler DA, Ivinson A, Rimmler J, Gregory SG, Schmidt S, Pericak-Vance MA, Akesson E, Hillert J, Datta P, Oturai A, Ryder LP, Harbo HF, Spurkland A, Myhr KM, Laaksonen M, Booth D, Heard R, Stewart G, Lincoln R, Barcellos LF, Hauser SL, Oksenberg JR, Kenealy SJ, Haines JL (2005) A high-density screen for linkage in multiple sclerosis. Am J Hum Genet 77:454–467

114. Sawcer S, Jones HB, Feakes R, Gray J, Smaldon N, Chataway J, Robertson N, Clayton D, Goodfellow PN, Compston A (1996) A genome screen in multiple sclerosis reveals susceptibility loci on chromosome 6p21 and 17q22. Nat Genet 13:464–468

115. Sawcer S, Maranian M, Setakis E, Curwen V, Akesson E, Hensiek A, Coraddu F, Roxburgh R, Sawcer D, Gray J, Deans J, Goodfellow PN, Walker N, Clayton D, Compston A (2002) A whole genome screen for linkage disequilibrium in multiple sclerosis confirms disease associations with regions previously linked to susceptibility. Brain 125:1337–1347

116. Seldin MF, Shigeta R, Villoslada P, Selmi C, Tuomilehto J, Silva G, Belmont JW, Klareskog L, Gregersen PK (2006) European population substructure: clustering of northern and southern populations. PLoS Genet 2:e143

117. Shinar Y, Pras E, Siev-Ner I, Gamus D, Brautbar C, Israel S, Achiron A (1998) Analysis of allelic association between D6S461 marker and multiple sclerosis in Ashkenazi and Iraqi Jewish patients. J Mol Neurosci 11:265–269

118. Sospedra M, Muraro PA, Stefanova I, Zhao Y, Chung K, Li Y, Giulianotti M, Simon R, Mariuzza R, Pinilla C, Martin R (2006) Redundancy in antigen-presenting function of the HLA-DR and -DQ molecules in the multiple sclerosis-associated HLA-DR2 haplotype. J Immunol 176:1951–1961

119. Spurkland A, Ronningen KS, Vandvik B, Thorsby E, Vartdal F (1991) HLA-DQA1 and HLA-DQB1 genes may jointly determine susceptibility to develop multiple sclerosis. Hum Immunol 30:69–75

120. Stoevring B, Frederiksen JL, Christiansen M (2007) CRYAB promoter polymorphisms: influence on multiple sclerosis susceptibility and clinical presentation. Clin Chim Acta 375:57–62

121. Swanberg M, Lidman O, Padyukov L, Eriksson P, Akesson E, Jagodic M, Lobell A, Khademi M, Borjesson O, Lindgren CM, Lundman P, Brookes AJ, Kere J, Luthman H, Alfredsson L, Hillert J, Klareskog L, Hamsten A, Piehl F, Olsson T (2005) MHC2TA is associated with differential MHC molecule expression and susceptibility to rheumatoid arthritis, multiple sclerosis and myocardial infarction. Nat Genet 37:486–494

122. The International MS Genetics Consortium (2007) Risk alleles for multiple sclerosis identified by a genomewide study. N Engl J Med 357:851–862

122. TMSGC (2001) A meta-analysis of genomic screens in multiple sclerosis. The Transatlantic Multiple Sclerosis Genetics Cooperative. Mult Scler 7:3–11

123. van Baarsen LG, van der Pouw Kraan TC, Kragt JJ, Baggen JM, Rustenburg F, Hooper T, Meilof JF, Fero MJ, Dijkstra CD, Polman CH, Verweij CL (2006) A subtype of multiple sclerosis defined by an activated immune defense program. Genes Immun 7:522–531

124. Vandenbroeck K, Fiten P, Heggarty S, Goris A, Cocco E, Hawkins SA, Graham CA, Marrosu MG, Opdenakker G (2002) Chromosome 7q21–22 and multiple sclerosis: evidence for a genetic susceptibility effect in vicinity to the protachykinin-1 gene. J Neuroimmunol 125:141–148

125. Vyshkina T, Banisor I, Shugart YY, Leist TP, Kalman B (2005) Genetic variants of complex I in multiple sclerosis. J Neurol Sci 228:55–64

126. Vyshkina T, Kalman B (2005) Haplotypes within genes of beta-chemokines in 17q11 are associated with multiple sclerosis: a second phase study. Hum Genet 118:67–75

127. Weber A, Infante-Duarte C, Sawcer S, Setakis E, Bellmann-Strobl J, Hensiek A, Rueckert S, Schoenemann C, Benediktsson K, Compston A, Zipp F (2003) A genome-wide German screen for linkage disequilibrium in multiple sclerosis. J Neuroimmunol 143:79–83

128. Whitney LW, Becker KG, Tresser NJ, Caballero-Ramos CI, Munson PJ, Prabhu VV, Trent JM, McFarland HF, Biddison WE (1999) Analysis of gene expression in mutiple sclerosis lesions using cDNA microarrays. Ann Neurol 46:425–428

129. Whitney LW, Ludwin SK, McFarland HF, Biddison WE (2001) Microarray analysis of gene expression in multiple sclerosis and EAE identifies 5-lipoxygenase as a component of inflammatory lesions. J Neuroimmunol 121:40–48

130. Wise LH, Lanchbury JS, Lewis CM (1999) Meta-analysis of genome searches. Ann Hum Genet 63:263–272

131. Xu C, Dai Y, Fredrikson S, Hillert J (1999) Association and linkage analysis of candidate chromosomal regions in multiple sclerosis: indication of disease genes in 12q23 and 7ptr-15. Eur J Hum Genet 7:110–116

132. Xu C, Dai Y, Lorentzen JC, Dahlman I, Olsson T, Hillert J (2001) Linkage analysis in multiple sclerosis of chromosomal regions syntenic to experimental autoimmune disease loci. Eur J Hum Genet 9:458–463

133. Yamasaki K, Horiuchi I, Minohara M, Kawano Y, Ohyagi Y, Yamada T, Mihara F, Ito H, Nishimura Y, Kira J (1999) HLA-DPB1*0501-associated opticospinal multiple sclerosis: clinical, neuroimaging and immunogenetic studies. Brain 122:1689–1696

134. Yeo TW, Roxburgh R, Maranian M, Singlehurst S, Gray J, Hensiek A, Setakis E, Compston A and Sawcer S (2003) Refining the analysis of a whole genome linkage disequilibrium association map: the United Kingdom results. J Neuroimmunol 143:53–59

135. Zhou Q, Rammohan K, Lin S, Robinson N, Li O, Liu X, Bai XF, Yin L, Scarberry B, Du P, You M, Guan K, Zheng P, Liu Y (2003) CD24 is a genetic modifier for risk and progression of multiple sclerosis. Proc Natl Acad Sci U S A 100:15041–15046

# Imaging of Remyelination and Neuronal Health

B.J. Erickson

## Contents

**Abstract** Remyelination of axons that have been demyelinated due to multiple sclerosis (MS) may be a critical step in restoring the damaged axons and reversing the disease process. While it is possible to establish the presence of remyelination with microscopy of tissue samples, it is important to have noninvasive or minimally invasive methods to measure remyelination in living

B.J. Erikson
Department of Radiology, Mayo Clinic, 200 First St. SW, Rochester, MN 55905, USA
e-mail: BJE@mayo.edu

M. Rodriguez (ed.), *Advances in Multiple Sclerosis and Experimental*
*Demyelinating Diseases. Current Topics in Microbiology and Immunology 318.*
© Springer-Verlag Berlin Heidelberg 2008

animals and humans. Such tools are critical to establishing the efficacy of agents purported to promote or enhance remyelination. This chapter reviews the technology of imaging of the brain, its application to MS, and the current state of imaging techniques for measuring remyelination and the health of the associated neurons in the setting of MS.

# Abbreviations

| | |
|---|---|
| BBB | Blood–brain barrier |
| BMB | 1,4-Bis(p-aminostyryl)-2-methoxy benzene |
| CT | Computed tomography |
| FA | Fractional anisotropy |
| Gd | Gadolinium |
| MRI | Magnetic resonance imaging |
| MRS | Magnetic resonance spectroscopy |
| MS | Multiple sclerosis |
| MT | Magnetization transfer |
| MTR | Magnetization transfer ratio |
| NAA | N-acetyl aspartate |
| NAWM | Normal-appearing white matter |
| ppm | Parts per million |
| SPMS | Secondary progressive multiple sclerosis |
| RRMS | Relapsing-remitting multiple sclerosis |

# 1 Introduction

## 1.1 The Rationale for Imaging Remyelination

While imaging has played a major role in the assessment of putative therapies in MS, little is known about the appearance of remyelination on either standard or nonstandard imaging methods as applied to human or animal models. Imaging is a widely valued method for learning about processes in vivo because it is either non- or minimally invasive. The earliest in vivo neuroimaging technology capable of showing the effects of MS was computed tomography (CT), where areas of demyelination were identified by loss of radio-opacity. While some of this low density was attributed to edema and inflammation, it was also known that some lesions would continue to have low signal, reflecting chronic demyelination. Some lesions would regain a portion of their density, raising the possibility of remyelination. However, CT is relatively insensitive to demyelination and quickly fell out of favor when magnetic resonance imaging (MRI) became available [26, 30].

Imaging is of great interest for the study of MS because of its ability to localize lesions, which in turn allows correlation with clinical symptoms. In the case of MS, the lesions visible with standard MRI methods are locations of frank demyelination. For many years, it was believed that the best in vivo measure of disease activity was the sum total of these focal lesions. Now we also know of an element of diffuse disease not readily apparent with standard MRI. It is unclear if or how these two components (that which is visible on conventional MRI and that which is not visible on conventional MRI) of demyelination reflect the overall state of disease. However, if imaging findings could be correlated with the disease and disease repair, it would be a powerful tool for developing and evaluating putative therapies.

While demyelination of axons was first believed to be the primary cause of the clinical deficits seen in MS, recent pathologic studies suggest neuronal loss may be better correlated with clinical course [1, 24]. This is a critical point: if a lesion is demyelinated and the neuron dies, myelin deposition (if possible) would be of no benefit. If the neuron or axon is so severely injured that it does not function properly, remyelination may occur but probably without restoration of function.

A related point is the distinction between myelin deposition and remyelination, which requires that axons be wrapped with at least one layer of myelin in order to restore normal or near normal axonal function. This distinction is obviously essential to development of a method that correlates with restoration of a function and is a critical component when evaluating imaging methods. Simply depositing myelin is not sufficient – it must also be functionally equivalent to the state prior to demyelination. The full volume of myelin present prior to demyelination may not be necessary to restore function. In that case, however, the imaging method must be able to differentiate between two axons where each has two wraps, and two axons in which one has no wraps and the other has four. While imaging is capable of spatial localization, current methods have a resolution of about 1 mm, limiting the ability to resolve regional variations.

Pathologists use myelin thickness as a marker of remyelination; areas with thin myelin layers presumably represent previously demyelinated areas that had been subsequently remyelinated [34]. This distinction is not possible with current imaging, but complete normalcy of myelin may not be a necessary or appropriate expectation for evaluation of remyelination.

Another puzzle is the possibility that brain plasticity results in clinical restoration of function even without repair of a portion of the brain. This plasticity could make it difficult to correlate imaging markers of remyelination with clinical functional status. Functional MRI can localize some, but not all, brain functions, and some localization paradigms require a high degree of patient cooperation. Therefore, it is unlikely that imaging will be able to correct for brain plasticity that hides the effects of demyelination.

Given all these factors, it is almost certain that conventional MRI methods lack the spatial resolution and contrast properties that allow complete characterization of the remyelination process. However, newer methods that have been engineered to more accurately characterize the presence and state of myelin appear quite promising.

This chapter will outline currently available methods reflecting components of remyelination helpful in understanding the natural history of the disease and reflect on the mechanisms and biology of putative remyelinating agents.

## 2    Conventional MRI of Remyelination

### 2.1    *Physics of Conventional MRI*

As mentioned previously, MRI is the primary tool for evaluating MS and proposed therapeutic agents. MRI is an extremely flexible tool that can provide images with a broad range of contrast properties. Understanding the physical basis for how an MRI produces images with specific contrast properties may help the reader to understand how remyelination might be visualized and some of the pitfalls and barriers.

MRI employs a strong magnetic field to align a (small) majority of hydrogen protons in a body. A radiofrequency pulse is then emitted into the body; if it is of the correct frequency, it will cause the aligned protons to be temporarily flipped out of alignment. How far they are tipped depends on the strength and duration of the radiofrequency pulse. When the pulse stops, the protons move back into alignment with the strong field. The rate at which they re-align is called the T1 time. Much like tops, protons also process around the axis of the main magnetic field (though protons process less with time, while tops process more with time) and will process at slightly different rates than their neighbors, depending on the local environment. How long they take to lose synchrony with their neighbors is called the T2 time.

An image is composed of picture elements or pixels. The numerical value of the pixel reflects the amount of signal generated by the protons in the tissue corresponding with that pixel. A typical MRI image is composed of a matrix of 256 pixels in the X direction and 256 pixels in the Y direction. MRI allows this matrix to be changed fairly easily, along with the thickness of the slice of tissue that image represents. One could collect images with very small pixels (so-called high-resolution images), which may allow better characterization of the tissues at a certain location. However, higher resolution increases the amount of noise in the image and/or the time needed to acquire the image. A longer acquisition time allows more chance for patient motion, possibly resulting in a blurry, useless image, and consumes time that could be used to collect other, more useful images.

The images used in clinical practice are weighted to reflect the T1 or T2 times of tissues in the image but are not quantitative. That is, the pixel value does not equal the actual T1 or T2 time. T1-weighted images are bright for tissues with short T1 times, and T2 weighted images are bright for tissues with long T2 times. Proton density or intermediate weighted images reflect the number of signal-producing hydrogen protons but also are not quantitative. Mobile hydrogen protons from water and some lipids provide the vast majority of the visible MR signal in the head. Air and bone are dark on MRI because they lack mobile protons, although the marrow fat within bone can produce signal.

## 2.2   T2 Images of Multiple Sclerosis

While it is possible to see brain lesions in patients with MS on CT, T2-weighted MRI is substantially more sensitive for MS lesions [26]. Early studies correlating MRI with histology demonstrate areas of increased T2 signal representing areas of greater demyelination [24]. An MS lesion appears on T2 images early in its course, usually expands to its maximum size over a few days, and then decreases in size over the next 4–6 weeks. This increased signal is primarily due to an increased fraction of water (edema) in the tissue. The extent of decrease is variable. In some cases, it decreases very little, and in other cases, it completely disappears. If a lesion continues to be visible, it likely reflects continued high fraction of water with tissue destruction and gliosis. Areas of largely restored signal may reflect minimal demyelination, or remyelination, which means there is little available room for excess water. An existing lesion can also undergo reactivation, which causes enlargement. T1-weighted images may show decreased signal where T2 images show increased signal, and the degree of signal loss varies among lesions. After the acute phase, the lesion may have partial or complete restoration of the signal.

MS patients have an average annual increase of T2 lesion load of about 10% [22, 43] albeit with significant individual variation. This increased T2 signal is due to the increased fraction of mobile water protons in lesions where myelin is replaced with gliosis; myelin has fewer mobile water protons, and the water that is present tends to be restricted in motion by the tight myelin wraps. However, there are other reasons for increased T2 signal, including the presence of edema within tissue with or without normal myelination. Conversely, T2-weighted images can appear entirely normal despite the presence of microscopic plaques.

Given this understanding of T2-weighted image appearance, a reasonable hypothesis is that T2 signal is reduced, if not normal, in areas of remyelination. Many of the early efforts to establish therapeutic efficacy of MS agents utilized T2-weighted imaging of the brain. In particular, measurement of the volume of abnormal T2-weighted tissue was used to gain FDA approval for agents such as interferon beta-1b [31]. Those MRI studies demonstrated a reduced rate of accumulation of abnormal T2 tissue compared with patients receiving placebo. This was taken as reasonable evidence of efficacy despite the lack of a demonstrated difference in clinical measures.

### 2.2.1   Quantitative T2 Images of MS

While most people are very familiar with T2-weighted imaging, some have experimented with creating images that reflect actual T2 times. This may be of value because conventional T2-weighted imaging does not have a reproducible intensity scale. Rather, it is necessary to express values relative to some other value – usually another tissue on the image – when reporting or measuring the size and intensity of lesions. If a tissue is not affected by the disease, one may compare the ratio over time or between individuals. True T2 images have pixel values where the T2 decay time is the actual pixel value at that location. True T2 images can therefore be compared across time and subjects. However, they are difficult to obtain and not a part of routine clinical practice. They do not appear to provide different information from T2-weighted images, even if they are reproducible.

### 2.2.2   Imaging of T2 Components

While there is a single intensity value for each pixel in an image including the T2 time images just described, the intensity actually represents the weighted sum of many protons located within the pixel. For clinical brain imaging, water protons are the dominant source of signal. However, the signal from water is not uniform, and the local environment of each water proton affects the signal produced. Since the size of a pixel is much larger than a single molecule of water, its signal is a combination of all the water molecules within that pixel. Some have looked at these components of T2 signal in the context of multiple sclerosis [27]. Some components (like bulk water) have a relatively long T2 time (seconds). In other regions, the T2 time is much shorter (milliseconds). In regions where myelin wraps around an axon, it results in thin layers of water. In this case, water exchanges protons with non-water molecules, and the T2 time of these protons differs greatly from that of bulk water protons. The study noted above found a short T2 component of the signal to correspond with the distribution of myelin in the brain. In areas of myelin destruction, there was a relative lack of the short T2 component. This included areas where axons were preserved despite complete loss of myelin. Because this was a single time point study, the authors did not address the impact of remyelination on this short T2 component. If enough remyelination occurred, one would expect to see a partial restoration of the short T2 component as more water interacted with myelin sheaths. It is unclear if remyelinated areas might have a different T2 time compared with normal myelination; if true, it may be due to the thinner and relatively fewer wraps in remyelinated areas.

## 2.3   T2-Weighted Imaging of Remyelination

While the trials of MS therapies have shown differences in the accumulation of T2 lesions, they have not focused on demonstrating remyelination. However, clinical trials have shown a difference in the rate of accumulation of T2 lesion load for some agents, but it is not clear that the therapies are promoting remyelination. They may simply be decreasing the rate of demyelination. In addition, although remyelination should improve the clinical status of patients in theory, several studies have shown that the volume of lesions on T2-weighted images does not correlate well with patient disability.

Can a T2-weighted image prove remyelination? Given the discussion above, it is unlikely that a T2-weighted image can show remyelination at a single point in time. Given our current understanding and current imaging methods, it would be difficult for any single-point-in-time image to be specific for remyelination. It is easier to imagine the demonstration of remyelination by serial imaging in which there is reduction of abnormality in a previously demyelinated area. For that to be true, it is necessary for the studies to be specific for demyelination and not sensitive to the associated inflammatory changes that later resolve and mimic remyelination.

A recent study of mice undergoing demyelination and then remyelination of the spinal cord suggests that T2 images show remyelination-associated changes [32]. Mice were treated with either placebo or rHIgM22, an antibody demonstrated to promote remyelination. The authors found that mice treated with rHIgM22 and demonstrating remyelination had smaller lesions on T2-weighted images, and less T2 intensity. In another study of the mouse/cuprizone model, where demyelination and remyelination have a very predictable time course, the authors [25] also found that T2 increased in the demyelination phase and declined (though not back to normal) after remyelination. While this may not prove that decreased T2 signal in human brain correlates with remyelination, it fits with our understanding of how T2 imaging works and is provocative.

## 2.4 T1-Weighted Imaging of MS and Remyelination

T1-weighted images also show lesions in MS but are less sensitive than T2 images. Previous pathologic studies have shown T1 hypointensity correlated with myelin destruction [40] and axonal loss [39]. In fact, T1 hypointensities appear to correlate better with clinical disability than T2 lesion load [41]. It is less well documented that restoration of T1 intensity correlates with remyelination or axonal preservation. As with T2 images, it is possible to create T1 images reflecting actual T1 times and, therefore, with a reproducible intensity scale, but these are not used in clinical care. They are largely used for research purposes, and there is no documentation that restoration of the T1 time is due to remyelination.

In many respects, the known data about T1-weighted images is similar to that of T2-weighted images. In a study, of mice treated with cuprizone [25], T1 signal loss correlated with demyelination, and T1 signal showed some recovery but not to baseline (expressed as a ratio of intensity to CSF).

Distinct from T2-weighted images, no one has demonstrated whether restoration of T1 signal is due to myelin deposition (functional or not) or to gliosis. While it is appealing to think that the T1 signal better reflects the higher lipid composition of myelin compared to gliotic tissue, this has not been shown.

Exogenous MRI contrast agents are available for intravenous injection, and the most popular agents are chelates of the rare-earth gadolinium (Gd). Gadolinium causes the T1 time of water to shorten, resulting in bright signal on T1-weighted images. When the blood–brain barrier (BBB) is intact, Gd is not able to interact with water protons in the brain, resulting in no signal enhancement. However, if the BBB allows leakage of plasma, the Gd agent will leak into brain tissue. This results in shortened T1 times for water in the immediate vicinity and bright lesions on T1-weighted images. MS lesions cause disruption of the BBB early on and will persist for 2–6 weeks. Examples of a gadolinium-enhanced T1-weighted image of an MS lesion and its corresponding T2-weighted image are provided in Fig. 1. Due to the lack of correlation between BBB disruption and remyelination, however, the role for Gd imaging of remyelination is doubtful.

At present, conventional MRI (T1- and T2-weighted images) has been the most extensively studied imaging technique in MS. It has been used for tracking the disease process and may show changes correlated with remyelination. However, human studies are lacking, and the confounding factors indicate caution in ascribing changes seen in either image type to remyelination.

## 3    Magnetization Transfer Imaging of Remyelination

### 3.1    Physics of Magnetization Transfer Imaging

Magnetization transfer (MT) imaging is a relatively new development in MRI. As mentioned previously, routine clinical brain imaging primarily reflects mobile water protons. If the proton is part of a large molecule that cannot move freely, the signal decays too rapidly for detection on conventional MRI. However, a fraction of water protons do interact with the protons of large molecules such as proteins, and this interaction does impact the magnetization state of the water protons. This

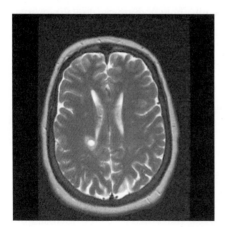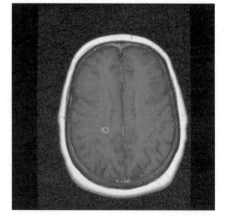

**Fig. 1** Conventional T2-weighted (**a**) and post-gadolinium T1-weighted images (**b**) of a demyelinating lesion in a patient multiple sclerosis. The ring of enhancement is classic for MS, and the rim of darker T2 signal is also commonly seen in demyelinating disease

exchange of magnetization can be detected with MT imaging. In regions with more macromolecules and less bulk water (both conditions being present with myelin sheets), there is more opportunity for MT to occur. By combining images with and without the suppression pulse, one may compute an image reflecting the fraction of MT, the so-called magnetization transfer ratio (MTR) image:

$$MTR = 100\% \times \frac{\left(M_0 - M_s\right)}{M_0}$$

where

$M_0$ = pixel intensity without the MT saturation pulse
$M_s$ = pixel intensity with the MT saturation pulse

## 3.2   Magnetization Transfer Imaging of MS

The early 1990s witnessed the first reports of MT imaging in animal models and patients. Those reports documented the expected finding that the MTR was lower in areas of demyelination than in subjects without demyelination or in normal areas. Shortly thereafter, reports documented that the so-called normal-appearing white matter (NAWM) had slightly abnormal values in patients with demyelinating disease compared with normal controls [12, 23]. This was exciting news for two reasons. First, it proposed a reliable way to diagnose demyelinating disease in patients with otherwise equivocal findings [14]. Second, although it was already known that NAWM was not normal on histological examination, this was one of the first in vivo imaging methods to corroborate this finding. MTR is relatively insensitive to edema compared with T2-weighted images, although one spinal imaging report suggests lower specificity [8]. Postmortem studies have also documented a semi-quantitative relationship between the degree of demyelination and the MTR [39]. Figure 2 shows the MT image and non-MT image in an MS patient and the resulting MTR image.

## 3.3   MT Imaging of Remyelination

Most reports of MT imaging and remyelination are in the guinea pig model of EAE [11] and the cuprizone mouse model. In both models, the MTR values drop during the demyelination phase and then increase, but not to baseline levels, during the remyelination phase. Studies also suggest a quantitative connection between the amount of remyelination and the MTR.

However, it is important to recognize that the remyelination process in humans may not match the two models mentioned above. In particular, the spotty, stochastic nature of remyelination may result in many myelin wraps around axons in one

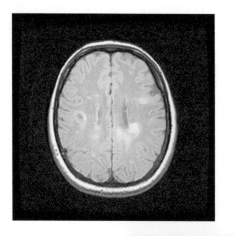
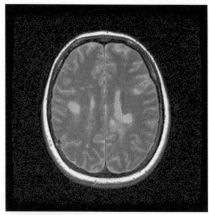
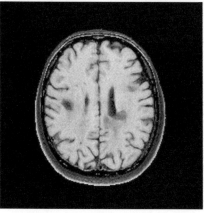

**Fig. 2** Magnetization transfer images in a patient with MS. **a** Image without MT suppression; **b** the same image but with MT suppression added. **c** the MTR image, which is computed from (**a**) and (**b**)

region, while others are denuded. The animal models described above with a predictable demyelination and remyelination may not accurately reflect MS.

There is little documentation of MTR correlation with remyelination in humans. In a clinical trial of interferon β-1b vs glatiramer acetate for relapsing remitting MS (RRMS), whole-brain MTR values showed some recovery for both agents, greater for glatiramer acetate [35]. Of course, it is not known if either agent actually promotes remyelination or if the alteration in signal is due to some other effect. A similar trial for secondary-progressive MS (SPMS) patients showed no such recovery [20]. If the agents do result in some remyelination in RRMS, but not SPMS, it suggests that increased MTR is due to remyelination. There has been and continues to be great excitement about the role of MT imaging in monitoring MS. This has resulted in the recommendation that MT imaging be included in MS trials [19].

# 4   Diffusion Imaging of Remyelination

## 4.1   *Physics of Diffusion MRI*

Diffusion imaging is the ability to measure the motion of water molecules and the restriction of water motion due to membranes. Based on Einstein's equation for diffusion:

$$r^2 = 2Dt$$

where

$\langle r^2 \rangle$ is mean squared displacement
D is diffusivity
t is diffusion time.

The commonly applied techniques are based on suppressing signal resulting from water proton movement in the magnetic field, using the Stejskal-Tanner [38] method. In that case, the signal observed is

$$I = I_0 e^{-TE/T2} e^{-bD}$$

where

I = observed signal intensity
$I_0$ is the observed signal in absence of diffusion weighting
TE is echo time
T2 is T2 decay time
b is diffusion sensitization
D is diffusivity.

If an image is collected without and with the diffusion pulses and all other factors remain constant, one can compute a diffusion-weighted image. Standard diffusion imaging methods apply diffusion pulses in three directions: the X, Y, and Z directions. Thus, including the image with no diffusion sensitivity, four images are acquired during routine diffusion imaging; from these four, the diffusion-weighted image, as well as apparent diffusion images, can be created. The term "apparent" is used because the diffusivity of water is not truly different, but structures like myelin are limiting its motion, resulting in an apparent reduction in diffusivity. Figure 3 shows the four images collected as well as the diffusion-weighted or trace image and the apparent diffusion coefficient image.

   One weakness of routine diffusion imaging is that it is not rotationally invariant. In other words, if four images were acquired in a patient and then the patient rotated her head and the same images acquired, the pixel values for a certain piece of tissue in the brain would be different. That is because fibers that restrict motion in a certain direction may be more or less aligned with the gradients depending on head position. For that

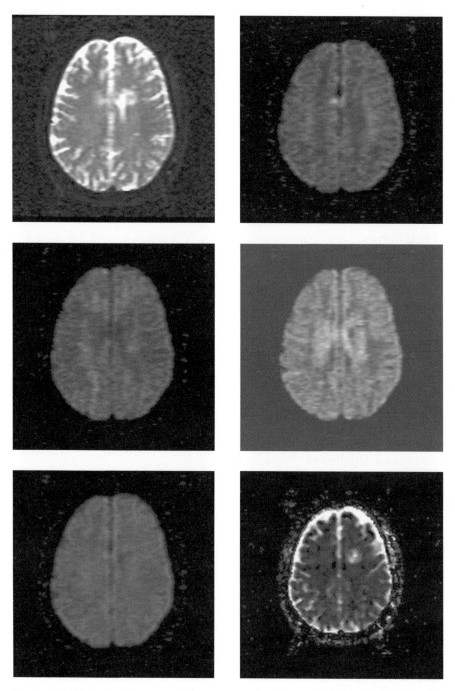

**Fig. 3** Diffusion images in a patient with MS. **a–d** Nondiffusion, X-sensitive, Y-sensitive, and Z-sensitive images respectively. **e** Diffusion-weighted image; **f** the apparent diffusion coefficient image

reason, a more sophisticated diffusion measurement is made, the diffusion tensor. One must acquire at least seven images (the four described previously, plus xy, xz, and yz) to compute the diffusion tensor images. These images can produce rotationally invariant metrics that reflect diffusion of water. A complete description is beyond the scope of this chapter, but Jones et al. provides an excellent review [21].

## 4.2 Diffusion Imaging of MS

In bulk water, diffusion of water is isotropic; that is, the amount of diffusion is equal in all directions. But in a fiber tract with a large number of myelin sheaths all coursing in the same direction, the water motion in the direction of the fibers will be much greater than in the two perpendicular directions. This difference is referred to as anisotropy, and the ratio of the amount of diffusion in the dominant direction to the amount of diffusion in the least dominant direction is called fractional anisotropy (FA). Moseley [28] was one of the first to demonstrate regional variations in the anisotropy of water diffusion in brain tissues. Of interest, the investigators showed normal white matter to have a higher FA than normal gray matter, in keeping with the expectation that myelin constrains the diffusion of water perpendicular to the direction of the axon it encloses.

In areas of myelin loss, the mean diffusivity increases while the FA decreases [13]. The exact changes in a given lesion, however, appear less predictable. An acute lesion tends to have reduced FA values [2], but the chronic course of diffusion measurement is variable [7].

Another interesting finding is that comparison of diffusion imaging (both FA and mean diffusivity) is abnormal in the area of T2 abnormality as well as in the surrounding region. It is not clear if this is due to greater sensitivity of diffusion imaging to MS lesions or if there are two separate phenomena occurring and T2 images are sensitive only to the one occurring centrally [18].

## 4.3 Diffusion Imaging of Remyelination

Based on the preceding discussion, diffusion seems to be a superb method to measure remyelination. Areas of gliosis that fail to remyelinate should have low FA and relatively high mean diffusivity. If and when remyelination occurs, FA should increase and mean diffusivity decrease. While it may indeed be this simple, there are some potential pitfalls to consider.

In addition to the variability of a lesion's course, it is also important to note that myelin is not the only important determinant of the anisotropy of water diffusion in the CNS. In studies of nonmyelinated neural structures, the fractional anisotropy is nearly as high as in myelinated structures (about 3.5 vs 4.5, respectively) [3]. Further studies [4] have found that neurofilaments do not have a significant impact on diffusion anisotropy, suggesting membranes in axons are likely the primary factor.

Neuron injury and Wallerian degeneration reduce anisotropy [5], as does induced injury in the spinal cord of rats [15].

While these studies suggest that diffusion may not be useful for detecting myelination, they do not prove its inefficacy in detecting remyelination. Rather, it indicates that detection is not as simple as initially thought. While a neuron may contribute to the fractional anisotropy, remyelination is likely to increase that value above that of an intact axon alone. Furthermore, in the human with demyelination, substantial unoccupied space that previously contained myelin would contribute to the diffusion signal, unlike the case where the tissue developed normally with little or no myelin. Therefore, there is hope that serial diffusion imaging could still be useful in measuring remyelination.

# 5    Spectroscopy of Remyelination

## 5.1    Physics of Magnetic Resonance Spectroscopy

Magnetic resonance spectroscopy (MRS) actually predates MRI, and early efforts focused on characterizing uniform samples of substances in test tubes. As with conventional imaging, most MRS work in humans is focused on proton signals, but it is possible to get spectroscopic signals from other elements. In the brain, the primary signal-producing molecules on proton spectroscopy are N-acetyl aspartate (NAA), choline, creatine, myoinositol, glutamine and glutamate, lactate as well as some lipids and amino acids. Figure 4 shows both a sample spectrum of normal white matter and a demyelinating lesion. The NAA peak is located at 2.02 parts per million (ppm) shift (the standard way that MRS spectra are described) and is a marker for healthy neurons [36]. However, its exact role in the neuron is not known. Choline is located at 3.2 ppm and is primarily found in membranes. It reflects more white matter than gray matter and tends to reflect myelin concentration, although many other diseases can affect it. Creatine is located at 3.0 ppm and is used in energy transfer. It apparently has a fairly constant concentration and is used to normalize MRS values; it is common to report the ratio of the metabolite of interest divided by creatine concentration.

There are two forms of MRS available on clinical MRI scanners. The more basic form provides a spectrum from a single sample of tissue. These samples are rectangular samples of 2–8 cm$^3$. This method is widely available and easily executed, with high reproducibility. However, only one sample is obtained; given the heterogeneity of MS, being able to obtain many samples is very useful. Magnetic resonance spectroscopic imaging or chemical shift imaging are terms that describe the techniques for acquiring a matrix of spectra. The disadvantages of MRS imaging are longer acquisition times (as long as 30 min) and lower quality of spectra. The matrix is commonly on the order of 32×32 for commonly applied methods, with two to four slices being acquired, so current methods do not cover the entire brain with the resolution available with conventional imaging.

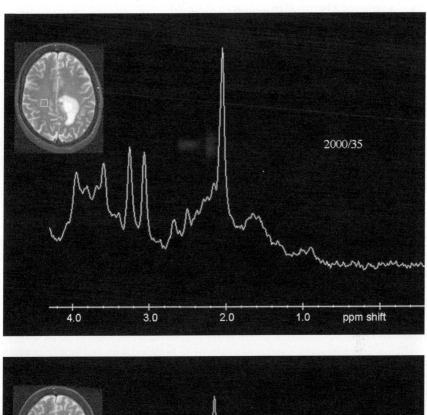

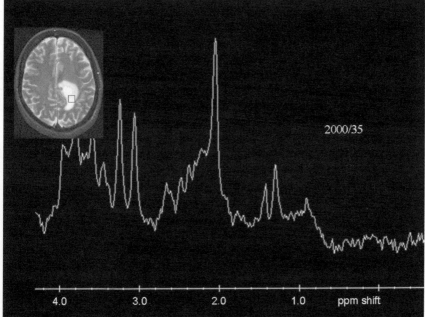

**Fig. 4** Spectroscopy in a patient with a demyelinating lesion. **a** From an area of normal-appearing white matter; **b** from the leading edge of the demyelination

## 5.2   MRS of MS and Remyelination

There are several chemicals of potential interest in MS [29, 42]. Given that choline is a
component of myelin, one might expect choline to be a primary target for evaluation.
However, the challenge is that the choline measured reflects only the forms of choline
with mobile protons. Therefore, during demyelination, and probably during remyelination, one will likely see elevation of the choline peak. However, when that is not in
process, such as in chronically demyelinated areas, one typically sees decreased choline
[9]. Furthermore, while choline is present in the myelin membranes, it is also present in
the membranes of all cells, including gliotic tissue present in MS lesions. Therefore, as
with other MRI methods, it is likely not specific for remyelination [16].

NAA is another chemical of interest. NAA is decreased in areas of chronic demyelination and has been shown to be inversely correlated with disability in MS [10].
This likely reflects the important role of myelin in the health of the axon and neuron.
Therefore, while NAA does not directly show the presence or absence of myelin, it
may be an accurate marker of neuronal health. This, in turn, may be a marker of
myelination, and, more importantly, a marker of effectiveness of myelination. An
increase in NAA levels, perhaps in combination with other imaging markers demonstrating increased myelin, may be the best marker of effective remyelination.

Some investigators have developed a technique for measuring the NAA level of
the entire brain, essentially a single voxel that encompasses the head [6, 17]. By
combining other imaging sequences to calculate brain volume, one is able to calculate the mean NAA concentration for the subject's brain. This may be a useful global marker of neuronal health and may be a good marker of global myelin repair.
While whole-brain NAA does appear to be related to T2 lesion load and disability
[6], no studies yet demonstrate remyelination on whole brain NAA.

Lactate is not detectable in normal brain tissue, but small amounts of lactate are
present in regions of demyelination, probably due to altered metabolism (glycolytic
pathways) in some of the associated inflammatory cells. As such, it is unlikely to
be a good marker for remyelination.

Lipids and amino acids below the NAA peak (<2 ppm shift) are also not normally observed in brain tissue except in pathologic conditions. Breakdown of
membranes will release detectable lipids. One might detect lipids as they are transported for remyelination, but lipids are unlikely to be a useful marker, given the
nonspecificity and low sensitivity.

## 6   Other Imaging Modalities

### 6.1   Radionuclide Imaging of MS

Not surprisingly, MS lesions, and particularly, chronic lesions with much tissue
destruction, undergo less local perfusion than normal brain tissue. Nuclear medicine methods reflecting perfusion and metabolic activity can also display the effects

of demyelination but, like CT, are not terribly sensitive. No agents specifically label myelin, either native or from remyelination. Therefore, no nuclear agents have played a major role in MS imaging to date.

However, there is growing interest in a future role for nuclear medicine agents, especially an agent that would unequivocally mark myelin. If the myelin wraps in remyelinated areas are thinner than native myelin, these areas might have even greater labeling, thus potentially representing a specific marker of remyelination. Of course, this is purely theoretical, and no such agent is available today for human use.

Stankoff et al. have reported [37] a positron-emitting agent (suitable for positron emission tomography imaging) based on Congo red that may identify remyelination more specifically. The agent, 1,4-bis(p-aminostyryl)-2-methoxy benzene (BMB), crosses the BBB and specifically binds to myelin. Therefore, it decreases in demyelinated regions and increases when remyelination occurs. However, as described above, it may not clearly differentiate between, for example, two axons with minimally adequate remyelination and another axon pair in which one has no myelin and the other has a surplus. The spatial resolution of PET is inherently limited to a bit less than 1 cm, and may also be an impediment to its use.

## 6.2   Molecular Imaging of MS

Molecular imaging is a popular new concept in medical imaging. Molecular imaging creates agents that interact with specific molecular targets, which substantially increases the usefulness of imaging. Traditional imaging, in contrast, largely focuses on demonstrating anatomic structures and pathology. The agent described in Sect. 6.1 is an example of a molecular imaging agent. In the past, most molecular agents have had radionuclides attached because there are many more options for synthesizing chemicals with radionuclides attached rather than requiring properties that make it visible for MRI or CT, and the low background of noise allows rather small concentrations of labeled agents to be detected.

The disadvantage, particularly for research purposes, is the risk of radiation. The exposure is low, but MS patients are particularly susceptible to radiation, at least at higher doses. However, once a certain molecular target is identified, it can be linked with atoms or molecules detectable with other modalities, such as MRI. For example, antibodies to Alzheimer-related plaques have been linked with gadolinium, making them detectable on MRI [33]. The identification of a remyelination-specific marker linked to an MRI-detectable agent would be a tremendous step toward direct measurement of remyelination.

Another novel approach has been applied to demyelinating disease [32]. In this study, biotin was attached to an antibody thought to promote remyelination. Subsequently, streptavidin attached to ultrasmall particles of iron oxide (USPIOs) was injected into the mice. Streptavidin has a strong affinity for biotin, and hence, the USPIOs attached to it would mark the location of the antibody. Antibody-injected mice showed enhancement, while a control group that did not have the antibody injected showed no localized enhancement. This experiment strongly indicated that the antibodies localized to the demyelinating lesion, which provided additional evidence of a direct role in the remyelination seen histopathologically. It is also an excellent example of the use of molecular agents to demonstrate mechanisms of action in vivo.

## Conclusions

MRI is the primary tool used today for evaluating demyelinating disease. It is useful in making the diagnosis, although conventional methods are not highly specific. Diffusion and MT imaging are methods that reflect how myelin alters the water signal detectable on MRI. Each holds promise of showing more normal alteration of water signal due to myelin. Both may require serial imaging to demonstrate remyelination.

Spectroscopy may also play a role. Although it may not directly reflect myelination, it may reflect the health of the neurons and axons. As such, it may reflect both remyelination potential and the actual efficacy of remyelination that has occurred.

Radio-labeled agents or other agents with antibodies or chemical affinities specific to a remyelination antigen could also reflect remyelination. While there is not currently an agent specific to newly deposited myelin, clever, accurate alternatives may be devised to demonstrate remyelination and/or restoration of neuronal health. Alternatively, myelin-specific agents combined with serial imaging may allow accurate characterization of remyelination.

## References

1. Arnold DL, Matthews PM, Francis G, Antel J (1990) Proton magnetic resonance spectroscopy of human brain in vivo in the evaluation of multiple sclerosis: Assessment of the load of disease. Magn Reson Med 14:154–159
2. Bammer R, Augustin M, Strasser-Fuchs S, Seifert T, Kapeller P, Stollberger R, Ebner F, Hartung H, Fazekas F (2000) Magnetic resonance diffusion tensor imaging for characterizing diffuse and focal white matter abnormalities in multiple sclerosis. J Magn Reson Imaging 15:583–589
3. Beaulieu C (2002) The basis of anisotropic water diffusion in the nervous system – a technical review. NMR Biomed 15:435–455
4. Beaulieu C, Allen P (1994) Water diffusion in the giant axon of the squid: Implications for diffusion-weighted MRI of the nervous system. Magn Reson Imaging 32:579–583
5. Beaulieu C, Does M, Snyder R, Allen P (1996) Changes in water diffusion due to Wallerian degeneration in peripheral nerve. Magn Reson Imaging 36:627–631
6. Bonneville F, Moriarty D, Li B, Babb J, Grossman R, Gonen O (2002) Whole-brain n-acetylaspartate concentration: Correlation with T2-weighted lesion volume and expanded disability status scale score in cases of relapsing-remitting multiple sclerosis. AJNR Am J Neuroradiol 23:371–375
7. Castriota-Scanderberg A, Sabatini U, Fasano F, Floris R, Fraracci L, Mario M, Nocentini U, Caltagirone C (2002) Diffusion of water in large demyelinating lesions: A follow-up study. Neuroradiology 44:764–767

8. Cook L, Foster P, Mitchell J, Karlik S (1994) In vivo 4.0 t magnetic resonance investigation of spinal cord inflammation, demyelination, and axonal damage in chronic-progressive experimental allergic encephalomyelitis. J Magn Reson Imaging 20:563–571

9. Davie CA, Barker GJ, Tofts PS et al (1993) Detection of myelin breakdown products by proton magnetic resonance spectroscopy. Lancet 341:630–631

10. De Stefano N, Narayanan S, Francis G, Arnaoutelis R, Tartaglia M, Antel J, Matthews P, Arnold D (2001) Evidence of axonal damage in the early stages of multiple sclerosis and its relevance to disability. Arch Neurol 58:65–70

11. Dousset V, Grossman RI, Ramer KN, Schnall MD, Young LH et al (1992) Experimental allergic encephalomyelitis and multiple sclerosis: Lesion characterization with magnetization transfer imaging. Radiology 182:483–491

12. Filippi M, Campi A, Dousset V, Baratti C, Martinelli V, Canal N, Scotti G, Comi G (1995) A magnetization transfer imaging study of normal-appearing white matter in multiple sclerosis. Neurology 45:478–482

13. Filippi M, Cercignani M, Inglese M, Horsfield M, Comi G (2001) Diffusion tensor magnetic resonance imaging in multiple sclerosis. Neurology 56:304–311

14. Filippi M, Rocca M, Minicucci L, Martinelli V, Ghezzi A, Bergamaschi R, Comi G (1999) Magnetization transfer imaging of patients with definite MS and negative conventional MRI. Neurology 52:845–848

15. Ford J, Hackney D, Alsop D, Jara H, Joseph P, Hand C, Black P (1994) MRI characterization of diffusion coefficients in a rat spinal cord injury model. Magn Reson Imaging 31:488–494

16. Gill S, Small R, Thomas D, Patel P, Porteous R, Van Bruggen N, Gadian D, Kauppinen R, Williams S (1989) Brain metabolites as 1H NMR markers of neuronal and glial disorders. NMR Biomed 2:196–200

17. Gonen O, Catalaa I, Babb J, Ge Y, Mannon L, Kolson D, Grossman R (2000) Total brain n-acetylaspartate: A new measure of disease load in MS. Neurology 54:15–19

18. Guo A, MacFall J, Provenzale J (2002) Multiple sclerosis: Diffusion tensor MR imaging for evaluation of normal-appearing white matter. Radiology 222:729–736

19. Horsfield M, Barker G, Barkhof F, Miller D, Thompson A, Filippi M (2003) Guidelines for using quantitative magnetization transfer magnetic resonance imaging for monitoring treatment of multiple sclerosis. J Magn Reson Imaging 17:389–397

20. Inglese M, van Waesberghe J, Rovaris M, Beckmann K, Barkhof F, Hahn D, Kappos L, DH, Polman C, Pozzilli C, Thompson A, Yousry T, Wagner K, Comi G, Filippi M (2003) The effect of interferon beta-1b on quantities derived from MT MRI in secondary progressive MS. Neurology 60:853–860

21. Jones D (2005) Fundamentals of diffusion MR imaging. In: Gillard J, Waldman A, Barker P (eds) Clinical MR neuroimaging. Cambridge, UK: Cambridge University Press, London, pp 54–85.

22. Koopmans R, Li D, Redekop W, Zhao G, Palmer M, Kastrukoff L, Paty D (1993) The use of magnetic resonance imaging in monitoring interferon therapy of multiple sclerosis. J Neuroimaging 3:163–168

23. Loevner L, Grossman R, Cohen J, Lexa F, Kessler D, Kolson D (1995) Microscopic disease in normal-appearing white matter on conventional MR images in patients with multiple sclerosis: Assessment with magnetization-transfer measurements. Radiology 196:511–515

24. Matthews PM, Pioro E, Narayanan S, De Stefano N, Fu L, Francis G, Antel J, Wolfson C, Arnold DL (1996) Assessment of lesion pathology in multiple sclerosis using quantitative MRI morphometry and magnetic resonance spectroscopy. Brain 119:715–722

25. Merkler D, Boretius S, Stadelmann C, Ernsting T, Michaelis T, Frahm J, Bruck W (2005) Multicontrast MRI of remyelination in the central nervous system. NMR Biomed 18:395–403

26. Miller DH, McDonald WI (1994) Neuroimaging in multiple sclerosis. Clin Neurosci 2:215–224

27. Moore G, Leung E, MacKay A, Vavasour I, Whittall K, Cover K, Li D, Hashimoto S, Oger J, Sprinkle T, Paty D (2000) A pathology-MRI study of the short-T2 component in formalin-fixed multiple sclerosis brain. Neurology 55:1506–1510

28. Moseley M, Cohen Y, Kucharczyk J, Asgari H, Wendland M, Tsuruda J, Norman D (1990) Diffusion-weighted MR imaging of anisotropic water diffusion in cat central nervous system. Radiology 176:439–445
29. Narayana P (2005) Magnetic resonance spectroscopy in the monitoring of multiple sclerosis. J Neuroimaging 15S:46S–57S
30. Nesbit GM, Forbes GS, Scheithauer BW, Okazaki H, Rodriguez M (1991) Multiple sclerosis: Histopathologic and MR and/or CT correlation in 37 cases at biopsy and three cases at autopsy. Radiology 180:467–474
31. Paty DW, Li DKB (1993) Interferon beta-1b is effective in relapsing-remitting multiple sclerosis. II. MRI analysis of a multicenter, randomized, double-blind, placebo-controlled trial. Neurology 43:662–667
32. Pirko I, Ciric B, Gamez J, Bieber AJ, Warrington AE, Johnson AJ, Hanson DP, Pease LR, Macura SI, Rodriguez M (2004) A human antibody that promotes remyelination enters the CNS and decreases lesion load as detected by T2-weighted spinal cord MRI in a virus-induced murine model of MS. FASEB J 18:1577–1579
33. Poduslo J, Curran G, Peterson J, McCormick D, Fauq A, Khan M, Wengenack T (2004) Design and chemical synthesis of a magnetic resonance contrast agent with enhanced in vitro binding, high blood-brain barrier permeability, and in vivo targeting to Alzheimer's disease amyloid plaques. Biochemistry 43:6064–6075
34. Raine C, Wu E (1993) Multiple sclerosis: Remyelination in acute lesions. J Neuropathol Exp Neurol 52:199–204
35. Richert N, Bagnato F, Howard T (2003) Whole brain magnetization transfer analysis of relapsing-remitting multiple sclerosis patients treated with ifnb-1b or glatiramer acetate (abstract P273). Mult Scler 9:S64
36. Simmons M, Frondoza C, Coyle J (1991) Immunocytochemical localization of n-acetyl-aspartate with monoclonal antibodies. Neuroscience 45:37–45
37. Stankoff B, Wang Y, Bottlaender M, Aigrot M, Dolle F, Wu C, Feinstein D, Huang G, Mathis C, Klunk W, Gould R, Lubetzki C, Zalc B (2006) Imaging of CNS myelin by positron-emitting tomography. Proc Natl Acad Sci U S A 103:9304–9309
38. Stejskal E, Tanner J (1965) Spin diffusion measurements: Spin echoes in the presence of a time-dependent field gradient. J Chem Phys 42:288–292
39. Van Waesberghe J, Kamphorst W, De Groot C, van Walderveen M, Castelijns J, Ravid R, Lycklama G, van der Valk P, Polman C, Thompson A, Barkhof F (1999) Axonal loss in multiple sclerosis lesions: Magnetic resonance imaging insights into substrates of disability. Ann Neurol 46:747–754
40. Van Walderveen M, Kamphorst W, Scheltens P, van Waesberghe J, Ravid R, Valk J, Polman C, Barkhof F (1998) Histopathologic correlate of hypointense lesions on T1-weighted spin-echo MRI in multiple sclerosis. Neurology 50:1282–1288
41. Van Walderveen MAA, Barkhof F, Hommes OR, Polman CH et al (1995) Correlating MRI and clinical disease activity in multiple sclerosis relevance of hypointense lesions on short-TR/short-TE (T1-weighted) spin-echo images. Neurology 45:1684–1690
42. Wolinsky JS, Narayana PA, Fenstermacher MJ (1990) Proton magnetic resonance spectroscopy in multiple sclerosis. Neurology 40:1764–1769
43. Zhao G, Li D, Wolinsky J, Koopmans R, Mietlowski W, Redekop W, Riddehough A, Cover K, Paty D (1997) Clinical and magnetic resonance imaging changes correlate in a clinical trial monitoring cyclosporine therapy for multiple sclerosis. The MS study group. J Neuroimaging 7:1–7

# Immunological Aspects of Axon Injury in Multiple Sclerosis

C.L. Howe

**Abstract**  The role of immune-mediated axonal injury in the induction of nonremitting functional deficits associated with multiple sclerosis is an area of active research that promises to substantially alter our understanding of the pathogenesis of this disease and modify or change our therapeutic focus. This review summarizes the current state of research regarding changes in axonal function during demyelination, provides evidence of axonal dysmorphia and degeneration associated with demyelination, and identifies the cellular and molecular effectors of immune-mediated axonal injury. Finally, a unifying hypothesis that links neuronal stress associated with demyelination-induced axonal dysfunction to immune recognition and immunopathology is provided in an effort to shape future experimentation.

C.L. Howe
Departments of Neuroscience and Neurology, Translational Immunovirology and Biodefense Program, Molecular Neuroscience Program, Mayo Clinic College of Medicine, Guggenheim 442-C, 200 First Street SW, Rochester, MN 55905, USA
e-mail: howe.charles@mayo.edu

M. Rodriguez (ed.), *Advances in Multiple Sclerosis and Experimental*                93
*Demyelinating Diseases. Current Topics in Microbiology and Immunology 318.*
© Springer-Verlag Berlin Heidelberg 2008

# 1 Introduction

Since the earliest characterizations of multiple sclerosis (MS) in the mid-1800s, the predominant pathological hallmark of the disease has been inflammatory injury to myelin with relatively little attention paid to axonal injury associated with the demyelinating process. Indeed, many early MS clinicians and researchers considered axonal preservation within the context of extensive demyelination a neuropathological criterion for the definition of the disease [58, 130]. While the axon preservation dogma was challenged early by scientists such as Babinski [15] and Marburg [151], it was largely eclipsed by the plethora of experimental studies focusing on demyelination associated with experimental autoimmunity induced against myelin antigens [97, 141]. Fortunately, the concept of axonal injury in MS, with a particular emphasis on the injured axon as the locus of nonremitting functional deficits associated with the disease, has experienced a recent resurgence, based largely on imaging studies that provided evidence for axonal loss in the demyelinated central nervous system (CNS) [263]. Herein, I will review the current evidence in support of MS as an immunopathological neurodegenerative disease and I will offer a unifying hypothesis for demyelination as a factor that predisposes axons to immune-mediated injury.

# 2 Changes in Axon Function During Demyelination

## 2.1 Conduction Block and Conduction Slowing

### 2.1.1 Acute Conduction Disruption

Myelinated axons rely upon saltatory action potential conduction conferred by the nodal architecture of the myelin sheath [57]. Complete loss or extensive thinning of the insulating myelin over an internode exposes regions of axolemma that are essentially devoid of sodium channels, resulting in action potential failure and loss of axonal information transfer [211, 260]. Thus, immediately following a segmental demyelinating event (i.e., loss of myelin over an individual internode) conduction blockade is complete and persists for at least several days [156]. Resolution of complete conduction block during persistent demyelination requires an adaptive redistribution of axonal sodium channels to compensate for current loss at the electrophysiologically silent region of axolemma (see Sect. 2.2 below). Of note, the conduction blockade is specific to the demyelinated internode and normally myelinated regions of the axon maintain the ability to transmit an action potential [155]. Therefore, conduction competence can be restored by factors acting locally at the site of demyelination. For example, even limited remyelination in the form of multiple short and thin internodes at the site of a demyelinated lesion can confer significant electrophysiological benefit and permit the action potential to pass through the demyelinated domain [235].

### 2.1.2   Slow Conduction Sequelae

Unfortunately, restoration of conduction due to sodium channel redistribution or remyelination does not return the axon to normal. While conduction under optimal conditions in restored axons facilitates substantial functional improvement over the acutely demyelinated state, such conduction is generally slower than normal and is more prone to intermittent and abrupt failure [156]. Likewise, while function associated with transmission of single action potentials is largely unaffected by conduction slowing, paired impulses and spike trains are far more sensitive to the lag effect of a slow conduction zone [156]. As one spike slows down at the demyelinated region it triggers a traffic jam that slows or blocks subsequent action potentials. This refractory period results in either exaggeration of the spike train interspike interval and truncation of the maximum spike frequency [156] or intermittent conduction failure when the demyelinated zone becomes hyperpolarized in response to potentiated activity of the sodium–potassium exchanger triggered by stacking of action potentials [36]. Functionally, frequency capping and intermittent conduction failure manifest as progressive weakening during even short duration motor activities [154] and vision blurring during prolonged gaze fixation [261].

### 2.1.3   Nodal Capacitance

Finally, not all demyelination is segmental. Rather, paranodal demyelination, in which the node of Ranvier is widened by retraction or peeling away of the paranodal loops, results in a substantial increase in the axolemmal membrane capacitance [245]. Because nodal capacitance is a factor of nodal area and because the area of a cylinder is a factor of circumference, even a small change in the radial length of a node on a large diameter axon results in a dramatic increase in nodal capacitance. This capacitance increase translates into an increase in the amount of current required to depolarize the node to firing threshold [237]. If the most proximal upstream node (the driving node for the action potential) is relatively far away from the site of paranodal demyelination, the local current generated when the action potential reaches the demyelinated node may be insufficient to overcome the elevated firing threshold, resulting in conduction block or intermittent conduction failure.

## 2.2   Sodium Channel Redistribution

### 2.2.1   Sodium Channel Subtypes and Normal Distribution

The nonuniform distribution of sodium channels within the axolemma associated with normal myelination generates the saltatory conduction pattern required for rapid transmission of action potentials by focusing the inward sodium current at the nodes [262]. Under normal circumstances, sodium channels are highly concentrated at the node of Ranvier (about 1,000–1,500 channels per square micrometer), while the sodium channel density in paranodal and internodal regions of the axon is two orders of magnitude lower (<50 channels per square micrometer) [49, 189, 229]. Of the nine sodium channel subtypes (designated $Na_v1.1$–$Na_v1.9$), $Na_v1.6$ is the predominant subtype localized to mature nodes of Ranvier [45], though $Na_v1.2$ and $Na_v1.8$ are also occasionally found in mature nodes [195]. Developmentally, $Na_v1.2$ channels are initially expressed in a diffuse manner across the premyelinated axolemma. Concomitant with the onset of myelination, these $Na_v1.2$ channels redistribute to nascent nodal regions and then undergo a switch to the $Na_v1.6$ subtype as the myelin sheath is completed [34, 120]. This subtype switch may control the ability of neurons to exhibit high-frequency firing and is intimately related to myelination. In dysmyelinated Shiverer mutant mice with a deletion of myelin basic protein (MBP), for example, axons do not switch from $Na_v1.2$ to $Na_v1.6$ sodium channels [34], and in normally nonmyelinated axons within the hippocampal mossy fiber and Schaffer collateral pathways, $Na_v1.2$ is the major channel subtype [195].

### 2.2.2 Sodium Channel Reorganization During Demyelination

Acute demyelination recapitulates several features of the axolemma observed developmentally during the premyelinated state. For example, following inflammatory demyelination of the optic nerve in experimental autoimmune encephalomyelitis (EAE) induced by myelin oligodendrocyte glycoprotein (MOG) immunization, there is widespread loss of $Na_v1.6$ at presumptive nodes of Ranvier and a drastic increase in the expression of $Na_v1.2$ sodium channels in a diffuse pattern along the entire extent of the demyelinated region [60]. Likewise, recent analysis of spinal cord and optic nerve tissue from patients with MS showed a similar increase in $Na_v1.2$ expression along extensive tracts of demyelinated axons [62]. The functional significance of this developmental recapitulation is perhaps best understood by comparing the acutely demyelinated axon to a normally unmyelinated axon – both must propagate an action potential in the absence of a nodal architecture. As discussed above, the functional sequelae of such a reversion to nonsaltatory conduction across the demyelinated zone mediated by a diffuse $Na_v1.2$ sodium channel distribution include frequency truncation, elongation of the refractory period, and loss of coherent spike trains. Nonetheless, redistribution and upregulation of $Na_v1.2$ sodium channels does permit some information transfer to occur along the demyelinated axon, leading to a functional recovery when compared to the initial demyelinated, nonconducting, low-sodium channel density condition.

In parallel with the functionally protective compensatory upregulation and redistribution of $Na_v1.2$ channels along the demyelinated axon, there is evidence that axons that do not downregulate the $Na_v1.6$ sodium channel are more susceptible to subsequent axonal injury. In fact, $Na_v1.6$ channel association with the sodium–calcium exchange pump within demyelinated regions drives a persistent inward sodium current that increases calcium influx into the axon as the sodium–calcium exchanger works to maintain intra-axonal sodium concentrations [103, 247]. Elevated calcium levels in the axon activate a variety of calcium-dependent proteases, including calpain, which can degrade neurofilaments, spectrin, talin, and actin [206], leading to acute axonal injury. Indeed, elevated calpain activity was found in demyelinated white matter in patients with MS and in EAE mice [228], and analysis of axons in EAE and MS tissue revealed that $Na_v1.6$ and the sodium–calcium exchanger were almost exclusively co-localized on injured demyelinated axons, while uninjured demyelinated axons did not express these molecules [61, 62].

## 2.3   Hyperexcitability and Hyperactivity

### 2.3.1   Spontaneous Discharge

The persistent expression of $Na_v1.6$ channels along the demyelinated axon also contributes to spurious axon firing triggered by the slow, noninactivating inward sodium current associated with this channel subtype [121]. These spontaneous discharges occur as continuous 10- to 50-Hz impulse trains [236] and are more common in demyelinated sensory axons [165], where they may contribute to the tingling paraesthesia, paroxysmal itching, trigeminal neuralgia, and pain associated with positive symptoms in MS [220]. Likewise, spontaneous discharges arising along demyelinated thalamic and basal ganglia axons may contribute to the generation of phonic tics [139] and paroxysmal dystonia [268], while spontaneous activity along demyelinated corticobulbar or limbic system tracts may trigger the inappropriate laughter and/or crying associated with pseudobulbar affect in MS patients [224].

### 2.3.2   Postural Deformation and Mechanosensitivity

Demyelinated axons become sensitive to physical deformation caused by postural movements, generating impulse trains in a mechanoreceptor-like fashion [236]. While the underlying mechanism responsible for this axonal mechanosensitivity is unclear, the physical manifestation in patients with MS is striking. Patient's with Lhermitte's symptom experience nonpainful electrical tingling sensations that radiate along the limbs in response to neck flexion triggered by antidromic conduction from a cervical demyelinated lesion centrifugally to the cutaneous nerve fascicles [182]. Likewise, postural deformation of the optic nerve in patients with optic neuritis triggers phosphene discharge [66].

### 2.3.3   Ephaptic Transmission

Nonsynaptic ephaptic transmission of activity from one demyelinated axon to another or from a demyelinated axon to a myelinated axon within brainstem or spinal tracts may account for some of the brief paroxysmal manifestations of MS [187]. While experimental evidence for such a spread of activity is limited [203, 204], demyelinated regions may become susceptible to such transmission due to hyperexcitability induced by altered sodium channel expression. This may account for some symptoms observed in patients [147, 244]. The contribution of these hyperexcitability manifestations to progressive axonal injury remains to be studied, but in light of the strong correlation between an elevated sodium current caused by aberrant $Na_v1.6$ expression, association of $Na_v1.6$ with the sodium–calcium pump, and the presence of axon injury markers, it seems reasonable to predict that repetitive activation triggered by spontaneous activation, postural deformation, or ephaptic transmission would inevitably promote elevation of intra-axonal calcium levels and exacerbation of injury to axonal structural integrity. As discussed below, this ongoing injury process may trigger stress responses that ultimately make the demyelinated axon a target for additional injury mediated by the immune system. Thus, compensatory redistribution of sodium channels, while effective in the short-term in re-establishing axonal conduction to overcome the negative symptoms of demyelination, may ultimately fuel axonal changes that promote the positive symptoms of MS and trigger a cascade of events culminating in complete axonal transection.

## 2.4   Retrograde Transport Defects

### 2.4.1   Normal Control of the Axon Cytoskeleton by Myelin

While intra-axonal and interneuronal factors such as cytoskeletal protein synthesis, electrical activity, patterns of synaptic connectivity, and retrograde transmission of neurotrophic support clearly establish critical regulatory parameters for the maintenance of the axon cytoskeleton and determination of axonal caliber, recent studies have provided evidence that myelination crucially influences axon structural biology. The peripheral demyelination mutant Trembler mouse offered the earliest evidence for myelin-dependent control of axon diameter. As the result of a point mutation in peripheral myelin protein 22 (PMP22), Trembler mice exhibit continuous rounds of myelination and demyelination in the peripheral nervous system (PNS), while the CNS is unaffected [249]. Morphological analysis of Trembler peripheral nerves showed many axons either lacking myelin or in a state of active demyelination [148]. Moreover, mean axon diameter was smaller in Trembler mice at all ages as compared to controls [12], and this effect was specific to the axoglial interaction, as Trembler Schwann cell grafts integrated into the wild type sciatic nerve exhibited normal axon diameters both proximal and distal to the graft but reduced calibers within the graft [1]. Reciprocally, engraftment of wild type sciatic nerve Schwann cells into Trembler mice showed wild type axon diameters within the graft and Trembler diameters distal and proximal to the graft [1]. Importantly, the local effects on diameter correlated with reduced rates of slow axonal transport [69], reduced neurofilament phosphorylation [71], increased neurofilament compaction [70], decreased microtubule stability, decreased tau expression, and decreased phosphorylation of microtubule-associated proteins [126]. Likewise, a reduction in neurofilament phosphorylation localized to the small gap in compact myelin causes the reduction in axon caliber and the increase in neurofilament density normally associated with the short unmyelinated node of Ranvier [113, 153].

Similar observations within the CNS were made in the Shiverer mutant. In these mice, expression of MBP is abrogated due to a deletion of the coding regions downstream from the first exon [213], resulting in complete failure to ever form compacted myelin [46]. As with the Trembler mice, though to a variable extent, axonal diameter, neurofilament phosphorylation, and microtubule stability were reduced, and neurofilament and microtubule densities were increased in Shiverer optic nerve [37, 127]. At the same time, protein levels for the medium- and high-molecular-weight isoforms of neurofilament were significantly lower in Shiverer axons, while the low-molecular-weight isoform of neurofilament was unaffected [37]. Of note, transgenic reconstitution of Shiverer mice with MBP to levels 25% of wild type led to the formation of thin myelin sheaths and normalization of some axonal parameters, such as protein expression levels for the medium-weight neurofilament subunit. In contrast, the presence of the thin myelin wraps in the transgenic Shiverer mice did not affect the expression and phosphorylation of the heavy neurofilament subunit, indicating that some aspect of myelin thickness regulates the neurofilament heavy subunit at both the transcriptional and the post-translational modification level [37]. In parallel with these architectural changes, the expression of $Na_v1.2$ sodium channels was increased on Shiverer axons, and these channels were distributed across the entire axolemma, as in unmyelinated axons in wild type mice [264]. Little to no $Na_v1.6$ was expressed on Shiverer axons, consistent with the absence of normal nodes of Ranvier [34].

Likewise, analysis of axons within the CNS of mice with a null mutation in the proteolipid protein (PLP) showed numerous structural and transport defects. In these mice, the myelin sheath is relatively normal and intact [128], but the animals exhibit paranodal accumulations of membranous organelles, axonal spheroid formation [99], and an age- and axon length-dependent degeneration of long spinal tracts [90]. Similar length-dependent axonal degeneration was observed in humans with a null mutation in PLP, as assessed by in vivo magnetic resonance spectroscopy (MRS) for N-acetyl aspartate [90]. Moreover, transplantation of neurospheres from PLP-null mice or from wild type mice into Shiverer mice showed that grafts myelinated by PLP-null oligodendrocytes contained axons with substantial accumulation of membranous organelles, while wild type grafts looked normal [79]. Mechanistically, fast axonal transport as assessed by the retrograde movement of fluorescent cholera toxin B in the optic nerve was severely impaired in PLP-deficient mice, and this defect correlated with a several-fold increase in the levels of the dynein and dynactin retrograde motor proteins in the optic nerve and spinal cord [79]. As these motor proteins were not different at the transcriptional level in PLP-null mice, the elevated levels likely reflect the progressive accumulation of retrogradely moving organelles bound by these proteins. This interpretation is consistent with the observation of the complete absence of retrograde transport of fluorescent cholera toxin B in some axons and the frequently increased density of intensely fluorescent accumulations of cholera toxin B along the axon up to a point, after which transport was completely stalled [79].

### 2.4.2  Axonal Protein Accumulation and Loss of Retrograde Transport During Demyelination

The analysis of axonal damage following non-missile, indirect traumatic brain or spinal cord injury led to the observation that amyloid precursor protein (APP) accumulates specifically at the lesion site [92, 226, 234]. APP is a normal constituent of fast axonal transport, but the levels of expression in the absence of injury are below the detection threshold of standard immunohistochemical techniques. Following traumatic injury, however, the accumulation of APP at swollen sites along the axon permits very sensitive detection of axon transport defects [226]. The appearance of APP-positive spheroids precedes other markers of axon injury, such as end-bulb formation or axolemmal disruption, and is, in fact, an extremely early marker for a wide variety of nontransecting injuries culminating in spatially restricted sites of anterograde and retrograde axonal transport slowing or blockade [55]. A common feature of several neurodegenerative models is the formation of multiple spheroids and varicosities along the length of the same axon in the absence of axonal transection or axolemmal disruption [55], suggesting that a common mechanism of multifocal axon transport disruption contributes to neurodegenerative phenomena of diverse etiologies. Critically, the frequent localization of the transport traffic jams to the nodes of Ranvier, as described above in PLP-deficient mice, for example, suggests that the nodal or paranodal architecture is particularly sensitive to transport disruption. Indeed, other models of paranodal defects, such as mice deficient in 2 ,3 -cyclic nucleotide phosphodiesterase, also show axonal swellings and accumulation of APP at the paranodes that increase with age and precede the onset of motor dysfunction and neurodegeneration. A synthesizing hypothesis for the formation of APP-laden axonal spheroids at the nodes of Ranvier suggests that numerous axonal insults elicit a common multifocal failure of axon transport at sites of elevated neurofilament density. Further, this failure in transport reduces and/or abrogates the effective communication of target-derived trophic support from the distal end of the axon to the neuron cell body, eventually culminating in either neuronal apoptosis or the loss of neuronal luxury functions [26, 72, 109, 110].

That a transport-dependent neurodegenerative mechanism may be active in the demyelinated CNS is supported by several studies showing that APP accumulation occurs within areas of acute inflammation and demyelination in tissue sections collected from patients with MS [29, 61, 82, 131]. Moreover, the presence of many APP-laden axonal spheroids at the margins of active chronic plaques [82] suggests a correlation between active demyelination and axonal transport disruption. Of note, one study did not detect APP immunoreactive axons and axon spheroids in chronically demyelinated inactive plaques [82], while other studies found considerable evidence for ongoing axon injury within plaques [29, 131]. This discrepancy suggests that axons are predominantly injured episodically at the sites of active inflammation but that APP is only reliable as a marker for axon injury at sites proximal to the neuron cell body. For example, as the axon injury evolves through time at sites progressively closer to the cell body, the more distal accumulations of APP may undergo degradation or the distal axon may be physically lost, reducing the likelihood that APP immunoreactivity remains associated with inactive plaques. Obviously, our understanding of axon injury kinetics and mechanisms within the context of demyelination requires more analysis.

However, animal models of demyelinating disease do provide additional insights into the relationship between axon injury, axonal transport defects, and the ultimate fate of axons following the loss of myelin. For example, in a marmoset model of EAE, APP immunoreactive axons and axonal spheroids were observed in areas of acute inflammation and demyelination [150]. Of note, the occurrence of such spheroids was low in this model, and the absence of axonal transection and large-scale axonal transport defects suggested the possibility of an ongoing axonal repair process. Importantly, this model provided evidence of APP immunoreactivity within axons in regions of normal-appearing white matter (NAWM) [150], suggesting that axon injury distal to the site of analysis could disrupt transport over long distances and within regions of the axon that remain myelinated.

Similarly, immunoreactivity for APP was elevated in the spinal cord of C57Bl/6 mice during MOG-induced EAE, and this axonal injury correlated with severe functional impairment. Treatment of these mice with glatiramer acetate prevented the development of clinical symptoms and substantially reduced the density of APP-immunoreactive axons in the spinal cord [94]. Likewise, active MOG-induced EAE lesions in Lewis rats were associated with an elevated number of APP-positive axons, and this model exhibited a substantial number of APP-immunoreactive axons within inactive lesions that had active inflammation at the edges [131]. Finally, in a focally demyelinated cortical model of MOG-induced EAE in Lewis rats, APP-positive axons were only detected within the region of active inflammation, and there was a strong correlation between the presence of microglia/macrophages or CD4+ T cells and injured axons [160]. Significantly, despite the rapid appearance of APP-positive axons within the cortical lesions, the density of cortical axons did not decrease over the 2-week disease course in this model [160], suggesting that axon injury and axonal transport disruption, as marked by increased APP immunostaining, are mechanistically separable from the process that results in absolute loss of the axon.

Finally, several retrograde tracer studies have shown compromised axonal transport in demyelinated axons. Persistent infection of SJL/J mice with the Theiler's murine encephalomyelitis virus (TMEV) induces a state of chronic spinal cord demyelination with many of the functional and pathological hallmarks of MS [123, 163, 167, 186, 246]. FluoroGold labeling from the lower thoracic spinal cord to the midbrain and brainstem revealed the loss of more than half of the axons emanating from the rubrospinal nucleus and the reticulospinal/raphespinal nuclear complex and almost complete loss of the axons arising from the vestibulospinal nucleus in chronically demyelinated mice [255]. Of note, the number of vestibulospinal neurons was only reduced by one-third, and the number of rubrospinal neurons was essentially unchanged [255], suggesting that the loss of retrograde transport was due to an axonal defect rather than to the absolute loss of neurons. Likewise, the extent of retrograde labeling correlated with preservation of motor function, such that mice exhibiting demyelination with relatively little loss of neurologic function showed substantial preservation of FluoroGold labeling in the midbrain and brainstem as compared to demyelinated and functionally compromised mice [27, 256].

### 2.4.3 Mitochondrial Manifestations

Conduction recovery along the demyelinated axolemma initiated by $Na_v1.2$ and $Na_v1.6$ upregulation and redistribution requires a concomitant increase in activity of the sodium-potassium ATPase pump to maintain a normal resting membrane potential. Even under normal conditions, the sodium–potassium pump consumes up to 50% of the total energy available in the brain [7]. The enhanced energy demand driven by pump activity along the demyelinated axon results in recruitment of additional mitochondria to bear the increased load [9]. Indeed, axons in Shiverer mice contain significantly more mitochondria than controls, and cytochrome c immunoreactivity is twofold higher in Shiverer white matter tracts [8], suggesting that increased mitochondrial function may be an adaptive response to demyelination. Likewise, an increase in intra-axonal mitochondria has been observed within demyelinated lesions in the TMEV model of MS [222], in several EAE models [59, 135], and following antibody-mediated demyelination of the optic nerve in cats [174].

Increased energy demand may explain the increase in intra-axonal mitochondria during demyelination [9]. Unfortunately, the specific functional state of mitochondria has not been adequately assessed in the demyelinating models discussed above. However, recent findings indicate severely compromised mitochondrial function in MS patients entering the chronic secondary progressive phase of the disease. Mitochondrial preparations from the motor cortex of such patients showed half the level of respiratory chain complex I and III activity measured in normal controls [78], suggesting that the axons and neurons in these patients were experiencing large-scale ATP starvation. Of note, these patients had already experienced widespread axonal loss, averaging 68% fewer axons than controls in another study [31]. This suggests that mitochondrial accumulation and hyperactivity, as indicated in the animal models described above, precedes a progressive decline in mitochondrial function that is correlated with axon dropout.

One potential pathway to intra-axonal mitochondrial dysfunction may involve exposure to nitric oxide (NO) and other reactive oxygen species (ROS) generated by activated immune cells during the inflammatory phase of demyelination [9]. As discussed in more detail below, NO induces transient conduction block in axons, induces degeneration of activated axons [122], reversibly inhibits cytochrome c oxidase function [41, 54], enhances mitochondrial production of superoxide anion and peroxynitrite [166, 194], inhibits electron transfer at respiratory chain complex III [194], opens the large conductance mitochondrial permeability transition pore [107], and induces generalized failure of mitochondrial metabolism and the reduction or cessation of ATP production [39, 40]. Once ATP production is compromised, a self-perpetuating chain reaction of energy failure-dependent mechanisms leads to inevitable loss of the demyelinated axon.

# 3  Axonal Degeneration During Demyelination

## 3.1  Histopathological Evidence

### 3.1.1  Dysmorphia and Axonal Transection

Dysmorphic changes in axons following demyelination include reduced axon caliber, *en passant* and terminal spheroid formation, accumulation of electron-dense organelles, dephosphorylation of neurofilaments, and cytoskeletal discontinuity and disorganization [111, 190]. As discussed above, the absence of myelin leads to an acute loss of neurofilament phosphorylation and concomitant compression of the individual neurofilaments, leading to increased neurofilament density and a reduction in axon caliber. Thus, changes in diameter, alterations in neurofilament phosphorylation and density, accumulation of APP and electron-dense organelles, and reduction in axonal transport all likely reflect an acute response to the absence of positive myelin-derived cues that precedes physical disruption of the axolemma [30]. Likewise, the development of *en passant* spheroids is probably the end-stage of a severe axonal transport defect culminating in the accumulation of retrogradely and anterogradely transported organelles, cytoskeletal components, ion channels, and neurotransmitter receptors [82, 93, 132, 190, 253]. Similarly, the presence of cytoskeletal discontinuities and disorganization of neurofilaments and microtubules within the axon may reflect the proteolytic activity of caspases [3] and calcium-dependent proteases such as calpain [100] and may serve as pathological hallmarks for impending axon disintegration. Finally, the irreversible outcome of these injury processes and also the final stage in any cell-mediated axon attack process (see Sect. 4 below) is the complete transection of the axon and the formation of a terminal spheroid. Such terminal end-bulbs result from the rapid sealing of the proximal ends of mechanically transected axons and the accumulation of anterogradely transported proteins and organelles at the new termini [56]. Three-dimensional reconstruction of numerous axon spheroids within tissue sections collected from patients with MS revealed that the majority of dephosphorylated neurofilament-positive axonal spheroids were caused by complete transection of the axon bearing the structure [253].

### 3.1.2  Evidence of Axon Loss

Quantitative analysis of the number of axonal spheroids within the white matter of tissue collected from 47 lesions in 11 different patients revealed an average of 11,236 terminal spheroids per cubic millimeter within actively demyelinating lesions, 3138 spheroids at the edge of chronic active lesions, and 875 spheroids at the center of chronic lesions [253]. In stark contrast, less than one such spheroid was observed per cubic millimeter in white matter from control samples [253]. Other studies provide similar measurements, showing an average axon loss of 68% in ten chronically demyelinated inactive lesions collected from five paralyzed patients [31], and a reduction from approximately $8 \times 10^5$ corticospinal tract axons on average in the cervical spinal cord of control samples to approximately $4.5 \times 10^5$ corticospinal axons in tissue samples collected from 55 MS patients [73].

Comparable measurements have been made in several animal models of MS. For example, axons were reduced by 60% in the cervical spinal cord of irreversibly paralyzed end-stage mice during EAE induced by PLP [265], and large-diameter axons were reduced by 62% [222] or 78% [157] within the anterolateral columns of chronically demyelinated SJL/J mice infected with TMEV. Likewise, 40%–50% of corticospinal tract axons were lost by 90 days after induction of EAE with MOG in C57Bl/6 mice [32], and 63% of thoracic axons were lost by 40 days after induction of EAE with MOG in DA rats [188]. Finally, there was a reduction in large diameter spinal axons from 28,766 axons per square millimeter in nondemyelinated TMEV-infected wild type mice to 17,129 axons per square millimeter in chronically demyelinated TMEV-infected mice deficient in CD4 [112].

### 3.1.3   Axonal Slow Burn

Several authors have used the term "slow burn" or "slow burning" axon injury to refer to persistent axon damage within inactive demyelinated lesions [131, 141, 210, 239]. In particular, this concept intends to suggest a separation between overt and active inflammation-mediated axon injury and a noninflammatory injury process that either evolves as a chain reaction initiated during the active inflammatory phase or as the result of intra-axonal changes induced by energy depletion and/or axonal transport defects. The evidence in support of axon injury within inactive lesions is presented above, but the most compelling argument in favor of the relevance of such a smoldering injury process is the fact that such inactive lesions may persist for many years through the disease course and even a small amount of ongoing axon dropout within such lesions will progressively accumulate to the point of debilitation [142].

## 3.2   Magnetic Resonance Imaging and Spectroscopy Evidence

### 3.2.1   Atrophy

White matter in the brain and spinal cord consists of 46% axons, 24% myelin, 17% glia, and 13% vasculature, by volume [162], which means that axonal loss will significantly impact tissue volume. Indeed, atrophy is presently one of the most robust imaging parameters, revealing that the brain and spinal cord of MS patients atrophies at a rate that is two to ten times faster than in healthy age-matched controls

[162]. Obviously, gross measurement of atrophy lacks fine resolution and may overestimate axon loss in conditions of dehydration or acute reduction of inflammation or underestimate axon loss during acute inflammatory infiltration or tissue swelling, but tissue volume changes are likely to serve as a key diagnostic marker for the evaluation of therapies aimed at axon preservation. For example, the assessment of brain atrophy in a 2-year placebo-controlled trial of beta interferon in relapsing remitting MS revealed that tissue shrinkage was reduced in the 2nd year of treatment and that this reduction did not correlate with lesion load [217]. Moreover, subsequent follow-up suggested that those patients with the greatest progression of atrophy over the initial 2-year period had the greatest risk for developing subsequent severe disability [85]. Importantly, measures of atrophy appear to be largely separable from changes in inflammation, and little correlation exists between lesion load and atrophy. Many of the treatments in clinical use or in clinical trial robustly alter lesion load but do not impact atrophy, suggesting that therapeutic strategies aimed at reducing axon injury have yet to be identified [218].

### 3.2.2 Diffusion Tensor Imaging

Diffusion tensor imaging (DTI) uses the anisotropic properties of water diffusion within white matter tracts to extract structural information [168]. In particular, the measurement of water movement parallel to identified axon tracts, called axial diffusivity, and perpendicular to axon tracts, called radial diffusivity, may distinguish axon injury from myelin injury. Decreased axial diffusivity occurs when axons are injured or dysfunctional, while increased radial diffusivity occurs within a white matter tract when myelin is injured [240–243]. DTI analysis of C57Bl/6 mice during MOG-induced EAE revealed a significant reduction in spinal cord axial diffusivity that correlated with intense APP immunoreactivity following histological examination [125], suggesting that this technique may allow noninvasive measurement of axonal integrity in both demyelinated and NAWM regions. In fact, DTI of 39 MS patients with variable disease manifestations showed a substantial reduction in fractional anisotropy within the NAWM of the corpus callosum, which was interpreted as evidence in favor of axon injury elicited at lesions outside of the corpus callosum [52]. Unfortunately, this analysis did not distinguish between radial and axial diffusivity. However, the presence of reduced fractional anisotropy within the context of elevated mean diffusivity is suggestive of a reduction in coherent water diffusion along the axis of the axon tracts within the corpus callosum. Future application of the radial and axial DTI measurements may serve as a surrogate marker for axon injury within the demyelinated CNS.

### 3.2.3 *N*-Acetyl Aspartate

*N*-acetyl aspartate (NAA) is the second most abundant amino acid after glutamate within the CNS, and it contributes the major peak on water-suppressed proton magnetic resonance spectra of brain tissue [63]. NAA is present at levels up to 20 mM within neurons and is turned over every 1–2 days [22]. Numerous studies have confirmed that NAA is localized predominantly to neurons and axons, and long projection neurons such as cortical pyramidal neurons and motor neurons stain more intensely for NAA than local interneurons [164, 233], suggesting that it plays a role in the increased metabolic demand of these neurons. NAA is synthesized in mitochondria from L-aspartate and acetyl coenzyme A and transported into the cytoplasm, where it may function as an osmoregulator to drive the removal of intraneuronal and intra-axonal water against a water gradient [23, 24]. NAA may also participate in the metabolism of neurotransmitters such as aspartate and gluta-mate [53], or it may have other, currently unknown functions. In general, reduc-tions in NAA may signify either reversible neuronal and axonal injury, altered neuronal and axonal metabolism, or irreversible loss of axons [63]. However, despite the accepted correlation between NAA levels and axon injury, an important caveat to the exclusivity of this relationship is the proposal that NAA is effluxed by neurons and taken up by oligodendrocytes, where it is catabolized as part of a water balance adaptation to the presence of the extremely hydrophobic myelin sheath [22]. Of note, demyelination is associated with disrupted aspartoacylase-mediated NAA metabolism within oligodendrocytes in Canavan disease [133]. Likewise, transient NAA reductions may be associated with acute mitochondrial dysfunction during inflammatory attack [68, 232], and such levels may recover with resolution of the inflammation. Nonetheless, numerous experiments support a connection between reduced NAA lines as measured by magnetic resonance spectroscopy and loss of axons and neurologic function.

For example, the ratio of NAA to creatine was reduced by 20% in the cortex of the wobbler mutant mouse concomitant with increased immunohistochemical evi-dence of axonal injury [193]. Likewise, the ratio of NAA to choline was reduced by 30% in the guinea pig brain during acute EAE induced by whole spinal cord homogenate, but this change preceded the development of significant neurologic deficits [38]. In contrast, a significant accumulation of swollen axons correlated with suppression of absolute NAA values was observed in monkeys 4 weeks after induction of EAE with MBP [209]. Unfortunately, no detailed analysis of NAA spectroscopy has been correlated to APP accumulation, spheroid formation, or other markers of axon injury in either the TMEV model of MS or in an EAE model with progressive axonal injury and neurologic deficit.

On the other hand, numerous studies of NAA by magnetic resonance spectros-copy and other techniques have been performed in humans with MS, and substan-tial correlation between reduced NAA and axonal injury and functional deficits has been observed. For example, a comparison of 11 ataxic MS patients, 11 nonataxic MS patients, and 11 healthy controls showed that the mean concentration of NAA in the cerebellum of ataxic patients was reduced to 6.7 mM as compared to 9.7 mM in the nonataxic MS patients and 9.6 mM in the controls [65]. Likewise, comparison of spinal cord material collected from MS lesions, NAWM in MS patients, and healthy control white matter revealed that axon density as measured by neurofila-ment staining was reduced by 62% in the MS lesion compared to the other tissue sections while NAA as measured by HPLC was reduced by more than 50% as compared to non-lesion white matter in MS patients and by more than 60% as compared to healthy controls [31]. Finally, analysis of the ratio of NAA to creatine in 88 MS patients revealed not only a 20% reduction in the aggregate population ratio compared to healthy controls, but also a very strong correlation between the NAA-to-creatine ratio and the severity of disability as measured by the Expanded Disability Status Scale [67].

# 4  Immune-Mediated Mechanisms of Axon Injury During Demyelination

## 4.1  Cellular Effectors of Axon Injury

### 4.1.1  Cytotoxic CD8+ T Cells

Cytotoxic CD8+ T cells (CTLs) are the dominant T cell within MS lesions, outnumbering CD4+ T cells by almost tenfold [35, 91] at the sites of active axon injury [14, 29]. These cells kill targets either via the release of cytotoxic granules containing perforin, granzyme B, and serglycin [48, 200, 252] or via the activation of cell surface death receptors such as Fas [21]. Despite debate regarding the relevance of neuronal expression of MHC class I molecules (see Sect. 4.2.1 below), all CNS cells of neuroectodermal origin can be induced to express MHC class I and can be killed by CTLs in vitro [178]. The majority of studies have addressed direct CTL-mediated induction of apoptosis in target cells, but CTLs may also specifically attack and transect axons without damaging the neuron cell body [158]. The recruitment of CTLs to the CNS may depend upon chemokines secreted by astrocytes at the site of injury, infection, or inflammation [202], and CTL recruitment and homing to the CNS may actually be facilitated as compared to CD4+ T cells [43, 47]. A unique aspect of the blood–brain barrier is that only activated T cells are able to surveil the brain parenchyma, causing the CNS to have the lowest concentration of T cells per gram of tissue of any organ [266]. However, intravenous introduction of activated CD8+ T cells leads to rapid MHC restriction-dependent accumulation within the CNS, peaking 9–12 h after administration [87, 104], indicating that the concept of immune privilege must be interpreted cautiously [89]. Whether these CTLs recognize distinct antigenic epitopes presented on MHC class I and the identity of these epitopes has only recently gained attention. Single-cell PCR analysis showed that CD8+ T cells specifically isolated from actively demyelinating lesions in human MS brain tissue were represented by substantial expansion of a small number of single clones, with less than half of the isolated CD8+ cells characterized as polyclonal and with some individual clones accounting for up to 35% of the entire CD8+ population [14]. This finding suggests that CTLs recruited to lesion sites can undergo antigen-specific expansion and must therefore recognize such an antigenic target presented on some cell type within the lesion. Coupled with the possibility of MHC class I expression on neurons and axons (see Sect. 4.2.1 below), it is reasonable to speculate that at least a component of this CTL population may recognize and specifically injure axons. This speculation must be tempered by the fact that activated CD8+ T cells also undergo large clonal expansions in healthy individuals [105, 197, 225], although the presence of such expanded cells in the demyelinated CNS and specifically within active lesions does provide both motive and opportunity for these cells to participate in axon injury.

Moreover, several lines of investigation provide solid evidence in favor of a role for CTLs in direct injury to axons and neurons. For example, while mice that are genetically deficient in either $\beta_2$-microglobulin [212] or perforin [112, 172] develop extensive demyelination during chronic infection with TMEV, neither develops significant clinical signs of neurologic deficit as measured by hind-limb motor evoked potentials, spontaneous vertical and horizontal movement, activity wheel behavior, or rotarod performance [83, 112, 172, 198, 212, 214, 256]. In contrast, mice on the same background but deficient in MHC class II expression developed both extensive demyelination and severe functional impairment, with many of the mice paralyzed or moribund by 120 days after infection [181, 212]. Of note, preservation of motor function in $\beta_2$-microglobulin-deficient mice appeared to be related to the upregulation and redistribution of sodium channels along the axolemma, while such redistribution was not observed in chronically infected, significantly impaired SJL/J mice [212]. Likewise, while axons were preserved in the $\beta_2$-microglobulin-deficient mice as assessed by Bielschowski staining and neurofilament immunoreactivity [111, 212], there was widespread disruption and loss of axons in chronically infected SJL/J mice [212]. In addition, retrograde axon transport as measured by midbrain and brainstem neuronal accumulation of FluoroGold applied at the lower thoracic level of the spinal cord was preserved in $\beta_2$-microglobulin-deficient mice but was severely compromised in SJL/J mice [255, 256]. Finally, both genetic deletion of CD8+ T cells [173] and peptide-mediated depletion of the immunodominant CTL response [117] led to preservation of motor function, despite the presence of extensive demyelination, suggesting that a substantial component of axon injury is mediated by CTLs in these models.

Furthermore, a growing body of evidence supports direct cytotoxic attack of neurons and axons by CD8+ T cells in vitro and in vivo. For example, following the induction of MHC class I surface expression on cultured hippocampal neurons and the exogenous loading of these class I molecules with a peptide derived from the lymphochoriomeningitis virus (LCMV), the addition of anti-LCMV CTLs led to rapid formation of immunological synapses on neurites and segmental cytoskeletal damage that occurred within 15–30 min [158]. Lesioned neurites exhibited spheroids with accumulated cytoskeletal components proximal to the CTL attack site and complete loss of the neuron-specific $\beta$III tubulin isoform over a spatial domain of 3–6 μm at the attack site [158]. Importantly, the observed injury was selective for neurites, was not detectable at the neuron cell body, and occurred prior to any evidence of apoptosis. Live cell imaging of CTL interactions with neurites revealed that the injury was elicited within minutes of contact and that membrane disruption preceded cytoskeletal disintegration [158]. While the mechanism of injury in this study was dependent upon MHC class I antigen presentation, other experiments using cultured fetal human neurons have shown that polyclonal activation of T cells via anti-CD3 ligation is sufficient to elicit neuron death within hours of incubation [96]. Neither unactivated T cells nor activated monocytes killed the neurons, and the death initiated by activated T cells occurred in both allogeneic and syngeneic circumstances and could not be blocked by either an MHC class I or an MHC class II function-blocking antibody [96]. Finally, neither cytokines nor T cell-conditioned media were sufficient to kill the neurons, but the addition of an anti-FasL function blocking antibody substantially reduced the level of neuronal death [96]. This finding is similar to the observation that neuron cell bodies are resistant to perforin-mediated injury but are susceptible to Fas-mediated killing by a population of MHC class I-restricted $CD8^+$ T cells [159].

The in vivo imaging evidence for a direct association between CTLs and injured axons is less clear. One example of contact between a demyelinated axon and a CD3-positive lymphocyte exhibiting polarization of granzyme B-containing granules toward the immunological synapse was reported in an acute MS lesion [178], suggesting that CTLs may mediate at least some axon injury in the demyelinated human brain. However, further work will be required to show whether this type of contact is frequent, whether it produces axon injury, and whether interference with such contact leads to axon preservation. Nonetheless, other CNS inflammatory diseases provide compelling evidence for direct axon and neuron injury mediated by CTLs. For example, while Rasmussen's encephalitis is associated with autoantibodies against a glutamate receptor subunit [10], much of the disease pathology is consistent with a CTL-mediated process [25], and $CD8^+$ T cells are frequently found in contact with and polarized toward MHC class I-positive injured neurons within Rasmussen's brain lesions [28].

### 4.1.2 $CD4^+$ T Cells

While analysis of MHC class II-restricted $CD4^+$ T cells has dominated the study of inflammatory CNS diseases, the majority of this work has focused on anti-myelin responses and mediation of demyelination rather than axon injury. However, several studies do suggest that $CD4^+$ T cells may directly elicit axon injury, although the mechanisms of such injury remain largely unclear. For example, polyclonal activation of T cells via anti-CD3 ligation produced both $CD8^+$ and $CD4^+$ neuronotoxic T cells, and magnetic isolation of activated $CD4^+$ cells produced a population of effectors that was fully competent to kill fetal human neurons in culture [96]. However, this killing was not blocked by treatment with an anti-MHC class II function blocking antibody [96], indicating that the cytotoxic effect was not mediated by peptide recognition. As with the $CD8^+$ cytotoxic effect described in Sect. 4.1.1 above, the $CD4^+$ killing could be blocked with an anti-FasL function blocking antibody, suggesting that nonspecifically activated $CD4^+$ T cells can kill neurons via Fas [96]. In contrast, however, other investigators reported that $CD4^+$ T cells were unable to injure neurites under circumstances that promoted CTL-mediated injury [158], suggesting that irreversible axon-specific T cell-mediated attack may predominantly depend upon CTLs. On the other hand, a reversible axon injury was reported when MBP-specific encephalitogenic CD4+ T cells were incubated with YFP-expressing embryonic neurons [230]. These neurons continuously express YFP in the cell body and neurites under normal culture conditions, but following incubation with activated MBP-specific CD4+ T cells, there was a redistribution of YFP into an aggregated bead-like pattern suggestive of axon transport disruption [230]. In addition, there was evidence of cytoskeletal disruption in the neurites as marked by discontinuities in β-tubulin staining, and stabilization with paclitaxol prevented both the disruption of microtubules and the loss of YFP fluorescence. However, despite the presence of cytoskeletal disruption and loss of YFP, membrane integrity was not compromised, the neurons did not die, and following removal of the T cells the YFP fluorescence renormalized [230], suggesting that the T cell-mediated effect was localized to the neurite cytoskeleton and was not mediated by physical transection of the process. This is substantially different from the CTL-mediated effects on axons described in Sect. 4.1.1 above and may have been caused by release of cytokines or other toxic mediators rather than by direct cell-to-cell contact. For example, TNFα triggers microtubule dissolution in endothelial cells that is reversed by paclitaxol [191], while interferon γ treatment induces aberrant microtubule aggregation in KNS-62 cells [81], suggesting that these factors may have been released by the MBP-specific T cells co-cultured with the neurons. Indeed, these encephalitogenic T cells have been shown to produce both TNFα and interferon γ [76]. Induction of EAE in YFP transgenic mice by adoptive transfer of MBP-specific CD4+ T cells also led to the loss of YFP fluorescence in axons within inflammatory lesions in the lumbar spinal cord [230], indicating that transient axon destabilization may have relevance to axon injury during demyelination. This fluorescence loss paralleled the onset of clinical symptoms and reached its nadir at the peak of functional impairment, but returned to normal levels as the disease resolved [230], suggesting that the axon injury was transient and not due to physical transection. It is important to note that this EAE model is characterized by a monophasic disease course that resolves completely within 15 days of onset, which would suggest that axons are not lost anywhere within the neuraxis of these mice. Obviously, analysis of YFP fluorescence in axons in mice following EAE induction that does result in persistent deficits or in mice chronically infected with TMEV would provide valuable insight into the kinetics of axon loss rather than axon dysregulation.

### 4.1.3  Natural Killer Cells

Because genetic deletion of perforin protects axons during demyelination induced by chronic TMEV infection, it is possible that either CTLs or natural killer (NK) cells are involved in axon injury following the loss of myelin [111, 112]. Likewise, the role of $\beta_2$-microglobulin in the same model system is compatible with either effector cell type, since NK cells recognize MHC class I molecules as well as several nonclassical MHC class Ib molecules that require $\beta_2$-microglobulin for surface expression [140, 183]. NK cell recognition of MHC class Ia and Ib molecules is more complex than CTL recognition, in that subsets of NK cells express a variety of activating and inhibiting surface receptors that engage specific MHC class I molecules in a finely tuned balance of positive and negative signaling in response to the presence or absence of MHC class I molecules. The fact that under specific circumstances NK cells will kill cells that do not express surface class Ia molecules [205] is interesting in light of the normally low or absent expression of MHC class Ia molecules on neurons [118, 119]. For example, NK cells may recognize demyelinated, class Ia-free axons as non-self following recruitment to sites of inflammatory demyelination. However, the NK cell response to targets is considerably more complex than the missing self model suggests [205] and depends upon crosstalk between a host of cell surface receptors that probe targets for both positive and negative recognition cues [140]. One of the primary activating receptors constitutively expressed by NK cells is the C-type lectin NKG2D, which stimulates cytotoxicity following binding to a family of stress-regulated MHC class Ib ligands that includes Rae-1, H60, and Mult-1 in the mouse (see Sect. 4.3.2 below) [140]. The role of NK cells and NKG2D receptors in axon injury within the context of CNS demyelination is currently unclear, but NK cells do have the capacity to recognize and kill syngeneic dorsal root ganglion neurons in a perforin-dependent manner in vitro [16, 17]. This death was apoptotic, rapidly induced, and depended upon expression of the NKG2D ligand Rae-1 [16, 17]. Cytotoxicity only occurred when glial cell protection of axons was limited, and the NK cells preferentially attacked unmyelinated portions of the axon, producing fragmentation and spheroid formation similar to that described above for CTL-mediated transection of axons [16, 158]. NK cells did not kill cultured hippocampal neurons, and this protection was correlated with the absence of Rae-1 expression in this population of neurons [17]. Moreover, MHC class I-deficient neurons prepared from $\beta_2$-microglobulin-deficient mice were resistant to NK cell-mediated lysis, suggesting that simply the absence of surface MHC class I molecules cannot stimulate cytotoxicity against neurons [17]. Finally, NK cell-mediated killing of DRG neurons was prevented by a function blocking anti-NKG2D antibody but not by control IgG [17].

### 4.1.4 Macrophages and Microglia

Microglia and monocyte-derived macrophages are the primary innate immune effectors within the CNS [19, 33, 98], and these cells produce numerous cytotoxic effector molecules upon activation (see Sect. 4.2 below). In addition to a critical role in phagocytosis and debris removal during demyelination [116], microglia and macrophages may directly induce axon injury. For example, stereotactic injection of the microglial and macrophage activator zymosan into the rat spinal cord produced focal areas of decreased neurofilament immunostaining that directly correlated with the density of activated macrophages [196]. As zymosan is not directly toxic to neurons or glia [86] but conditioned media from zymosan-stimulated microglia and macrophages kills neurons in vitro [95], it is likely that these activated cells released a cytotoxic factor or factors that specifically injured axons. In parallel, activated microglia and macrophages may injure axons via direct contact. For example, the number of injured axons within an MS lesion correlates very well with the number of macrophages present in the lesion [82, 253], and terminal axonal spheroids are frequently found engulfed by microglia or macrophages within the center of active lesions [253]. Of note, robust axonal injury was observed in $\beta_2$-microglobulin-deficient mice following induction of either a predominantly inflammatory EAE with MBP or a predominantly demyelinating EAE induced by MOG, and this injury was specifically associated with massive macrophage infiltration into the spinal cord [146]. While the mechanism of axon injury was not clarified in this study, other experiments suggest that macrophages exhibit a cytotoxic phenotype characterized by expression of perforin, granzyme B, and the NKG2D receptor [13, 75]. In fact, macrophages appear to be the final cytotoxic effector in the death of pancreatic $\beta$ cells induced by adoptive transfer of diabetogenic CD4[+] T cells, and this cytotoxicity is likely perforin-dependent and mediated by NKG2D or other activating NK receptors on the macrophages [44]. It is tempting to speculate that the perforin- and $\beta_2$-microglobulin-dependent axon injury described in Sect. 4.1.1 above in the TMEV model involves cytotoxic macrophages, but the functional role of these cells in the demyelinated CNS remains to be determined.

## 4.2 Molecular Effectors of Axon Injury

### 4.2.1 Perforin and Granzymes

The dominant mechanism for NK cell- and CTL-mediated killing of target cells is the release of cytolytic granules containing the pore-forming protein perforin, the proteoglycan serglycin, and a family of serine proteases known as the granzymes [145, 251, 258]. Granzyme B, a known mediator of caspase-dependent apoptosis, is packaged within the cytolytic granule in complex with serglycin. Following T cell receptor recognition of the appropriate peptide:MHC class I complex on target cells and the formation of the immune synapse, the granzyme:serglycin complex and perforin are exocytosed by the CTL [145, 251, 258]. Confusion currently exists regarding the role of perforin in the steps subsequent to cytolytic granule exocytosis, but the current model suggests that granzymes, either free or in complex with serglycin, bind to the surface of the target cell and are endocytosed. This event appears to occur in the absence of perforin [88, 192, 227]. However, once endocytosed, perforin may facilitate the transfer of granzymes from target cell endosomes to the cytosol via endosomolysis, apparently without plasma membrane pore formation [42, 88, 161]. The finding that genetic deletion of this cytotoxic effector results in almost complete preservation of large-diameter spinal axons despite the presence of persistent demyelination and robust immune cell infiltration into the spinal cord suggests a clear role for perforin in axon injury [112]. In addition, both cytotoxic granule extracts and purified granzyme A induced rapid and complete neurite retraction when added to cultures of a mouse neuron cell line [248] and T cell-mediated killing of neurons in live brain slices was prevented by the inhibition of perforin with concanamycin A [180]. Finally, granzyme B itself, in the absence of perforin, kills neurons via the stimulation of $G_{i\alpha}$ protein-coupled receptors [259].

## 4.2.2   Fas/FasL

Fas ligand (FasL) is a member of the tumor necrosis factor (TNF) family of proteins present on activated cytotoxic T cells. Binding of FasL to the Fas receptor (CD95) on the surface of target cells induces apoptosis via the recruitment of the Fas-associated death domain (FADD) adaptor protein to the death domain located on the intracellular portion of Fas [250]. Clustering of FADD results in recruitment of pro-caspase 8 to Fas via its interaction with the death effector domain in FADD, generating the death-inducing signaling complex (DISC) at the plasma membrane. Recruitment of pro-caspase 8 to the DISC results in autocleavage and activation of caspase 8 [221], which in turn activates effector caspases such as caspase 3 [84]. Little evidence exists for a role of Fas/FasL in axon injury within the demyelinated CNS, but it has been shown that neutralization of FasL improves spinal axon regeneration following spinal cord transection [74]. It is unclear whether this is due to specific preservation of axons, acute protection of neurons from apoptosis, or changes in the inhibitory myelin milieu.

## 4.2.3   Interferon γ and Tumor Necrosis Factor α

Interferon γ (IFNγ) and tumor necrosis factor α (TNFα) are $T_H1$ cytokines that exert pleiotropic effects within the CNS [169]. IFNγ, in particular, is important for the upregulation of MHC class I expression by target cells and it plays a critical role in the activation of microglia and macrophages [177]. The direct effect of IFNγ and TNFα on demyelinated axons is unknown. However, in addition to the microtubule effects discussed above, both IFNγ [124] and TNFα [179] inhibit neurite outgrowth and induce neurite retraction in cultured neurons. At the same time, other investigators have reported that these cytokines synergistically promote neurite outgrowth [50] and are individually neuroprotective [215, 254]. This discrepancy suggests that the interaction of IFNγ or TNFα with axons is complicated and depends upon the health status of the axon and neuron [6]. For example, genetic deletion of TNFα leads to the preservation of more axons in the sciatic nerve following the induction of Wallerian degeneration by transection [231], suggesting that within the context of an axon injured by another means, TNFα exacerbates the injury process.

## 4.2.4   Nitric Oxide

Nitric oxide (NO) is a freely diffusible, reactive, soluble gas produced both physiologically and pathologically by the action of nitric oxide synthase (NOS) on

L-arginine [51]. NOS occurs in three major forms: neuronal NOS (nNOS), endothelial NOS (eNOS), and inducible NOS (iNOS; also inflammatory, immunological, or independent of calcium). Both nNOS and eNOS are constitutively expressed and generate low levels of NO in response to transient intracellular calcium signals in either the brain (nNOS) or the vasculature (eNOS). Low nanomolar concentrations of NO produced under normal physiological conditions by nNOS and eNOS generate signals to control synaptic function or regulate blood flow by binding to soluble guanylate cyclase and stimulating the production of cyclic guanosine 3,5′-monophosphate (cGMP) [170]. In contrast, iNOS is not constitutively expressed in the CNS and is only found following inflammatory induction in microglia, macrophages, and astrocytes [171], where it continuously generates toxic high levels of NO and NO-derived reactive nitrogen species such as peroxynitrite (ONOO⁻) [80]. Peroxynitrite, formed by the diffusion-limited interaction of NO with the superoxide anion ($O_2^-$), is a powerful oxidizing agent that can evolve into several toxic radicals, such as nitrogen dioxide and the carbonate radical anion, which concomitantly trigger widespread tissue damage via the oxidation and nitration of tyrosines and lipids [11]. Moreover, while NO and peroxynitrite have half-lives in tissue measured in milliseconds to seconds, nitrosation products such as nitrosothiol adducts exhibit half-lives measured in hours and days, and these products can therefore diffuse over much greater distances, spreading injury via transnitrosation of additional tyrosines, lipids, and thiol groups [199].

The best evidence for the production of NO and reactive nitrogen injury products in MS is the presence of elevated nitrotyrosine in CSF [267], the abundant expression of iNOS mRNA within MS lesions [18], and the expression of iNOS protein within macrophages and microglia in acute MS lesions [185]. Likewise, iNOS mRNA [129] and protein [64] are expressed within inflammatory lesions in EAE in a manner that correlates with the severity of neurological deficit [184], and iNOS expression is associated with the inflammatory infiltrate present within the demyelinated spinal cord in the TMEV model of MS [115].

NO production by macrophages and microglia within demyelinated lesions may play a major role in the acute suppression of axonal conduction and in the eventual exacerbation of axonal injury and loss [238]. Demyelinated axons are exquisitely sensitive to reversible NO-mediated axon conduction blockade [207], and the relatively low concentrations of NO that may be associated with a persistent residual microglial- and macrophage-mediated inflammatory response within chronically demyelinated lesions may selectively impair demyelinated axons [238]. Mechanistically, NO directly impairs axon function in myriad ways, including inhibition of sodium and calcium channels [2, 134, 208], disruption of the sodium–potassium electrogenic pump [101], and aberrant depolarization mediated by cGMP [20]. NO is also reported to inhibit mitochondrial function (see Sect. 2.4.3 above), resulting in reduced ATP production that compromises the ability to maintain axonal ion gradients [7]. In support of such mitochondrial dysfunction within demyelinated lesions, oxidative damage to mitochondrial DNA and impaired NADH dehydrogenase activity occur within active MS lesions [149, 257], while decreased mitochondrial respiratory chain function has been observed in macrophages and microglia isolated from rats 12–15 days after induction of EAE with MBP [269]. Since the density of activated macrophages within MS lesions appears to predict the extent of axonal injury [82], and since activated macrophages are closely associated with such injured axons [253], the production of inflammatory mediators such as NO by these cells may contribute prominently to the acute suppression of axonal function and may play a central role as the trigger for consequent degenerative mechanisms.

### 4.2.5  Proteases

One such downstream mechanism of axonal destruction may involve the activation of axonal proteases and the disruption and degradation of the axonal cytoskeleton [206]. In addition to calcium-dependent calpain-mediated axonal injury, as described in Sect. 3.1.1 above, caspases, cathepsins, plasminogen activators, and matrix metalloproteinases (MMPs) may also participate in the final degradation and destruction of demyelinated axons. For example, caspase-3 activation within axons was correlated to the development of substantial axon degeneration in an IL-12-induced model of EAE [3], while intra-axonal cathepsin D has been implicated in axon destruction at sites of impaired retrograde transport [219]. Finally, tissue plasminogen activator (tPA), a fibrinolytic enzyme significantly upregulated within neurons [5] and in the CSF of MS patients [4], was intensely associated with large diameter demyelinated axons and axonal ovoids along the borders of acute MS lesions [102], suggesting that this enzyme may contribute to axonal degradation associated with demyelination.

## 4.3  Neuronal and Axonal Expression of Immune-Related Molecules

### 4.3.1  The MHC Class I Controversy

The concept of the CNS as an immune-privileged organ, while correct in the strictest definition of privilege, has come to be incorrectly interpreted by many investigators to mean immune-deficient, immune-compromised, or immune-protected [89]. This is nowhere more true than in the widespread notion that neurons are incapable of expressing MHC class I or are only competent to produce nonfunctional, unloaded surface class I molecules under the artificial conditions of in vitro culture [77, 108, 118, 119, 136–138, 143, 152, 201]. It is certainly the case that neurons express no or very little functional MHC class I, $\beta_2$-microglobulin, or TAP1/2 peptide transporter under normal, nonpathological conditions [119] (though expression is observed in neurons during specific developmental time windows [114, 144]), but mounting evidence indicates that induction of functional MHC class I expression on neurons is not only possible but likely pathologically relevant. For example, while even high doses of IFNγ failed to upregulate MHC class I or $\beta_2$-microglobulin expression in cultured, electrically active hippocampal neurons, the combination of electrophysiological silencing by tetrodotoxin (TTX) and IFNγ treatment induced such expression in 100% of neurons analyzed [175]. Moreover, this treatment paradigm induced the expression of MHC class I on the surface of 93% of neurons analyzed, as assessed by live-cell immunostaining [175], and led to the upregulation of TAP1 and TAP2 genes in 95% and 90% of hippocampal neurons analyzed, respectively [176]. Surface expression of MHC class I was not restricted to the neuron cell body in these cultures, but was also observed on presumptive axons [158]. That this surface MHC class I was functional and physiologically relevant is supported by the finding that peptide loading with an H-2D$^b$-specific peptide induced neurite transection by CTLs bearing T cell receptors restricted to this peptide epitope [158]. Finally, in addition to axonal and neuronal expression of MHC class I associated with virus infection of the CNS, a recent study provides unequivocal evidence of MHC class I expression on neurons and axons associated with actively demyelinating lesions within tissue samples collected from patients with MS [106]. Thus, these findings support a model in which the electrical silencing induced by demyelination combined with the localized release of IFNγ by inflammatory cells infiltrating the demyelinated lesion leads to the upregulation of neuronal and axonal MHC class I that can be recognized by CTLs to initiate axonal transection. The identity of peptides presented by such axonal MHC class I remains a mystery but may range from virus-derived epitopes [216, 223] to self-epitopes derived from the active degradation of proteins accumulated within the axon at sites of demyelination, as discussed in Sect. 4.2.5 above.

### 4.3.2 Nonclassical MHC Class I Molecules

In addition to the expression of MHC class Ia molecules, neurons may also express a variety of MHC class Ib molecules following demyelination and/or electrical silencing. While there is currently no evidence that neurons differentially regulate the expression of NKG2D ligands such as Rae-1, H-60, and Mult-1, the fact that some populations of neurons, such as DRG neurons, are susceptible to NK cell-mediated killing via recognition of NKG2D ligands, while other populations, such as hippocampal

---

**Fig. 1** Proposed model for demyelination-dependent immune-mediated axon injury. **A** Healthy myelinated axon. Phosphorylated neurofilaments (*gray lines with protrusions*) maintain axon caliber. Sodium channels (Na$_v$1.6) are only distributed at the nodes of Ranvier (*gray ovals*). Vesicles and proteins are shuttled along microtubules (*dashed central line*) both anterogradely and retrogradely – normal neuronal function and communication of trophic support depend upon this intra-axonal traffic. **B** Acutely demyelinated axon. Neurofilaments at the site of myelin loss are dephosphorylated, leading to a reduction in axon caliber and accumulative disruption of intra-axonal transport. New sodium channel isoforms (Na$_v$1.2) are redistributed along the denuded axolemma to compensate for the loss of saltatory conduction (*black ovals*). Aberrant maintenance of Na$_v$1.6 channels (*light gray ovals in the axolemma*) associated with heightened sodium–calcium exchanger activity initiates pathologic changes in ionic homeostasis at the site of demyelination.

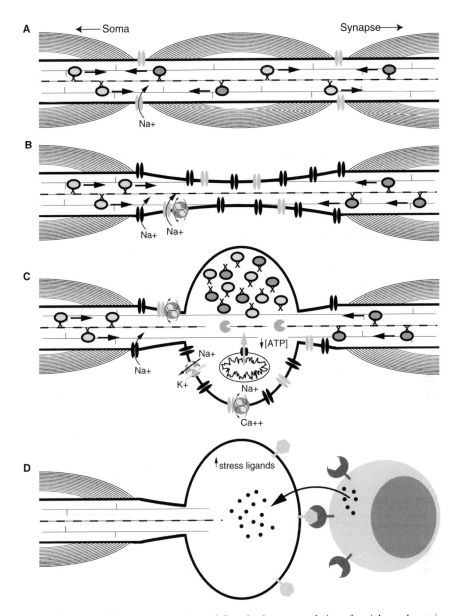

**Fig. 1** (continued) **C** Progressive transport defects lead to accumulation of vesicles and proteins at the demyelinated site; such accumulation exacerbates the transport problems, leads to a decrease or loss of retrograde trophic support to the neuron cell body, and creates *en passant* spheroids. At the same time, loss of ionic homeostasis and increased metabolic demand lead to mitochondrial injury, loss of energy production, and activation of calcium-dependent proteases such as calpain, which further injures the cytoskeleton and worsens the transport defect. **D** Eventually, the stress of trophic factor withdrawal, energy imbalance, and loss of ionic homeostasis lead to the upregulation of immune ligands on the surface of the denuded axolemma that activate or co-stimulate immune effector cells such as cytotoxic T cells, natural killer cells, and macrophages. These effectors release various cytotoxic molecules such as perforin granules, toxic cytokines, and reactive oxygen species that trigger axonal transection and potentially neuronal apoptosis

neurons, are not [17], suggests that such regulation may be possible. It would be interesting to know whether TTX and IFNγ, in addition to inducing MHC class Ia expression on hippocampal neurons, also made them susceptible to NK cell-mediated killing via recognition of upregulated NKG2D ligand expression.

## 5   Stress and the Naked Axon – A Hypothesis

Simply stated, our current working hypothesis is that the stress of demyelination, manifested as retrograde transport defects, intra-axonal protein aggregation, retrograde trophic support withdrawal, mitochondrial dysfunction, and electrical dysregulation and silencing, results in the induction of aberrant neuronal and axonal expression of MHC class Ia and Ib molecules that serve as molecular recognition cues for the engagement of CTL- and NK cell-dependent attack, injury, transection, and killing of neurons and axons (Fig. 1). While much work remains to prove this model, our unifying hypothesis may help filter the currently available data and may provide a rationale for the construction of future experiments. Of note, it may also provide a basis for the rational design of new therapeutics aimed at thwarting the immune recognition of MHC molecules on demyelinated axons. Ultimately, any therapy that preserves axons will preserve neurologic function in demyelinated patients and will also promote the maintenance of a substrate upon which remyelinating strategies can work. In the absence of axonal protection and preservation, no amount of remyelination induction will ever matter to patients with multiple sclerosis.

**Acknowledgements**  The author is supported by grants from the National Multiple Sclerosis Society (RG3636) and the National Institutes of Health (NS32129), and by a generous gift from Donald and Frances Herdrich. Many of the synthesizing concepts of this review were the result of fruitful conversations with Dr. Chandra Deb, Nikilyn Kinzel, Kevin Pavelko, Dr. Larry Pease, and Dr. Moses Rodriguez.

## References

1. Aguayo AJ, Attiwell M, Trecarten J, Perkins S, Bray GM (1977) Abnormal myelination in transplanted Trembler mouse Schwann cells. Nature 265:73–75
2. Ahern GP, Hsu SF, Klyachko VA, Jackson MB (2000) Induction of persistent sodium current by exogenous and endogenous nitric oxide. J Biol Chem 275:28810–18815
3. Ahmed Z, Doward AI, Pryce G, Taylor DL, Pocock JM, Leonard JP, Baker D, Cuzner ML (2002) A role for caspase-1 and -3 in the pathology of experimental allergic encephalomyelitis: inflammation versus degeneration. Am J Pathol 161:1577–1586
4. Akenami FO, Siren V, Koskiniemi M, Siimes MA, Teravainen H, Vaheri A (1996) Cerebrospinal fluid activity of tissue plasminogen activator in patients with neurological diseases. J Clin Pathol 49:577–580
5. Akenami FO, Siren V, Wessman M, Koskiniemi M, Vaheri A (1999) Tissue plasminogen activator gene expression in multiple sclerosis brain tissue. J Neurol Sci 165:71–76

6. Allan SM, Rothwell NJ (2001) Cytokines and acute neurodegeneration. Nat Rev Neurosci 2:734–744
7. Ames A 3rd (2000) CNS energy metabolism as related to function. Brain Res Brain Res Rev 34:42–68
8. Andrews H, White K, Thomson C, Edgar J, Bates D, Griffiths I, Turnbull D, Nichols P (2006) Increased axonal mitochondrial activity as an adaptation to myelin deficiency in the Shiverer mouse. J Neurosci Res 83:1533–1539
9. Andrews HE, Nichols PP, Bates D, Turnbull DM (2005) Mitochondrial dysfunction plays a key role in progressive axonal loss in multiple sclerosis. Med Hypotheses 64:669–677
10. Andrews PI, McNamara JO (1996) Rasmussen's encephalitis: an autoimmune disorder? Curr Opin Neurobiol 6:673–678
11. Augusto O, Bonini MG, Amanso AM, Linares E, Santos CC, De Menezes SL (2002) Nitrogen dioxide and carbonate radical anion: two emerging radicals in biology. Free Radic Biol Med 32:841–859
12. Ayers MM, Anderson RM (1976) Development of onion bulb neuropathy in the Tremebler mouse. Morphometric study. Acta Neuropathol (Berl) 36:137–152
13. Baba T, Ishizu A, Iwasaki S, Suzuki A, Tomaru U, Ikeda H, Yoshiki T, Kasahara M (2006) CD4+/CD8+ macrophages infiltrating at inflammatory sites: a population of monocytes/macrophages with a cytotoxic phenotype. Blood 107:2004–2012
14. Babbe H, Roers A, Waisman A, Lassmann H, Goebels N, Hohlfeld R, Friese M, Schroder R, Deckert M, Schmidt S, Ravid R, Rajewsky K (2000) Clonal expansions of CD8(+) T cells dominate the T cell infiltrate in active multiple sclerosis lesions as shown by micromanipulation and single cell polymerase chain reaction. J Exp Med 192:393–404
15. Babinski J (1885) Recherche sur l'anatomie pathologique de la sclérose en plaque et étude comparative des diverses variétés de sclérose de la moelle. Archives de Physiologie Normale et Pathologique 2:186–207
16. Backstrom E, Chambers BJ, Kristensson K, Ljunggren HG (2000) Direct NK cell-mediated lysis of syngenic dorsal root ganglia neurons in vitro. J Immunol 165:4895–4900
17. Backstrom E, Chambers BJ, Ho EL, Naidenko OV, Mariotti R, Fremont DH, Yokoyama WM, Kristensson K, Ljunggren HG (2003) Natural killer cell-mediated lysis of dorsal root ganglia neurons via RAE1/NKG2D interactions. Eur J Immunol 33:92–100
18. Bagasra O, Michaels FH, Zheng YM, Bobroski LE, Spitsin SV, Fu ZF, Tawadros R, Koprowski H (1995) Activation of the inducible form of nitric oxide synthase in the brains of patients with multiple sclerosis. Proc Natl Acad Sci USA 92:12041–12045
19. Bailey SL, Carpentier PA, McMahon EJ, Begolka WS, Miller SD (2006) Innate and adaptive immune responses of the central nervous system. Crit Rev Immunol 26:149–188
20. Bains JS, Ferguson AV (1997) Nitric oxide depolarizes type II paraventricular nucleus neurons in vitro. Neuroscience 79:149–159
21. Barry M, Bleackley RC (2002) Cytotoxic T lymphocytes: all roads lead to death. Nat Rev Immunol 2:401–409
22. Baslow MH (2002) Evidence supporting a role for N-acetyl-L-aspartate as a molecular water pump in myelinated neurons in the central nervous system. An analytical review. Neurochem Int 40:295–300
23. Baslow MH (2003) N-acetylaspartate in the vertebrate brain: metabolism and function. Neurochem Res 28:941–953
24. Baslow MH (2003) Brain N-acetylaspartate as a molecular water pump and its role in the etiology of Canavan disease: a mechanistic explanation. J Mol Neurosci 21:185–190
25. Bauer J, Bien CG, Lassmann H (2002) Rasmussen's encephalitis: a role for autoimmune cytotoxic T lymphocytes. Curr Opin Neurol 15:197–200
26. Beattie EC, Zhou J, Grimes ML, Bunnett NW, Howe CL, Mobley WC (1996) A signaling endosome hypothesis to explain NGF actions: potential implications for neurodegeneration. Cold Spring Harb Symp Quant Biol 61:389–406
27. Bieber AJ, Ure DR, Rodriguez M (2005) Genetically dominant spinal cord repair in a murine model of chronic progressive multiple sclerosis. J Neuropathol Exp Neurol 64:46–57

28. Bien CG, Bauer J, Deckwerth TL, Wiendl H, Deckert M, Wiestler OD, Schramm J, Elger CE, Lassmann H (2002) Destruction of neurons by cytotoxic T cells: a new pathogenic mechanism in Rasmussen's encephalitis. Ann Neurol 51:311–318

29. Bitsch A, Schuchardt J, Bunkowski S, Kuhlmann T, Bruck W (2000) Acute axonal injury in multiple sclerosis. Correlation with demyelination and inflammation. Brain 123:1174–1183

30. Bjartmar C, Yin X, Trapp BD (1999) Axonal pathology in myelin disorders. J Neurocytol 28:383–395

31. Bjartmar C, Kidd G, Mork S, Rudick R, Trapp BD (2000) Neurological disability correlates with spinal cord axonal loss and reduced N-acetyl aspartate in chronic multiple sclerosis patients. Ann Neurol 48:893–901

32. Black JA, Liu S, Hains BC, Saab CY, Waxman SG (2006) Long-term protection of central axons with phenytoin in monophasic and chronic-relapsing EAE. Brain 129:3196–3208

33. Block ML, Zecca L, Hong JS (2007) Microglia-mediated neurotoxicity: uncovering the molecular mechanisms. Nat Rev Neurosci 8:57–69

34. Boiko T, Rasband MN, Levinson SR, Caldwell JH, Mandel G, Trimmer JS, Matthews G (2001) Compact myelin dictates the differential targeting of two sodium channel isoforms in the same axon. Neuron 30:91–104

35. Booss J, Esiri MM, Tourtellotte WW, Mason DY (1983) Immunohistological analysis of T lymphocyte subsets in the central nervous system in chronic progressive multiple sclerosis. J Neurol Sci 62:219–232

36. Bostock H, Grafe P (1985) Activity-dependent excitability changes in normal and demyelinated rat spinal root axons. J Physiol 365:239–257

37. Brady ST, Witt AS, Kirkpatrick LL, de Waegh SM, Readhead C, Tu PH, Lee VM (1999) Formation of compact myelin is required for maturation of the axonal cytoskeleton. J Neurosci 19:7278–7288

38. Brenner RE, Munro PM, Williams SC, Bell JD, Barker GJ, Hawkins CP, Landon DN, McDonald WI (1993) The proton NMR spectrum in acute EAE: the significance of the change in the Cho:Cr ratio. Magn Reson Med 29:737–745

39. Brookes PS, Bolanos JP, Heales SJ (1999) The assumption that nitric oxide inhibits mitochondrial ATP synthesis is correct. FEBS Lett 446:261–263

40. Brorson JR, Schumacker PT, Zhang H (1999) Nitric oxide acutely inhibits neuronal energy production. The Committees on Neurobiology and Cell Physiology. J Neurosci 19:147–158

41. Brown GC, Cooper CE (1994) Nanomolar concentrations of nitric oxide reversibly inhibit synaptosomal respiration by competing with oxygen at cytochrome oxidase. FEBS Lett 356:295–298

42. Browne KA, Blink E, Sutton VR, Froelich CJ, Jans DA, Trapani JA (1999) Cytosolic delivery of granzyme B by bacterial toxins: evidence that endosomal disruption, in addition to transmembrane pore formation, is an important function of perforin. Mol Cell Biol 19:8604–8615

43. Cabarrocas J, Bauer J, Piaggio E, Liblau R, Lassmann H (2003) Effective and selective immune surveillance of the brain by MHC class I-restricted cytotoxic T lymphocytes. Eur J Immunol 33:1174–1182

44. Calderon B, Suri A, Unanue ER (2006) In CD4+ T-cell-induced diabetes, macrophages are the final effector cells that mediate islet beta-cell killing: studies from an acute model. Am J Pathol 169:2137–2147

45. Caldwell JH, Schaller KL, Lasher RS, Peles E, Levinson SR (2000) Sodium channel Na(v)1.6 is localized at nodes of ranvier, dendrites, and synapses. Proc Natl Acad Sci USA 97:5616–5620

46. Campagnoni AT (1988) Molecular biology of myelin proteins from the central nervous system. J Neurochem 51:1–14

47. Carson MJ, Reilly CR, Sutcliffe JG, Lo D (1999) Disproportionate recruitment of CD8+ T cells into the central nervous system by professional antigen-presenting cells. Am J Pathol 154:481–494

48. Catalfamo M, Henkart PA (2003) Perforin and the granule exocytosis cytotoxicity pathway. Curr Opin Immunol 15:522–527

49. Chiu SY, Schwarz W (1987) Sodium and potassium currents in acutely demyelinated inter-nodes of rabbit sciatic nerves. J Physiol 391:631–649
50. Cho SG, Yi SY, Yoo YS (2005) IFNgamma and TNFalpha synergistically induce neurite outgrowth on PC12 cells. Neurosci Lett 378:49–54
51. Christopherson KS, Bredt DS (1997) Nitric oxide in excitable tissues: physiological roles and disease. J Clin Invest 100:2424–2429
52. Ciccarelli O, Werring DJ, Barker GJ, Griffin CM, Wheeler-Kingshott CA, Miller DH, Thompson AJ (2003) A study of the mechanisms of normal-appearing white matter damage in multiple sclerosis using diffusion tensor imaging – evidence of Wallerian degeneration. J Neurol 250:287–292
53. Clark JF, Doepke A, Filosa JA, Wardle RL, Lu A, Meeker TJ, Pyne-Geithman GJ (2006) N-acetylaspartate as a reservoir for glutamate. Med Hypotheses 67:506–512
54. Cleeter MW, Cooper JM, Darley-Usmar VM, Moncada S, Schapira AH (1994) Reversible inhibition of cytochrome c oxidase, the terminal enzyme of the mitochondrial respiratory chain, by nitric oxide. Implications for neurodegenerative diseases. FEBS Lett 345:50–54
55. Coleman M (2005) Axon degeneration mechanisms: commonality amid diversity. Nat Rev Neurosci 6:889–898
56. Coleman MP, Perry VH (2002) Axon pathology in neurological disease: a neglected thera-peutic target. Trends Neurosci 25:532–537
57. Coman I, Aigrot MS, Seilhean D, Reynolds R, Girault JA, Zalc B, Lubetzki C (2006) Nodal, paranodal and juxtaparanodal axonal proteins during demyelination and remyelination in multiple sclerosis. Brain 129:3186–3195
58. Compston A, Lassmann H, McDonald I (2006) The story of multiple sclerosis. In: Confavreux C, Lassmann H, McDonald I, Miller D, Noseworthy J, Smith K, Wekerle H (eds) McAlpine's Multiple Sclerosis. Elsevier, Philadelphia, pp. 3–68
59. Condie RM, Good RA (1959) Experimental allergic encephalomyelitis: its production, pre-vention, and pathology as studied by light and electron microscopy. Prog Neurobiol 4:321–392
60. Craner MJ, Lo AC, Black JA, Waxman SG (2003) Abnormal sodium channel distribution in optic nerve axons in a model of inflammatory demyelination. Brain 126:1552–1561
61. Craner MJ, Hains BC, Lo AC, Black JA, Waxman SG (2004) Co-localization of sodium channel Nav1.6 and the sodium-calcium exchanger at sites of axonal injury in the spinal cord in EAE. Brain 127:294–303
62. Craner MJ, Newcombe J, Black JA, Hartle C, Cuzner ML, Waxman SG (2004) Molecular changes in neurons in multiple sclerosis: altered axonal expression of Nav1.2 and Nav1.6 sodium channels and Na+/Ca2+ exchanger. Proc Natl Acad Sci USA 101:8168–8173
63. Criste GA, Trapp BD (2006) N-acetyl-L-aspartate in multiple sclerosis. Adv Exp Med Biol 576:199–214; discussion 361–363
64. Cross AH, Manning PT, Stern MK, Misko TP (1997) Evidence for the production of perox-ynitrite in inflammatory CNS demyelination. J Neuroimmunol 80:121–130
65. Davie CA, Barker GJ, Webb S, Tofts PS, Thompson AJ, Harding AE, McDonald WI, Miller DH (1995) Persistent functional deficit in multiple sclerosis and autosomal dominant cere-bellar ataxia is associated with axon loss. Brain 118:1583–1592
66. Davis FA, Bergen D, Schauf C, McDonald I, Deutsch W (1976) Movement phosphenes in optic neuritis: a new clinical sign. Neurology 26:1100–1104
67. De Stefano N, Narayanan S, Francis GS, Arnaoutelis R, Tartaglia MC, Antel JP, Matthews PM, Arnold DL (2001) Evidence of axonal damage in the early stages of multiple sclerosis and its relevance to disability. Arch Neurol 58:65–70
68. De Stefano N, Narayanan S, Francis SJ, Smith S, Mortilla M, Tartaglia MC, Bartolozzi ML, Guidi L, Federico A, Arnold DL (2002) Diffuse axonal and tissue injury in patients with multi-ple sclerosis with low cerebral lesion load and no disability. Arch Neurol 59:1565–1571
69. de Waegh S, Brady ST (1990) Altered slow axonal transport and regeneration in a myelin-deficient mutant mouse: the trembler as an in vivo model for Schwann cell-axon interactions. J Neurosci 10:1855–1865

70. de Waegh SM, Brady ST (1991) Local control of axonal properties by Schwann cells: neuro-filaments and axonal transport in homologous and heterologous nerve grafts. J Neurosci Res 30:201–212
71. de Waegh SM, Lee VM, Brady ST (1992) Local modulation of neurofilament phosphoryla-tion, axonal caliber, and slow axonal transport by myelinating Schwann cells. Cell 68:451–463
72. Delcroix JD, Valletta J, Wu C, Howe CL, Lai CF, Cooper JD, Belichenko PV, Salehi A, Mobley WC (2004) Trafficking the NGF signal: implications for normal and degenerating neurons. Prog Brain Res 146:3–23
73. DeLuca GC, Ebers GC, Esiri MM (2004) Axonal loss in multiple sclerosis: a pathological survey of the corticospinal and sensory tracts. Brain 127:1009–1018
74. Demjen D, Klussmann S, Kleber S, Zuliani C, Stieltjes B, Metzger C, Hirt UA, Walczak H, Falk W, Essig M, Edler L, Krammer PH, Martin-Villalba A (2004) Neutralization of CD95 ligand promotes regeneration and functional recovery after spinal cord injury. Nat Med 10:389–395
75. Diefenbach A, Hsia JK, Hsiung MY, Raulet DH (2003) A novel ligand for the NKG2D recep-tor activates NK cells and macrophages and induces tumor immunity. Eur J Immunol 33:381–391
76. Dittel BN, Merchant RM, Janeway CA Jr (1999) Evidence for Fas-dependent and Fas-independent mechanisms in the pathogenesis of experimental autoimmune encephalomyelitis. J Immunol 162:6392–400
77. Drew PD, Lonergan M, Goldstein ME, Lampson LA, Ozato K, McFarlin DE (1993) Regulation of MHC class I and beta 2-microglobulin gene expression in human neuronal cells. Factor binding to conserved cis-acting regulatory sequences correlates with expression of the genes. J Immunol 150:3300–3310
78. Dutta R, McDonough J, Yin X, Peterson J, Chang A, Torres T, Gudz T, Macklin WB, Lewis DA, Fox RJ, Rudick R, Mirnics K, Trapp BD (2006) Mitochondrial dysfunction as a cause of axonal degeneration in multiple sclerosis patients. Ann Neurol 59:478–489
79. Edgar JM, McLaughlin M, Yool D, Zhang SC, Fowler JH, Montague P, Barrie JA, McCulloch MC, Duncan ID, Garbern J, Nave KA, Griffiths IR (2004) Oligodendroglial modulation of fast axonal transport in a mouse model of hereditary spastic paraplegia. J Cell Biol 166:121–131
80. Espey MG, Miranda KM, Thomas DD, Xavier S, Citrin D, Vitek MP, Wink DA (2002) A chemical perspective on the interplay between NO, reactive oxygen species, and reactive nitrogen oxide species. Ann N Y Acad Sci 962:195–206
81. Everding B, Wilhelm S, Averesch S, Scherdin U, Holzel F, Steffen M (2000) IFN-gamma-induced change in microtubule organization and alpha-tubulin expression during growth inhibition of lung squamous carcinoma cells. J Interferon Cytokine Res 20:983–990
82. Ferguson B, Matyszak MK, Esiri MM, Perry VH (1997) Axonal damage in acute multiple sclerosis lesions. Brain 120:393–399
83. Fiette L, Aubert C, Brahic M, Rossi CP (1993) Theiler's virus infection of beta 2-microglob-ulin-deficient mice. J Virol 67:589–592
84. Fischer U, Janicke RU, Schulze-Osthoff K (2003) Many cuts to ruin: a comprehensive update of caspase substrates. Cell Death Differ 10:76–100
85. Fisher E, Rudick RA, Simon JH, Cutter G, Baier M, Lee JC, Miller D, Weinstock-Guttman B, Mass MK, Dougherty DS, Simonian NA (2002) Eight-year follow-up study of brain atrophy in patients with MS. Neurology 59:1412–1420
86. Fitch MT, Doller C, Combs CK, Landreth GE, Silver J (1999) Cellular and molecular mecha-nisms of glial scarring and progressive cavitation: in vivo and in vitro analysis of inflamma-tion-induced secondary injury after CNS trauma. J Neurosci 19:8182–8198
87. Flugel A, Berkowicz T, Ritter T, Labeur M, Jenne DE, Li Z, Ellwart JW, Willem M, Lassmann H, Wekerle H (2001) Migratory activity and functional changes of green fluores-cent effector cells before and during experimental autoimmune encephalomyelitis. Immunity 14:547–560

88. Froelich CJ, Orth K, Turbov J, Seth P, Gottlieb R, Babior B, Shah GM, Bleackley RC, Dixit VM, Hanna W (1996) New paradigm for lymphocyte granule-mediated cytotoxicity. Target cells bind and internalize granzyme B, but an endosomolytic agent is necessary for cytosolic delivery and subsequent apoptosis. J Biol Chem 271:29073–29079

89. Galea I, Bechmann I, Perry VH (2007) What is immune privilege (not)? Trends Immunol 28:12–18

90. Garbern JY, Yool DA, Moore GJ, Wilds IB, Faulk MW, Klugmann M, Nave KA, Sistermans EA, van der Knaap MS, Bird TD, Shy ME, Kamholz JA, Griffiths IR (2002) Patients lacking the major CNS myelin protein, proteolipid protein 1, develop length-dependent axonal degeneration in the absence of demyelination and inflammation. Brain 125:551–561

91. Gay FW, Drye TJ, Dick GW, Esiri MM (1997) The application of multifactorial cluster analysis in the staging of plaques in early multiple sclerosis. Identification and characterization of the primary demyelinating lesion. Brain 120:1461–1483

92. Gentleman SM, Nash MJ, Sweeting CJ, Graham DI, Roberts GW (1993) Beta-amyloid precursor protein (beta APP) as a marker for axonal injury after head injury. Neurosci Lett 160:139–144

93. Geurts JJ, Wolswijk G, Bo L, van der Valk P, Polman CH, Troost D, Aronica E (2003) Altered expression patterns of group I and II metabotropic glutamate receptors in multiple sclerosis. Brain 126:1755–1766

94. Gilgun-Sherki Y, Panet H, Holdengreber V, Mosberg-Galili R, Offen D (2003) Axonal damage is reduced following glatiramer acetate treatment in C57/bl mice with chronic-induced experimental autoimmune encephalomyelitis. Neurosci Res 47:201–207

95. Giulian D, Vaca K, Corpuz M (1993) Brain glia release factors with opposing actions upon neuronal survival. J Neurosci 13:29–37

96. Giuliani F, Goodyer CG, Antel JP, Yong VW (2003) Vulnerability of human neurons to T cell-mediated cytotoxicity. J Immunol 171:368–379

97. Gold R, Linington C, Lassmann H (2006) Understanding pathogenesis and therapy of multiple sclerosis via animal models: 70 years of merits and culprits in experimental autoimmune encephalomyelitis research. Brain 129:1953–1971

98. Gordon S, Taylor PR (2005) Monocyte and macrophage heterogeneity. Nat Rev Immunol 5:953–964

99. Griffiths I, Klugmann M, Anderson T, Yool D, Thomson C, Schwab MH, Schneider A, Zimmermann F, McCulloch M, Nadon N, Nave KA (1998) Axonal swellings and degeneration in mice lacking the major proteolipid of myelin. Science 280:1610–1633

100. Guyton MK, Wingrave JM, Yallapragada AV, Wilford GG, Sribnick EA, Matzelle DD, Tyor WR, Ray SK, Banik NL (2005) Upregulation of calpain correlates with increased neurodegeneration in acute experimental auto-immune encephalomyelitis. J Neurosci Res 81:53–61

101. Guzman NJ, Fang MZ, Tang SS, Ingelfinger JR, Garg LC (1995) Autocrine inhibition of Na+/K(+)-ATPase by nitric oxide in mouse proximal tubule epithelial cells. J Clin Invest 95:2083–2088

102. Gveric D, Hanemaaijer R, Newcombe J, van Lent NA, Sier CF, Cuzner ML (2001) Plasminogen activators in multiple sclerosis lesions: implications for the inflammatory response and axonal damage. Brain 124:1978–1988

103. Herzog RI, Cummins TR, Ghassemi F, Dib-Hajj SD, Waxman SG (2003) Distinct repriming and closed-state inactivation kinetics of Nav1.6 and Nav1.7 sodium channels in mouse spinal sensory neurons. J Physiol 551:741–750

104. Hickey WF (1999) Leukocyte traffic in the central nervous system: the participants and their roles. Semin Immunol 11:125–137

105. Hingorani R, Choi IH, Akolkar P, Gulwani-Akolkar B, Pergolizzi R, Silver J, Gregersen PK (1993) Clonal predominance of T cell receptors within the CD8+ CD45RO+ subset in normal human subjects. J Immunol 151:5762–5769

106. Hoftberger R, Aboul-Enein F, Brueck W, Lucchinetti C, Rodriguez M, Schmidbauer M, Jellinger K, Lassmann H (2004) Expression of major histocompatibility complex class I molecules on the different cell types in multiple sclerosis lesions. Brain Pathol 14:43–50

107. Horn TF, Wolf G, Duffy S, Weiss S, Keilhoff G, MacVicar BA (2002) Nitric oxide promotes intracellular calcium release from mitochondria in striatal neurons. Faseb J 16:1611–1622

108. Horwitz MS, Evans CF, Klier FG, Oldstone MB (1999) Detailed in vivo analysis of interferon-gamma induced major histocompatibility complex expression in the central nervous system: astrocytes fail to express major histocompatibility complex class I and II molecules. Lab Invest 79:235–242

109. Howe CL, Mobley WC (2004) Signaling endosome hypothesis: A cellular mechanism for long distance communication. J Neurobiol 58:207–216

110. Howe CL, Mobley WC (2005) Long-distance retrograde neurotrophic signaling. Curr Opin Neurobiol 15:40–48

111. Howe CL, Rodriguez M (2005) Remyelination as neuroprotection. In: Waxman SG (ed) Multiple Sclerosis as a Neuronal Disease. Elsevier, Burlington, MA, pp. 389–419

112. Howe CL, Adelson JD, Rodriguez M (2007) Absence of perforin expression confers axonal protection despite demyelination. Neurobiol Dis 25:354–359

113. Hsieh ST, Kidd GJ, Crawford TO, Xu Z, Lin WM, Trapp BD, Cleveland DW, Griffin JW (1994) Regional modulation of neurofilament organization by myelination in normal axons. J Neurosci 14:6392–6401

114. Huh GS, Boulanger LM, Du H, Riquelme PA, Brotz TM, Shatz CJ (2000) Functional requirement for class I MHC in CNS development and plasticity. Science 290:2155–2159

115. Iwahashi T, Inoue A, Koh CS, Shin TK, Kim BS (1999) Expression and potential role of inducible nitric oxide synthase in the central nervous system of Theiler's murine encephalomyelitis virus-induced demyelinating disease. Cell Immunol 194:186–193

116. Jack C, Ruffini F, Bar-Or A, Antel JP (2005) Microglia and multiple sclerosis. J Neurosci Res 81:363–373

117. Johnson AJ, Upshaw J, Pavelko KD, Rodriguez M, Pease LR (2001) Preservation of motor function by inhibition of CD8+ virus peptide-specific T cells in Theiler's virus infection. FASEB J 15:2760–2762

118. Joly E, Mucke L, Oldstone MB (1991) Viral persistence in neurons explained by lack of major histocompatibility class I expression. Science 253:1283–5

119. Joly E, Oldstone MB (1992) Neuronal cells are deficient in loading peptides onto MHC class I molecules. Neuron 8:1185–1190

120. Kaplan MR, Cho MH, Ullian EM, Isom LL, Levinson SR, Barres BA (2001) Differential control of clustering of the sodium channels Na(v)1.2 and Na(v)1.6 at developing CNS nodes of Ranvier. Neuron 30:105–119

121. Kapoor R, Li YG, Smith KJ (1997) Slow sodium-dependent potential oscillations contribute to ectopic firing in mammalian demyelinated axons. Brain 120:647–652

122. Kapoor R, Davies M, Blaker PA, Hall SM, Smith KJ (2003) Blockers of sodium and calcium entry protect axons from nitric oxide-mediated degeneration. Ann Neurol 53:174–180

123. Kim BS, Lyman MA, Kang BS, Kang HK, Lee HG, Mohindru M, Palma JP (2001) Pathogenesis of virus-induced immune-mediated demyelination. Immunol Res 24:121–130

124. Kim IJ, Beck HN, Lein PJ, Higgins D (2002) Interferon gamma induces retrograde dendritic retraction and inhibits synapse formation. J Neurosci 22:4530–4539

125. Kim JH, Budde MD, Liang HF, Klein RS, Russell JH, Cross AH, Song SK (2006) Detecting axon damage in spinal cord from a mouse model of multiple sclerosis. Neurobiol Dis 21:626–632

126. Kirkpatrick LL, Brady ST (1994) Modulation of the axonal microtubule cytoskeleton by myelinating Schwann cells. J Neurosci 14:7440–7450

127. Kirkpatrick LL, Witt AS, Payne HR, Shine HD, Brady ST (2001) Changes in microtubule stability and density in myelin-deficient shiverer mouse CNS axons. J Neurosci 21:2288–2297

128. Klugmann M, Schwab MH, Puhlhofer A, Schneider A, Zimmermann F, Griffiths IR, Nave KA (1997) Assembly of CNS myelin in the absence of proteolipid protein. Neuron 18:59–70

129. Koprowski H, Zheng YM, Heber-Katz E, Fraser N, Rorke L, Fu ZF, Hanlon C, Dietzschold B (1993) In vivo expression of inducible nitric oxide synthase in experimentally induced neurologic diseases. Proc Natl Acad Sci USA 90:3024–3027

130. Kornek B, Lassmann H (1999) Axonal pathology in multiple sclerosis. Brain Pathol 9:651–656
131. Kornek B, Storch MK, Weissert R, Wallstroem E, Stefferl A, Olsson T, Linington C, Schmidbauer M, Lassmann H (2000) Multiple sclerosis and chronic autoimmune encephalomyelitis: a comparative quantitative study of axonal injury in active, inactive, and remyelinated lesions. Am J Pathol 157:267–276
132. Kornek B, Storch MK, Bauer J, Djamshidian A, Weissert R, Wallstroem E, Stefferl A, Zimprich F, Olsson T, Linington C, Schmidbauer M, Lassmann H (2001) Distribution of a calcium channel subunit in dystrophic axons in multiple sclerosis and experimental autoimmune encephalomyelitis. Brain 124:1114–1124
133. Kumar S, Mattan NS, de Vellis J (2006) Canavan disease: a white matter disorder. Ment Retard Dev Disabil Res Rev 12:157–165
134. Kurenny DE, Moroz LL, Turner RW, Sharkey KA, Barnes S (1994) Modulation of ion channels in rod photoreceptors by nitric oxide. Neuron 13:315–324
135. Lampert P, Carpenter S (1965) Electron microscopic studies on the vascular permeability and the mechanism of demyelination in experimental allergic encephalomyelitis. J Neuropathol Exp Neurol 24:11–24
136. Lampson LA, Fisher CA, Whelan JP (1983) Striking paucity of HLA-A, B, C and beta 2-microglobulin on human neuroblastoma cell lines. J Immunol 130:2471–2478
137. Lampson LA, Whelan JP (1983) Paucity of HLA-A,B,C molecules on human cells of neuronal origin: microscopic analysis of neuroblastoma cell lines and tumor. Ann NY Acad Sci 420:107–114
138. Lampson LA (1995) Interpreting MHC class I expression and class I/class II reciprocity in the CNS: reconciling divergent findings. Microsc Res Tech 32:267–285
139. Lana-Peixoto MA, Teixeira AL (2002) Simple phonic tic in multiple sclerosis. Mult Scler 8:510–511
140. Lanier LL (2005) NKG2D in innate and adaptive immunity. Adv Exp Med Biol 560:51–56
141. Lassmann H (2003) Axonal injury in multiple sclerosis. J Neurol Neurosurg Psychiatry 74:695–697
142. Lassmann H, Wekerle H (2005) The pathology of multiple sclerosis. In: Waxman SG (ed) Multiple Sclerosis as a Neuronal Disease. Elsevier, Burlington, MA, pp. 557–599
143. Lawrence JM, Morris RJ, Wilson DJ, Raisman G (1990) Mechanisms of allograft rejection in the rat brain. Neuroscience 37:431–462
144. Leinders-Zufall T, Brennan P, Widmayer P, S PC, Maul-Pavicic A, Jager M, Li XH, Breer H, Zufall F, Boehm T (2004) MHC class I peptides as chemosensory signals in the vomeronasal organ. Science 306:1033–1037
145. Lieberman J (2003) The ABCs of granule-mediated cytotoxicity: new weapons in the arsenal. Nat Rev Immunol 3:361–370
146. Linker RA, Rott E, Hofstetter HH, Hanke T, Toyka KV, Gold R (2005) EAE in beta-2 microglobulin-deficient mice: axonal damage is not dependent on MHC-I restricted immune responses. Neurobiol Dis 19:218–228
147. Love S, Coakham HB (2001) Trigeminal neuralgia: pathology and pathogenesis. Brain 124:2347–2360
148. Low PA (1976) Hereditary hypertrophic neuropathy in the trembler mouse. Part 2. Histopathological studies: electron microscopy. J Neurol Sci 30:343–368
149. Lu F, Selak M, O'Connor J, Croul S, Lorenzana C, Butunoi C, Kalman B (2000) Oxidative damage to mitochondrial DNA and activity of mitochondrial enzymes in chronic active lesions of multiple sclerosis. J Neurol Sci 177:95–103
150. Mancardi G, Hart B, Roccatagliata L, Brok H, Giunti D, Bontrop R, Massacesi L, Capello E, Uccelli A (2001) Demyelination and axonal damage in a non-human primate model of multiple sclerosis. J Neurol Sci 184:41–49
151. Marburg O (1906) Die sogenannte "akute multiple Sklerose" (Encephalomyelitis peraxialis scleroticans). Jahrb Neurol Psych 27:211–312
152. Massa PT, Ozato K, McFarlin DE (1993) Cell type-specific regulation of major histocompatibility complex (MHC) class I gene expression in astrocytes, oligodendrocytes, and neurons. Glia 8:201–207

153. Mata M, Kupina N, Fink DJ (1992) Phosphorylation-dependent neurofilament epitopes are reduced at the node of Ranvier. J Neurocytol 21:199–210

154. McDonald I, Compston A (2006) The symptoms and signs of multiple sclerosis. In: Confavreux C, Lassmann H, Mcdonald I, Miller, D, Noseworthy J, Smith K, Wekerle H (eds) McAlpine's Multiple Sclerosis. Elsevier, Philadelphia, pp. 287–346

155. McDonald WI (1963) The effects of experimental demyelination on conduction in peripheral nerve: a histological and electrophysiological study. II. Electrophysiological observations. Brain 86:501–524

156. McDonald WI, Sears TA (1970) The effects of experimental demyelination on conduction in the central nervous system. Brain 93:583–598

157. McGavern DB, Murray PD, Rivera-Quinones C, Schmelzer JD, Low PA, Rodriguez M (2000) Axonal loss results in spinal cord atrophy, electrophysiological abnormalities and neurological deficits following demyelination in a chronic inflammatory model of multiple sclerosis. Brain 123:519–531

158. Medana I, Martinic MA, Wekerle H, Neumann H (2001) Transection of major histocompatibility complex class I-induced neurites by cytotoxic T lymphocytes. Am J Pathol 159:809–815

159. Medana IM, Gallimore A, Oxenius A, Martinic MM, Wekerle H, Neumann H (2000) MHC class I-restricted killing of neurons by virus-specific CD8+ T lymphocytes is effected through the Fas/FasL, but not the perforin pathway. Eur J Immunol 30:3623–3633

160. Merkler D, Ernsting T, Kerschensteiner M, Bruck W, Stadelmann C (2006) A new focal EAE model of cortical demyelination: multiple sclerosis-like lesions with rapid resolution of inflammation and extensive remyelination. Brain 129:1972–1983

161. Metkar SS, Wang B, Aguilar-Santelises M, Raja SM, Uhlin-Hansen L, Podack E, Trapani JA, Froelich CJ (2002) Cytotoxic cell granule-mediated apoptosis: perforin delivers granzyme B-serglycin complexes into target cells without plasma membrane pore formation. Immunity 16:417–428

162. Miller DH, Barkhof F, Frank JA, Parker GJ, Thompson AJ (2002) Measurement of atrophy in multiple sclerosis: pathological basis, methodological aspects and clinical relevance. Brain 125:1676–1695

163. Miller SD, Olson JK, Croxford JL (2001) Multiple pathways to induction of virus-induced autoimmune demyelination: lessons from Theiler's virus infection. J Autoimmun 16:219–227

164. Moffett JR, Namboodiri MA, Cangro CB, Neale JH (1991) Immunohistochemical localization of N-acetylaspartate in rat brain. Neuroreport 2:131–134

165. Mogyoros I, Bostock H, Burke D (2000) Mechanisms of paresthesias arising from healthy axons. Muscle Nerve 23:310–320

166. Moncada S, Erusalimsky JD (2002) Does nitric oxide modulate mitochondrial energy generation and apoptosis? Nat Rev Mol Cell Biol 3:214–220

167. Monteyne P, Bureau JF, Brahic M (1997) The infection of mouse by Theiler's virus: from genetics to immunology. Immunol Rev 159:163–176

168. Mori S, Zhang J (2006) Principles of diffusion tensor imaging and its applications to basic neuroscience research. Neuron 51:527–539

169. Munoz-Fernandez MA, Fresno M (1998) The role of tumour necrosis factor, interleukin 6, interferon-gamma and inducible nitric oxide synthase in the development and pathology of the nervous system. Prog Neurobiol 56:307–340

170. Murad F (2006) Shattuck Lecture. Nitric oxide and cyclic GMP in cell signaling and drug development. N Engl J Med 355:2003–2011

171. Murphy S, Simmons ML, Agullo L, Garcia A, Feinstein DL, Galea E, Reis DJ, Minc-Golomb D, Schwartz JP (1993) Synthesis of nitric oxide in CNS glial cells. Trends Neurosci 16:323–328

172. Murray PD, McGavern DB, Lin X, Njenga MK, Leibowitz J, Pease LR, Rodriguez M (1998) Perforin-dependent neurologic injury in a viral model of multiple sclerosis. J Neurosci 18:7306–7314

173. Murray PD, Pavelko KD, Leibowitz J, Lin X, Rodriguez M (1998) CD4(+) and CD8(+) T cells make discrete contributions to demyelination and neurologic disease in a viral model of multiple sclerosis. J Virol 72:7320–7329

174. Mutsaers SE, Carroll WM (1998) Focal accumulation of intra-axonal mitochondria in demyelination of the cat optic nerve. Acta Neuropathol (Berl) 96:139–143

175. Neumann H, Cavalie A, Jenne DE, Wekerle H (1995) Induction of MHC class I genes in neurons. Science 269:549–552

176. Neumann H, Schmidt H, Cavalie A, Jenne D, Wekerle H (1997) Major histocompatibility complex (MHC) class I gene expression in single neurons of the central nervous system: differential regulation by interferon (IFN)-gamma and tumor necrosis factor (TNF)-alpha. J Exp Med 185:305–316

177. Neumann H (2001) Control of glial immune function by neurons. Glia 36:191–199

178. Neumann H, Medana IM, Bauer J, Lassmann H (2002) Cytotoxic T lymphocytes in autoimmune and degenerative CNS diseases. Trends Neurosci 25:313–319

179. Neumann H, Schweigreiter R, Yamashita T, Rosenkranz K, Wekerle H, Barde YA (2002) Tumor necrosis factor inhibits neurite outgrowth and branching of hippocampal neurons by a rho-dependent mechanism. J Neurosci 22:854–862

180. Nitsch R, Pohl EE, Smorodchenko A, Infante-Duarte C, Aktas O, Zipp F (2004) Direct impact of T cells on neurons revealed by two-photon microscopy in living brain tissue. J Neurosci 24:2458–2464

181. Njenga MK, Pavelko KD, Baisch J, Lin X, David C, Leibowitz J, Rodriguez M (1996) Theiler's virus persistence and demyelination in major histocompatibility complex class II-deficient mice. J Virol 70:1729–1737

182. Nordin M, Nystrom B, Wallin U, Hagbarth KE (1984) Ectopic sensory discharges and paresthesiae in patients with disorders of peripheral nerves, dorsal roots and dorsal columns. Pain 20:231–245

183. Ogasawara K, Lanier LL (2005) NKG2D in NK and T cell-mediated immunity. J Clin Immunol 25:534–540

184. Okuda Y, Nakatsuji Y, Fujimura H, Esumi H, Ogura T, Yanagihara T, Sakoda S (1995) Expression of the inducible isoform of nitric oxide synthase in the central nervous system of mice correlates with the severity of actively induced experimental allergic encephalomyelitis. J Neuroimmunol 62:103–112

185. Oleszak EL, Zaczynska E, Bhattacharjee M, Butunoi C, Legido A, Katsetos CD (1998) Inducible nitric oxide synthase and nitrotyrosine are found in monocytes/macrophages and/or astrocytes in acute, but not in chronic, multiple sclerosis. Clin Diagn Lab Immunol 5:438–445

186. Oleszak EL, Chang JR, Friedman H, Katsetos CD, Platsoucas CD (2004) Theiler's virus infection: a model for multiple sclerosis. Clin Microbiol Rev 17:174–207

187. Ostermann PO, Westerberg CE (1975) Paroxysmal attacks in multiple sclerosis. Brain 98:189–202

188. Papadopoulos D, Pham-Dinh D, Reynolds R (2006) Axon loss is responsible for chronic neurological deficit following inflammatory demyelination in the rat. Exp Neurol 197:373–385

189. Peles E, Salzer JL (2000) Molecular domains of myelinated axons. Curr Opin Neurobiol 10:558–565

190. Peterson JW, Kidd GJ, Trapp BD (2005) Axonal degeneration in multiple sclerosis: the histopathological evidence. In Waxman SG (ed) Multiple Sclerosis as a Neuronal Disease. Elsevier, Burlington, MA, pp. 165–184

191. Petrache I, Birukova A, Ramirez SI, Garcia JG, Verin AD (2003) The role of the microtubules in tumor necrosis factor-alpha-induced endothelial cell permeability. Am J Respir Cell Mol Biol 28:574–581

192. Pinkoski MJ, Hobman M, Heibein JA, Tomaselli K, Li F, Seth P, Froelich CJ, Bleackley RC (1998) Entry and trafficking of granzyme B in target cells during granzyme B-perforin-mediated apoptosis. Blood 92:1044–1054

193. Pioro EP, Wang Y, Moore JK, Ng TC, Trapp BD, Klinkosz B, Mitsumoto H (1998) Neuronal pathology in the wobbler mouse brain revealed by in vivo proton magnetic resonance spectroscopy and immunocytochemistry. Neuroreport 9:3041–3046

194. Poderoso JJ, Carreras MC, Lisdero C, Riobo N, Schopfer F, Boveris A (1996) Nitric oxide inhibits electron transfer and increases superoxide radical production in rat heart mitochondria and submitochondrial particles. Arch Biochem Biophys 328:85–92

195. Poliak S, Peles E (2003) The local differentiation of myelinated axons at nodes of Ranvier. Nat Rev Neurosci 4:968–980

196. Popovich PG, Guan Z, McGaughy V, Fisher L, Hickey WF, Basso DM (2002) The neuropathological and behavioral consequences of intraspinal microglial/macrophage activation. J Neuropathol Exp Neurol 61:623–633

197. Posnett DN, Sinha R, Kabak S, Russo C (1994) Clonal populations of T cells in normal elderly humans: the T cell equivalent to "benign monoclonal gammapathy". J Exp Med 179:609–618

198. Pullen LC, Miller SD, Dal Canto MC, Kim BS (1993) Class I-deficient resistant mice intracerebrally inoculated with Theiler's virus show an increased T cell response to viral antigens and susceptibility to demyelination. Eur J Immunol 23:2287–2293

199. Radi R (2004) Nitric oxide, oxidants, and protein tyrosine nitration. Proc Natl Acad Sci USA 101:4003–4008

200. Raja SM, Metkar SS, Froelich CJ (2003) Cytotoxic granule-mediated apoptosis: unraveling the complex mechanism. Curr Opin Immunol 15:528–532

201. Rall GF, Mucke L, Oldstone MB (1995) Consequences of cytotoxic T lymphocyte interaction with major histocompatibility complex class I-expressing neurons in vivo. J Exp Med 182:1201–1212

202. Ransohoff RM, Tani M (1998) Do chemokines mediate leukocyte recruitment in post-traumatic CNS inflammation? Trends Neurosci 21:154–159

203. Rasminsky M (1978) Ectopic generation of impulses and cross-talk in spinal nerve roots of "dystrophic" mice. Ann Neurol 3:351–357

204. Rasminsky M (1980) Ephaptic transmission between single nerve fibres in the spinal nerve roots of dystrophic mice. J Physiol 305:151–169

205. Raulet DH (2006) Missing self recognition and self tolerance of natural killer (NK) cells. Semin Immunol 18:145–150

206. Ray SK, Banik NL (2003) Calpain and its involvement in the pathophysiology of CNS injuries and diseases: therapeutic potential of calpain inhibitors for prevention of neurodegeneration. Curr Drug Targets CNS Neurol Disord 2:173–189

207. Redford EJ, Kapoor R, Smith KJ (1997) Nitric oxide donors reversibly block axonal conduction: demyelinated axons are especially susceptible. Brain 120:2149–2157

208. Renganathan M, Cummins TR, Waxman SG (2002) Nitric oxide blocks fast, slow, and persistent Na+ channels in C-type DRG neurons by S-nitrosylation. J Neurophysiol 87:761–775

209. Richards TL, Alvord EC Jr, Peterson J, Cosgrove S, Petersen R, Petersen K, Heide AC, Cluff J, Rose LM (1995) Experimental allergic encephalomyelitis in non-human primates: MRI and MRS may predict the type of brain damage. NMR Biomed 8:49–58

210. Rieckmann P, Maurer M (2002) Anti-inflammatory strategies to prevent axonal injury in multiple sclerosis. Curr Opin Neurol 15:361–370

211. Ritchie JM, Rogart RB (1977) Density of sodium channels in mammalian myelinated nerve fibers and nature of the axonal membrane under the myelin sheath. Proc Natl Acad Sci USA 74:211–215

212. Rivera-Quinones C, McGavern D, Schmelzer JD, Hunter SF, Low PA, Rodriguez M (1998) Absence of neurological deficits following extensive demyelination in a class I-deficient murine model of multiple sclerosis. Nat Med 4:187–193

213. Roach A, Takahashi N, Pravtcheva D, Ruddle F, Hood L (1985) Chromosomal mapping of mouse myelin basic protein gene and structure and transcription of the partially deleted gene in Shiverer mutant mice. Cell 42:149–155

214. Rodriguez M, Dunkel AJ, Thiemann RL, Leibowitz J, Zijlstra M, Jaenisch R (1993) Abrogation of resistance to Theiler's virus-induced demyelination in H-2b mice deficient in beta 2-microglobulin. J Immunol 151:266–276
215. Rodriguez M, Zoecklein LJ, Howe CL, Pavelko KD, Gamez JD, Nakane S, Papke LM (2003) Gamma interferon is critical for neuronal viral clearance and protection in a susceptible mouse strain following early intracranial Theiler's murine encephalomyelitis virus infection. J Virol 77:12252–12265
216. Rodriguez M, Zoecklein L, Gamez JD, Pavelko KD, Papke LM, Nakane S, Howe C, Radhakrishnan S, Hansen MJ, David CS, Warrington AE, Pease LR (2006) STAT4- and STAT6-signaling molecules in a murine model of multiple sclerosis. FASEB J 20:343–345
217. Rudick RA, Fisher E, Lee JC, Simon J, Jacobs L (1999) Use of the brain parenchymal fraction to measure whole brain atrophy in relapsing-remitting MS. Multiple Sclerosis Collaborative Research Group. Neurology 53:1698–1704
218. Rudick RA, Fisher E (2005) Brain atrophy as a measure of neurodegeneration and neuroprotection. In: Waxman SG (ed) Multiple Sclerosis as a Neuronal Disease. Elsevier, Burlington, MA, pp. 201–214
219. Sahenk Z, Whitaker JN, Mendell JR (1990) Immunocytochemical evidence for the retrograde transport of intraaxonal cathepsin D: possible relevance to the dying-back process. Brain Res 510:1–6
220. Sakurai M, Kanazawa I (1999) Positive symptoms in multiple sclerosis: their treatment with sodium channel blockers, lidocaine and mexiletine. J Neurol Sci 162:162–168
221. Salvesen GS, Dixit VM (1999) Caspase activation: the induced-proximity model. Proc Natl Acad Sci USA 96:10964–10967
222. Sathornsumetee S, McGavern DB, Ure DR, Rodriguez M (2000) Quantitative ultrastructural analysis of a single spinal cord demyelinated lesion predicts total lesion load, axonal loss, and neurological dysfunction in a murine model of multiple sclerosis. Am J Pathol 157:1365–1376
223. Scarisbrick IA, Rodriguez M (2003) Hit-hit and hit-run: viruses in the playing field of multiple sclerosis. Curr Neurol Neurosci Rep 3:265–271
224. Schiffer R, Pope LE (2005) Review of pseudobulbar affect including a novel and potential therapy. J Neuropsychiatry Clin Neurosci 17:447–454
225. Schwab R, Szabo P, Manavalan JS, Weksler ME, Posnett DN, Pannetier C, Kourilsky P, Even J (1997) Expanded CD4+ and CD8+ T cell clones in elderly humans. J Immunol 158:4493–4499
226. Sherriff FE, Bridges LR, Sivaloganathan S (1994) Early detection of axonal injury after human head trauma using immunocytochemistry for beta-amyloid precursor protein. Acta Neuropathol (Berl) 87:55–62
227. Shi L, Mai S, Israels S, Browne K, Trapani JA, Greenberg AH (1997) Granzyme B (GraB) autonomously crosses the cell membrane and perforin initiates apoptosis and GraB nuclear localization. J Exp Med 185:855–866
228. Shields DC, Schaecher KE, Saido TC, Banik NL (1999) A putative mechanism of demyelination in multiple sclerosis by a proteolytic enzyme, calpain. Proc Natl Acad Sci USA 96:11486–11491
229. Shrager P (1987) The distribution of sodium and potassium channels in single demyelinated axons of the frog. J Physiol 392:587–602
230. Shriver LP, Dittel BN (2006) T-cell-mediated disruption of the neuronal microtubule network: correlation with early reversible axonal dysfunction in acute experimental autoimmune encephalomyelitis. Am J Pathol 169:999–1011
231. Siebert H, Bruck W (2003) The role of cytokines and adhesion molecules in axon degeneration after peripheral nerve axotomy: a study in different knockout mice. Brain Res 960:152–156
232. Signoretti S, Marmarou A, Tavazzi B, Lazzarino G, Beaumont A, Vagnozzi R (2001) N-acetylaspartate reduction as a measure of injury severity and mitochondrial dysfunction following diffuse traumatic brain injury. J Neurotrauma 18:977–991

233. Simmons ML, Frondoza CG, Coyle JT (1991) Immunocytochemical localization of N-acetyl-aspartate with monoclonal antibodies. Neuroscience 45:37–45

234. Smith DH, Uryu K, Saatman KE, Trojanowski JQ, McIntosh TK (2003) Protein accumulation in traumatic brain injury. Neuromolecular Med 4:59–72

235. Smith EJ, Blakemore WF, McDonald WI (1979) Central remyelination restores secure conduction. Nature 280:395–396

236. Smith KJ, McDonald WI (1980) Spontaneous and mechanically evoked activity due to central demyelinating lesion. Nature 286:154–155

237. Smith KJ (1994) Conduction properties of central demyelinated and remyelinated axons, and their relation to symptom production in demyelinating disorders. Eye 8:224–237

238. Smith KJ, Lassmann H (2002) The role of nitric oxide in multiple sclerosis. Lancet Neurol 1:232–241

239. Smith KJ (2006) Axonal protection in multiple sclerosis – a particular need during remyelination? Brain 129:3147–3149

240. Song SK, Sun SW, Ramsbottom MJ, Chang C, Russell J, Cross AH (2002) Dysmyelination revealed through MRI as increased radial (but unchanged axial) diffusion of water. Neuroimage 17:1429–1436

241. Song SK, Sun SW, Ju WK, Lin SJ, Cross AH, Neufeld AH (2003) Diffusion tensor imaging detects and differentiates axon and myelin degeneration in mouse optic nerve after retinal ischemia. Neuroimage 20:1714–1722

242. Song SK, Kim JH, Lin SJ, Brendza RP, Holtzman DM (2004) Diffusion tensor imaging detects age-dependent white matter changes in a transgenic mouse model with amyloid deposition. Neurobiol Dis 15:640–647

243. Song SK, Yoshino J, Le TQ, Lin SJ, Sun SW, Cross AH, Armstrong RC (2005) Demyelination increases radial diffusivity in corpus callosum of mouse brain. Neuroimage 26:132–140

244. Spissu A, Cannas A, Ferrigno P, Pelaghi AE, Spissu M (1999) Anatomic correlates of painful tonic spasms in multiple sclerosis. Mov Disord 14:331–335

245. Stephanova DI, Daskalova M (2005) Differences in potentials and excitability properties in simulated cases of demyelinating neuropathies. Part II. Paranodal demyelination. Clin Neurophysiol 116:1159–1166

246. Stohlman SA, Hinton DR (2001) Viral induced demyelination. Brain Pathol 11:92–106

247. Stys PK, Waxman SG, Ransom BR (1992) Ionic mechanisms of anoxic injury in mammalian CNS white matter: role of Na+ channels and Na(+)-Ca2+ exchanger. J Neurosci 12:430–439

248. Suidan HS, Bouvier J, Schaerer E, Stone SR, Monard D, Tschopp J (1994) Granzyme A released upon stimulation of cytotoxic T lymphocytes activates the thrombin receptor on neuronal cells and astrocytes. Proc Natl Acad Sci USA 91:8112–8116

249. Suter U, Welcher AA, Ozcelik T, Snipes GJ, Kosaras B, Francke U, Billings-Gagliardi S, Sidman RL, Shooter EM (1992) Trembler mouse carries a point mutation in a myelin gene. Nature 356:241–244

250. Thorburn A (2004) Death receptor-induced cell killing. Cell Signal 16:139–144

251. Trapani JA, Smyth MJ (2002) Functional significance of the perforin/granzyme cell death pathway. Nat Rev Immunol 2:735–747

252. Trapani JA, Sutton VR (2003) Granzyme B: pro-apoptotic, antiviral and antitumor functions. Curr Opin Immunol 15:533–543

253. Trapp BD, Peterson J, Ransohoff RM, Rudick R, Mork S, Bo L (1998) Axonal transection in the lesions of multiple sclerosis. N Engl J Med 338:278–285

254. Turrin NP, Rivest S (2006) Tumor necrosis factor alpha but not interleukin 1 beta mediates neuroprotection in response to acute nitric oxide excitotoxicity. J Neurosci 26:143–151

255. Ure D, Rodriguez M (2000) Extensive injury of descending neurons demonstrated by retrograde labeling in a virus-induced murine model of chronic inflammatory demyelination. J Neuropathol Exp Neurol 59:664–678

256. Ure DR, Rodriguez M (2002) Preservation of neurologic function during inflammatory demyelination correlates with axon sparing in a mouse model of multiple sclerosis. Neuroscience 111:399–411

257. Vladimirova O, O'Connor J, Cahill A, Alder H, Butunoi C, Kalman B (1998) Oxidative damage to DNA in plaques of MS brains. Mult Scler 4:413–418
258. Voskoboinik I, Smyth MJ, Trapani JA (2006) Perforin-mediated target-cell death and immune homeostasis. Nat Rev Immunol 6:940–952
259. Wang T, Allie R, Conant K, Haughey N, Turchan-Chelowo J, Hahn K, Rosen A, Steiner J, Keswani S, Jones M, Calabresi PA, Nath A (2006) Granzyme B mediates neurotoxicity through a G-protein-coupled receptor. FASEB J 20:1209–1211
260. Waxman SG (1977) Conduction in myelinated, unmyelinated, and demyelinated fibers. Arch Neurol 34:585–589
261. Waxman SG (1981) Clinicopathological correlations in multiple sclerosis and related diseases. Adv Neurol 31:169–182
262. Waxman SG, Ritchie JM (1993) Molecular dissection of the myelinated axon. Ann Neurol 33:121–136
263. Waxman SG (2005). Multiple Sclerosis as a Neuronal Disease. Elsevier, Burlington, MA.
264. Westenbroek RE, Noebels JL, Catterall WA (1992) Elevated expression of type II Na+ channels in hypomyelinated axons of Shiverer mouse brain. J Neurosci 12:2259–2267
265. Wujek JR, Bjartmar C, Richer E, Ransohoff RM, Yu M, Tuohy VK, Trapp BD (2002) Axon loss in the spinal cord determines permanent neurological disability in an animal model of multiple sclerosis. J Neuropathol Exp Neurol 61:23–32
266. Yeager MP, DeLeo JA, Hoopes PJ, Hartov A, Hildebrandt L, Hickey WF (2000) Trauma and inflammation modulate lymphocyte localization in vivo: quantitation of tissue entry and retention using indium-111-labeled lymphocytes. Crit Care Med 28:1477–1482
267. Zabaleta M, Marino R, Borges J, Camargo B, Ordaz P, De Sanctis JB, Bianco NE (2002) Activity profile in multiple sclerosis: an integrative approach. A preliminary report. Mult Scler 8:343–349
268. Zenzola A, De Mari M, De Blasi R, Carella A, Lamberti P (2001) Paroxysmal dystonia with thalamic lesion in multiple sclerosis. Neurol Sci 22:391–394
269. Zielasek J, Reichmann H, Kunzig H, Jung S, Hartung HP, Toyka KV (1995) Inhibition of brain macrophage/microglial respiratory chain enzyme activity in experimental autoimmune encephalomyelitis of the Lewis rat. Neurosci Lett 184:129–132

# The Multiple Sclerosis Degradome: Enzymatic Cascades in Development and Progression of Central Nervous System Inflammatory Disease

I.A. Scarisbrick

**Abstract**  An array of studies implicate different classes of protease and their endogenous inhibitors in multiple sclerosis (MS) pathogenesis based on expression patterns in MS lesions, sera, and/or cerebrospinal fluid (CSF). Growing evidence exists regarding their mechanistic roles in inflammatory and neurodegenerative aspects of this disease. Proteolytic events participate in demyelination, axon injury, apoptosis, and development of the inflammatory response including immune cell activation and extravasation, cytokine and chemokine activation/inactivation, complement activation, and epitope spreading. The potential significance of proteolytic activity to MS therefore relates not only to their potential use as important biomarkers of disease activity, but additionally as prospective therapeutic targets. Experimental data indicate that understanding the net physiological consequence of altered protease levels in MS development and progression necessitates understanding protease activity in the context of substrates, endogenous

I.A. Scarisbrick

Department of Physical Medicine and Rehabilitation, Neurology, Physiology and Biomedical Engineering, Mayo College of Medicine, 200 First St. SW Rochester, MN 55905, USA

e-mail: Scarisbrick.Isobel@Mayo.edu

M. Rodriguez (ed.), *Advances in Multiple Sclerosis and Experimental*
*Demyelinating Diseases. Current Topics in Microbiology and Immunology 318.*
© Springer-Verlag Berlin Heidelberg 2008

inhibitors, and proteolytic cascade interactions, which together make up the MS degradome. This review will focus on evidence regarding the potential physiologic role of those protease families already identified as markers of disease activity in MS; that is, the metallo-, serine, and cysteine proteases.


# 1   Introduction

Multiple Sclerosis (MS) is considered a complex and heterogeneous multifocal demyelinating disease of the central nervous system (CNS) which is of unde-termined origin. Several theories regarding the initiating event have emerged, and these include a viral, or autoimmune cause [61], or metabolically depend-ent neurodegenerative changes that promote inflammation, all on a background of genetic susceptibility [13, 28]. While the initiating event in MS is not known and likely a combination of factors participate, the prevailing view of patho-genesis is that it involves a pro-inflammatory assault on CNS white matter driven by autoreactive T cells and activated macrophages, among other immune cells, which results in myelin destruction, axon and neuron degeneration, and irreversible neurological deficits [24, 266]. Regardless of whether the trigger-ing event is viral, autoimmune, and/or metabolic, the effector processes pro-moting demyelination and axon injury are multifactorial and include cytokines, chemokines, and the focus of this review, proteases. The range of potential involvement of proteolytic activity in MS pathogenesis extends from parenchy-mal degenerative events, including myelin destruction and axon injury, to release of antigenic self epitopes, immune cell activation, and permeabilization of the blood–brain barrier (BBB).

Since the overall function of proteases involves hydrolytic breakdown of pro-teins and polypeptides, they have found functional roles in an array of physiologic activities including digestion, fertilization, cellular proliferation and differentiation, cell signaling and migration, wound healing, apoptosis, angiogenesis, and inflam-matory responses. While proteases were once viewed as nonspecific degradative enzymes associated with protein catabolism, it is now clear that many proteases hydrolyze highly specific peptide bonds, resulting in limited substrate modification. Limited proteolysis is dictated by protease specificity and activation, accessibility of substrate peptide bonds, and availability of protease inhibitors, or a combination of these, and represents an essential mechanism mediating precise control of cellu-lar processes. By processing bioactive molecules, proteases regulate the availability and function of a wide range of proteins responsible for initiation, modulation, and termination of important cellular activities. Physiologic roles in maintaining a healthy state and in driving inflammatory, respiratory, cardiovascular, neurodegen-erative, and immunological diseases, as well as certain types of cancer and viral infections, have been described. Widespread involvement in health and disease makes proteases very attractive targets for development of new drugs for treatment of a variety of conditions including MS.

## 2 Multiple Classes of Protease Implicated in MS

Proteases (proteinases, peptidases, proteolytic enzymes) catalyze the hydrolysis of covalent peptide bonds in proteins. As of 2007, more than 565 genes encoding proteases or protease-like proteins have been identified in human, and proteases are estimated to comprise 1.7% of the human genome [154, 198, 213]. Despite evidence for roles in a variety of pathological conditions, the biological activities of many proteases remain undefined, including their relevant substrates, activators, and endogenous inhibitors. Understanding *in vivo* roles is complicated by the fact that proteases generally operate in cascades with other proteases, substrates, binding proteins, and inhibitors in the cellular microenvironment.

Five distinct protease catalytic classes have been defined: metallo-, serine, cysteine, threonine, and aspartic. These five classes are further divided into families according to MEROPS database criteria, which include amino acid sequence and three-dimensional folding. Metallo- and serine protease families are the largest, known to consist of 187 and 176 members, respectively, followed by cysteine (143 members), threonine (27 members), and aspartic (21 members).

Protease activity is essential to life but must be tightly controlled to prevent damage to the producing cells and surrounding tissues. Proteases are produced as inactive zymogen precursors, and activation most commonly occurs by cleavage of a C-terminal pro-peptide with the arrival of a specific protease to intracellular compartments such as lysosomes, or in the extracellular environment in the case of secreted proteases. There is an additional level of control in most cases involving a series of endogenous inhibitors that bind and block catalytic activity. Approximately 18 protease inhibitor families have been identified. A delicate balance exists between proteases, their activating enzymes, and endogenous inhibitors, which control activation and catabolism of intracellular and extracellular proteins. To understand the contribution of proteases to development of pathology, individual proteases must therefore be viewed as part of a system which includes their specific activities, level of redundancy, temporal and spatial distribution and expression level, activation state, turnover, and inhibition properties [154, 170]. We propose the term "MS degradome" to encompass the set of proteases, substrates, and protease inhibitors involved in development and progression of MS.

### 2.1 *Matrix Metalloproteases*

Matrix metalloproteases (MMPs) have received most attention regarding their role in MS pathogenesis [298], and in experimental models of MS including experimental autoimmune encephalomyelitis (EAE) [48, 265, 288] and Theiler's murine encephalomyelitis virus (TMEV) [273] (Table 1). MMPs make up an expanding family of enzymes with a zinc-binding motif that degrade and remodel structural

**Table 1** Summary of matrix metalloproteases implicated in MS pathogenesis or in the pathogenesis of animal models

| Pathogenesis | Protease | Disease association |
|---|---|---|
| MS Sera | MMP-9 | Elevated prior to Gd-enhancing lesions [267, 286] |
| | TACE | Reduced by IFN-β [299] and methylpred-nisolone [220] |
| | ADAM-17 | Correlates with TNF-α during relapse [50] |
| | | Elevated fracktalkine levels [127] |
| MS CSF | MMP-9 | Elevated with Gd-enhancing lesions [164] |
| | MMP-9/TIMP-1 | Elevations predictive of new Gd-enhancing lesions [126, 287] |
| | MMP-2 | Constitutive |
| | ADAM-17 | Elevated fracktalkine levels [127] |
| MS PBMC | MMP-2 | Elevated in monocytes [14] |
| | MMP-2, -14, TIMP-1 | mRNA elevated [14] |
| | TACE | Levels correlate with new Gd-enhancing lesions [239] |
| MS lesions | MMP-3, -9 | Capillary endothelial cells [162] |
| | MMP-2, -3, -9 | Activated astrocytes and microglia [51, 103] |
| | MMP-2, -7, -9, 12 | Elevated in macrophages [6, 51, 281] |
| | MMP-2, -7, -9 | Elevated in plaque and NAWM [62, 151] |
| | MMP-3 | Elevated in acute lesions prior to demyelination [151] |
| | TACE | T lymphocytes in chronic active plaques |
| Animal models | MMP-9 | Elevated in EAE CNS [48, 201] |
| | | MMP-9$^{-/-}$ resistant to EAE [68] |
| | | Synthetic inhibitors block BBB damage and EAE [88, 107, 192] |
| | MMP-8 | Elevated in EAE CNS [194, 265] |
| | MMP-3 | Elevated 10-fold prior to demyelination in DM-20-overexpressing mice [67] |
| | MMP-3, TIMP-1 | Elevated early TMEV CNS [273] |
| | MMP-12 | Elevated late TMEV CNS, microglia, macrophages [273] |
| | MMP-2 | Elevated EAE CNS at peak disease [288] |
| | | MMP-12$^{-/-}$ EAE disease exacerbation [288] |
| | | MMP-2$^{-/-}$ EAE disease exacerbation [73] |

proteins in the extracellular matrix (ECM), such as collagens, aggrecan, fibronectin, and laminin. The 23 identified MMPs compose four major groups differing in structure and substrate specificity, the collagenases (MMP-1, -8, -13), gelatinases (MMP-2, -9), stromelysins (MMP-3, -7, -10, -11), and membrane-type MMPs (MMP-14, -15, -16, -24). In mature CNS, MMPs are low or nondetectable, but several become upregulated in cases of neurological disease including MS, malignant glioma, and stroke. In brain, the major MMPs identified include MMP-2 (gelatinase A), MMP-3 (stromelysin 1), MMP-7 (matrilysin), MMP-9 (gelatinase B), and membrane-type metalloproteases [298]. The proteolytic activity of MMPs is tightly controlled by transcription, activation, the tissue inhibitors of metalloproteases (TIMPs), and $\alpha_2$-macroglobulins. While traditionally viewed as effectors of ECM catabolism participating in tissue morphogenesis and wound healing, MMP activities are also linked to modification of matrix–integrin contacts, resulting in signaling events that alter cell survival [42, 169, 252]. Significantly, MMP-knockout mice are associated with relatively minor alterations in matrix turnover, suggesting MMPs are not essential to normal matrix remodeling. Emerging studies indicate MMPs are capable of cleaving a wide range of bioactive substrates including cytokines, growth factors, Fas ligand, and chemokines, and therefore MMPs may exert regulatory effects on cell responses involved in host defense [152, 170]. Abnormal expression of several MMP members has been linked not only to MS but also to arthritis, cancer, atherosclerosis, lung disease, and cardiac dysfunction [181, 252].

There is ample evidence that MMP-9 levels are elevated in sera and CSF of MS patients [87, 200, 220]. In sera, MMP-9 levels increase prior to an acute attack and the appearance of gadolinium-enhancing lesions [267, 286]. In primary progressive MS, interferon beta (IFN-$\beta$) treatment reduces sera MMP-9 levels [299]. High-dose intravenous methylprednisolone treatment, the first-line treatment for acute relapses, also returns MMP-9 to normal levels [220]. In CSF, MMP-9 levels are increased in MS patients with gadolinium-enhancing lesions, but not in CSF from Devic's neuromyelitis optica patients [164]. The availability of TIMPs plays an important role in determining MMP-9's effects, since a higher MMP-9/TIMP-1 ratio predicts new enhancing MRI lesions [126, 287].

The likely integral role of other MMPs in the MS degradome is underscored by the fact that MMP-9 can be activated by both MMP-2 [79] and MMP-3 [195], and each of these, among other MMPs, have been associated with MS pathogenesis. MMP-2 is constitutively found in CSF and elevated in monocytes from MS patients [14]. Both monocytes and neutrophils contribute to altered MMP activity [108], but endogenous CNS sources are also likely. For example, capillary endothelial cells of MS brain are both MMP-3- and MMP-9-positive [162], and isolated cerebral capillaries produce MMP-9 in response to inflammatory stimuli [51, 103]. Activated astrocytes and microglia also produce MMP-2, -3 and -9 [49, 90]. Real-time PCR analysis of 23 MMPs in subsets of human leukocytes indicates MMP-11, -26, and -27 are enriched in B cells, MMP-15, -16, -24, and -28 are prominent in T lymphocytes, and the majority of MMPs are detected in monocytes. Notably, these studies showed only MMP-2, MMP-14, and TIMP-1 to be elevated in peripheral blood monocytes isolated from MS patients [14]. In MS lesions, MMP-2, -7, -9, and -12 are each detected at elevated levels in macrophages [6, 51, 281]. Of interest, MMP-2, -7, and -9 proteins are expressed not only in plaques but also in adjacent normal-appearing white matter (NAWM) [62, 151]. MMP-3 mRNA has also been observed within early MS lesions, prior to demyelination [151].

Supporting findings in MS patients, the induction or enhanced expression of several MMP family members has been linked to promotion of disease in animal models of MS [48, 130]. For example, MMP-9 is elevated in brain of EAE mice [48, 201], and MMP-9-deficient young mice are resistant to EAE development

[68]. Further, synthetic inhibitors of MMP-9 activity partially block BBB damage and manifestation of EAE [88, 107, 192]. MMP-8 (neutrophil collagenase) likewise increases in CNS in response to EAE and correlates with symptom severity [194, 265]. A comprehensive examination of 11 MMPs, and all four TIMPs, in TMEV-infected SJL/J mouse spinal cord points to a prominent role for MMP-3 and TIMP-1 in early stages of disease, while MMP-12 is prominent in microglia/macrophages at more chronic stages, suggestive of a role in ongoing demyelination [273]. MMP-12, also known as macrophage metalloelastase, is known to promote ECM proteolysis and tissue invasion [243]. Of interest with regard to MMP-3, DM-20-overexpressing mice, a transgenic model of demyelination, upregulate MMP-3 in CNS by 10-fold prior to onset of demyelination [67]. MMP-3 can also be induced in CNS resident cells by lipopolysaccharide (LPS) [97]. As seen in TMEV, MMP-12 is dramatically upregulated in EAE at the peak of disease [201]. However, MMP-12-null mice have a significantly worse disease course, suggesting MMP-12 plays a protective role in EAE pathogenesis [288]. Notably, EAE is also exacerbated in MMP-2-null mice, and in this, disease exacerbation is associated with elevated MMP-9 [73]. Since proteases are generally members of activation/inactivation cascades, it is difficult to determine whether phenotype in knockout mice is due to alteration of a target protease or secondary to alteration of a down-stream effector protease or substrate.

### 2.1.1 A Disintegrin and Metalloproteases

The cell surface A disintegrin and metalloproteases (ADAMs), or secreted ADAMTS, are a subfamily of metalloproteases (Adamalysins). Over 40 ADAM family members are known, with characterized roles in modulation of cell adhesion molecule function [114]. The disintegrin domain is capable of interacting with integrins to modify adhesion. The metalloprotease domain cleaves membrane-bound adhesion molecules, thereby mediating anti-adhesive function. ADAMs also regulate shedding of cell surface-anchored cytokines, such as tumor necrosis factor (TNF-$\alpha$), cytokine receptors for interleukin (IL) -1, IL-6, and chemokines. Metalloprotease-mediated shedding can result in release of soluble ectodomains, which influence intracellular signaling pathways.

TNF-$\alpha$ converting enzyme (TACE), also known as ADAM-17, is responsible for release of the Th1 cytokine TNF-$\alpha$ from its cell-bound inactive precursor. In MS, TACE mRNA levels in peripheral blood mononuclear cells (PBMCs) are correlated with the number of new gadolinium-enhancing lesions [239]. TACE is localized to invading T lymphocytes in active and chronic active MS plaques [131]. Moreover, TACE levels in serum are correlated with TNF-$\alpha$ levels in relapsing-remitting MS patients during relapse [50]. ADAM-17 is also responsible for shedding of CX3CL1 (fractalkine), which is found in CSF and/or serum of patients with CNS inflammatory disease, as well as other inflammatory conditions, and may therefore serve as an inflammatory marker. CSF fractalkine levels are increased in

Guillain-Barre Syndrome, MS, and viral and bacterial meningitis, relative to controls; however, in serum, fractalkine levels are elevated only in MS [127]. Soluble fractalkine has several proposed functions, including activation of circulating leukocytes [160] in addition to anti-inflammatory actions in blocking adhesion of leukocytes to membrane-bound fractalkine [127].

## 2.2 Serine Proteases

There are a growing number of links between inflammation and the coagulation/ fibrinolytic systems governed by serine proteases. Serine protease activity depends on a catalytic triad comprising the active site, which includes serine, histidine, and aspartate residues. The major clans of serine protease include chymotrypsin-like, subtilisn-like (prokaryotes), alpha/beta hydrolases, and signal peptidases. Chymotrypsin-like proteases (S1 peptidases) include pancreatic digestive enzymes, chymotrypsin, trypsin and elastase, the clotting factors, factor Xa, factor XI, thrombin, plasmin, plasminogen activators, kallikreins, granzymes, cathepsin G, and complement factors including C1r, C1s, and the C3 convertases. In each case, serine proteases are produced as inactive zymogen precursors, requiring proteolytic removal of a pro-peptide for bioactivity. Serine protease activation/inactivation cascades are integrally involved in a diverse array of physiological functions ranging from digestive and degradative processes to blood clotting, fibrinolysis, cellular and humoral immunity, fertilization, embryogenesis, and tissue remodeling. Serine protease activity is further tightly regulated by serine protease inhibitors, or serpins, that mimic the 3D structure of the protease substrate and block substrate binding or result in protease destruction. Endogenous serpins include antithrombin, $\alpha$1-antitrypsin, complement 1-inhibitor, $\alpha$1-antichymotrypsin, plasminogen activator inhibitor 1 (PAI-1), and neuroserpin. Reflecting their importance, approximately 20% of proteins found in blood plasma are serpins. Underscoring the critical role of serpin inhibition is the fact that a small activating event, through cascade interactions, results in rapid amplification of serine protease activity.

As with MMPs, substantial evidence exists for alterations in serine protease levels in MS sera, CSF, and CNS lesions (Table 2). Indeed, alterations in serine protease activity are among the first detectable signs of inflammatory demyelination [55]. Importantly, with BBB breakdown, serum proteins such as thrombin and the plasminogen activators, tissue plasminogen activator (tPA), and urokinase plasminogen activator (uPA) are able to enter the CNS prior to signs of clinical disease and demyelination [129, 133, 282]. Considerable evidence suggests that the activities of these enzymes are altered in response to various injuries including ischemia, inflammation, and excitotoxicity. Cumulatively, data point to a functional loss in fibrinolytic potential in NAWM and in demyelinating MS lesions prior to CNS inflammation and clinical manifestation [129, 139, 282].

**Table 2** Summary of serine proteases implicated in MS pathogenesis or in the pathogenesis of animal models

| Pathogenesis | Protease Subfamily | Disease Association |
|---|---|---|
| MS Sera | **Elastase** | Elevated thrombomodulin [82] |
| MS CSF | **Plasminogen activator** | |
| | tPA | Elevated [4] |
| | PAI-1 | Elevated [4] |
| | uPA, $\alpha$2-antiplasmin | Detected [4, 55] |
| | **Elastase** | Elevated [222] |
| MS PBMC | NA | NA |
| MS lesions | **Plasminogen activator** | |
| | tPA | Elevated [55], localized to nonphosphorylated neurofilament positive axons [99, 100] |
| | PAI-1 | Elevated with fibrin deposition [47, 99] |
| | uPA, $\alpha$2-antiplasmin | Localized to neurons in areas of demyelination |
| | **Elastase** | Mast cells chronic active plaques [115, 136] |
| | **Tissue kallikreins** | |
| | K6 | Elevated [231] |
| Animal models | **Plasminogen activator** | |
| | tPA, PAI-1 | Elevated activated astrocytes EAE [261] |
| | uPA, uPAR | Inflammatory cells, EAE [261] |
| | | Fibrin deposition precedes clinical disease [118] |
| | | Fibrin removal suppresses EAE [3, 118, 204] |
| | tPA | tPA$^{-/-}$ more severe acute EAE, axon injury [70] |
| | uPAR | uPAR$^{-/-}$ delayed acute disease, exacerbated chronic disease [70] |
| | **Thrombin** | Fibrin deposition correlates with TMEV susceptibility [119] |
| | PN1, ATIII | Batroxobin, reduced TMEV clinical disease [119] |
| | | Elevated in EAE [18, 117] |
| | **Elastase** | Mast cell-deficient mice reduced EAE [235] |
| | **Tissue kallikreins** | Elevated in astrocytes, T cells, macrophages EAE and TMEV [26, 27, 45, 229] |
| | K6 | Elevated in oligodendroglia in EAE [262] |
| | K8 | K8$^{-/-}$ delayed demyelination in EAE [262] |

## 2.2.1 Plasminogen Activators

Tissue plasminogen activator is constitutively expressed by CNS neurons and microglia, and although experimental evidence supports a role in regulation of synaptic plasticity, deregulation is believed to contribute to neuronal degeneration [37, 236, 270]. Contributing to altered fibrinolytic activity in MS lesions are broad-spectrum protease inhibitors, such as α2-macroglobulin and α1-antitrypsin, which enter the CNS through the damaged BBB. Further, PAI-1, which inhibits tPA, while present in very low levels in plasma, is rapidly induced by pro-inflammatory cytokines IL-1β and TNF-α [159]. As a result, while tPA has been reported to be elevated in CSF of MS patients by 10-fold relative to controls [4], and in MS lesions [55], the concomitant increase in PAI-1, along with formation of tPA:PAI-1 complexes in MS tissues, serves to decrease active tPA, thereby decreasing fibrinolytic activity and contributing to fibrin deposition [47, 99]. Suggestive of a role in axon injury, tPA is co-localized in MS lesions with demyelinated axons that stain positively for nonphosphorylated neurofilament and fibrin [99, 100].

The other major fibrinolytic protease, uPA, along with its endogenous inhibitor α2-antiplasmin, is seen in MS CSF and is localized to neurons in areas of demyelination [4, 55]. High levels of uPA, uPA receptor (uPAR), and PAI-1 occur in acute MS lesions in association with mononuclear cells and foamy macrophages suggestive of a role in facilitation of CNS cellular infiltration [7, 55, 99]. uPAR is constitutively expressed by leukocytes, including monocytes and activated T cells, and plays a prominent role in adhesion and migration to sites of inflammation by interactions with vitronectin and integrins [259, 283].

Studies regarding the plasminogen activator system in animal models of MS support the idea that the level of fibrinolysis modulates both inflammatory and degenerative events in CNS. As in MS, fibrin deposition in EAE precedes clinical manifestation [118]. Removal of fibrin in EAE suppresses disease development and neurological deficits [3, 118, 204]. Supporting the important role of fibrinolysis in CNS inflammatory disease, tPA$^{-/-}$ mice show early and more severe acute disease and incomplete recovery from EAE with significantly higher CNS levels of PAI-1 and fibrin accumulation in association with nonphosphorylated neurofilament axons [70, 155]. By contrast, uPAR$^{-/-}$ mice show delayed, less acute disease with delayed infiltration of inflammatory cells. However, uPAR$^{-/-}$ mice develop chronic disease as a result of steadily increasing inflammation, increased levels of uPA, and a greater degree of demyelination [70]. Combined results point to complex roles for tPA and uPA activity in development of CNS inflammatory disease with critical activities in regulating CNS levels of blood proteins, which may enter through a leaky BBB [155].

## 2.2.2 Thrombin

Thrombin is another serum protein that may enter the CNS through a damaged BBB, although both pro-thrombin and thrombin-receptor (PAR-1) are expressed by CNS resident cells [64]. Thrombin is a multifunctional serine protease best characterized for its role in cleaving fibrinogen to yield fibrin, but additional roles include hormone-like effects in numerous cell types mediated by activation of protease-activated receptors (PAR-1, -3, and -4), such as proliferation of astrocytes and neurite retraction [66, 98]. Thrombin also induces mast cell degranulation, monocyte and neutrophil chemotaxis, induction of cytokine expression, increased vascular permeability, and promotion of transendothelial migration of neutrophils [46]. Little information exists regarding the activity of thrombin in MS patients, but studies in animal models point to roles in pathogenesis, which like plasminogen activators, appears to be related in large part to altered fibrin levels. In the case of TMEV-induced disease, fibrin deposition is greater in susceptible SJL/J mice compared to the resistant C57BL/6 background. Moreover, batroxobin, a thrombin-like defibrinogenating enzyme, reduces clinical signs of disease but not perivascular monocular cell infiltration [119]. The important relationship between thrombin and serpins in disease pathogenesis is suggested by studies showing elevated endogenous inhibitors of thrombin, PN1 and ATIII in CNS of mice with EAE, with PN1 being most abundant prior to clinical disease and ATIII levels paralleling the peak of clinical disease [18, 117].

### 2.2.3 Elastase

Several other serine proteases associated with inflammatory cell subsets, including mast cell tryptase and neutrophil elastase, are also implicated in MS. Tryptase is the major secretory product of mast cells released in response to mast cell activation along with histamine, heparin, and other proteases. Tryptase is implicated in a number of different inflammatory and allergic conditions such as conjunctivitis, rhinitis, and asthma, and is elevated in CSF of MS patients [222]. While T cells and macrophages have long been established as the main effector cells in MS, a role for mast cells, traditionally associated with allergic reactions, is suggested, since mast cells are associated with chronic active plaques [115, 136] and mast cell-deficient mice exhibit markedly reduced EAE disease progression and severity [235]. Neutrophil elastase is released in response to inflammatory stimuli and rapidly degrades connective tissue proteins, thereby contributing to tissue destruction. Thrombomodulin is an endothelial cell transmembrane glycoprotein that is cleaved to its soluble form by neutrophil elastase. Soluble thrombomodulin can be used as a measure of damage to the BBB and has a role in binding thrombin and activation of the natural anticoagulant protein C [33]. Serum levels of thrombomodulin increase in acute relapsing MS and in chronic progressive MS, relative to controls [82]. Neutrophils are also rich in other serine proteases including cathepsin G, proteinase 3, and serprocidins, which have combined proteolytic and bactericidal activities.

### 2.2.4 Tissue Kallikreins

Tissue kallikreins are a serine protease subfamily with trypsin- or chymotrypsin-like enzymatic activity. Fifteen tissue kallikreins have been identified located in tandem on human chromosome 19q. The classical kallikreins were the first to be identified, K1 (tissue/renal/pancreatic kallikrein), K2 (prostate specific glandular kallikrein), and K3 (prostate-specific antigen). Evidence suggests that K1 participates in blood flow regulation, sodium equilibrium, tumor cell invasiveness, and inflammation [36], while K2 and K3 are widely used biomarkers for prostate cancer prognosis [183]. Far less is currently known regarding the newly identified neo-kallikreins, but value as disease biomarkers in steroid hormone-related cancers has been described [30]. Emerging studies link altered tissue, sera, or CSF kallikrein levels to neurological disorders with levels of K6 downregulated in brain lesions [302] and sera [174] of Alzheimer's patients but upregulated in active MS lesions [229] and stroke [272]. Other tissue kallikreins have also been implicated in CNS disease; for example, K8 has been linked to epileptogenesis in mice [57]. Kallikreins, like other serine proteases, may be involved in discrete proteolytic processing such as growth factor or cell surface receptor activation, and/or more nonselective degradative activities.

Investigators are only beginning to study the potential activity of kallikreins in the pathogenesis of MS because most members of this family have only been recently discovered [30]. A number of kallikreins are clearly in a position to participate in MS, since their expression bridges both the CNS and immune system, and several are transcriptionally regulated by immune cell activation [230]. Additionally, while not fully elucidated, kallikreins likely participate in activation/inactivation cascades with other serine proteases [25] and, indeed, may be regulated by overlapping endogenous inhibitors such as $\alpha$1-antichymotrypsin, $\alpha$1-antitrypsin, and $\alpha$2-macroglobulin [157]. Already, kallikrein 6 (K6), the most abundant kallikrein in CNS with preferential expression by neurons and oligodendroglia, has been shown to be upregulated at sites of active demyelination in MS lesions, in TMEV, and in EAE models [26, 27, 45, 229]. Importantly, inhibiting K6 enzymatic activity delays the onset of disease and reduces clinical and histological signs in EAE. Notably, disease attenuation parallels diminished Th1 responses, which points to a prominent role for K6 not only in lesion development but also in modulation of the inflammatory response [27]. Furthermore, it was recently demonstrated that kallikreins are not only capable of modifying the extracellular environment but, like other serine proteases, may serve in a hormone-like capacity by virtue of their ability to activate select PAR. Several lines of evidence indicate that K6 specifically activates PAR-2 [5], mediating intracellular $Ca^{2+}$ flux [196]. Of great interest in this regard, PAR-2 expression has been demonstrated in association with macrophages in MS lesions, and reduced clinical disease in association with EAE is observed in PAR-2 knockout mice [191]. Neuropsin, also known as K8, has a demonstrated role in neuronal plasticity and is elevated in oligodendroglia in EAE. Additionally, K8$^{-/-}$ mice show delayed onset and progression of clinical disease with reduced demyelination and oligodendroglial apoptosis [262]. Supporting the likely role of trypsin and chymotrypsin-like kallikreins in pathogenesis of CNS inflammatory disease, oral administration of Bowman-Birk Inhibitor, a soy-derived inhibitor of serine proteases with trypsin and chymotrypsin activities, suppresses clinical and histological signs of EAE including T cell autoreactivity [92].

## 2.3    Cysteine Proteases

Cysteine proteases have a nucleophilic cysteine thiol in the catalytic triad. Cysteine proteases include lysosomal cathepsins, cytosolic $Ca^{2+}$-activated calpains, and caspases. Like other proteases, cysteine proteases are produced as inactive precursor proteins requiring proteolytic processing for activation. In the case of caspases, this activation depends critically on recruitment platforms such as the apoptosome for caspase-9 and the inflammasome for caspase-1 [167].

### 2.3.1    Caspases

As a fundamental player in apoptosis, the caspase family is the subject of multiple studies regarding its role in both MS lesion pathogenesis and regulation of inflammatory cell turnover (Table 3). Additionally, a growing body of literature indicates that certain caspases have an important role in regulation of inflammatory responses beyond their actions in cell execution. The caspase family includes 13 members in humans. Both inflammatory caspases (-1, -4, -5 in humans, and -1, -11, and -12 in mouse), and apoptotic caspases (-7, -3, -6, -8, -10, -2, -9), are synthesized as inactive zymogen precursors. Cell death caspases are either initiators (caspases-2, -8, -9, and -10) or executioners (caspases-3, -6, and -7) of apoptosis. Caspase-mediated cell death is a final common pathway of many neurological and non-neurological disorders. Some caspases, such as caspase-8, have additional roles unrelated to cell death, including T cell homeostasis, proliferation and activation [227], and cell motility [105]. Not surprisingly, caspases have been shown to activate several kinases, including protein kinase C isoforms, mitogen-activated protein kinase/extracellular-signal regulated kinase (MAPK/ERK), and kinase kinase (MEKK-1), and to inactivate p53, focal adhesion kinase (FAK), transcription factors nuclear factor-kB (NF-kB), and signal transducer and activator of transcription-1 (STAT-1) [69].

Critical roles for inflammatory caspases have been demonstrated in maturation of pro-inflammatory cytokines, IL-1β, and IL-18 [188]. Caspase-1 (IL-1B converting enzyme (ICE)) is responsible for the proteolytic activation of the inflammatory mediator IL-1β, and blocking caspase-1 decreases neurological injury in several disease models [304]. Elevations in caspase-1 appear to play a prominent role in MS pathogenesis. Caspase-1 levels correlate with ongoing inflammatory responses as caspase-1 protein is found in CSF of patients with acute, but not stable, MS [78]. Moreover, both caspase-1 and IL-18 mRNA are significantly elevated in PBMCs derived from MS patients compared to controls [83, 112]. Caspase-1 is also upregulated in acute and chronic MS plaques, with expression associated with microglia, infiltrating perivascular mononuclear cells, and oligodendrocytes [173]. In EAE, caspase-1 mRNA is elevated in CNS, and caspase-1-deficient mice show reduced incidence and severity [84]. Caspase-1 is likely to participate both in inflammatory and cell death processes in the evolution of MS lesions, since a caspase-1 inhibitor, but not an inhibitor of caspase-3, reduced oligodendroglial death in response to cytokine challenge *in vitro* [173].

### 2.3.2 Calpain

Calpains are nonlysosomal $Ca^{2+}$-dependent intracellular proteases that promote limited cleavage of intracellular proteins involved in cell motility and adhesion. There are 14 human calpains that proteolyze many signaling-related substrates, including protein kinase C, a subunit of G-proteins, and protein tyrosine phosphatases. Calpains are upstream of the Rho GTPase family, Rac1 and RhoA, which promote lamellipodia formation. Calapin-1 is abundant in most tissues and well characterized in MS (Table 3). Under normal circumstances, Calpain-1 is associated with calpastatin, its specific endogenous inhibitor. Cytosolic calpain-1 is associated with cytoskeletal rearrangement, but calpain-1 may also be secreted from activated macrophages and T cells [60, 248] and degrades all major myelin proteins [10]. Calpain-1 expression occurs in MS plaques [62, 242] and in association with activated astrocytes, microglia, and infiltrating inflammatory cells in EAE [241]. Notably, the onset of calpain-1 expression and activity in CNS correlates with onset of clinical signs of EAE [231]. Cysteic-leucyl-argininal, a novel calpain-1 inhibitor that readily crosses the BBB, reduces CNS demyelination, inflammatory cell infiltration, and clinical signs of EAE [104].

### 2.3.3 Cathepsins

Eleven endosomal/lysosomal cathepsins are known in human: cathepsin B, C, F, H, K, L, O, S, V, X and W. Cathepsins are related to degranulation of cytotoxic lymphocytes [8], processing of MHC II antigens and maturation of MHC class II molecules [93], and activation of granzymes, neutrophil elastase, and trypsinogen [101, 147]. Cathepsin B levels are elevated in CSF [179], CNS [23], and peripheral blood monocytes of MS patients [22]. Cathepsin C is also upregulated in MS plaques [39]. Both cathepsin A and C increase in the spinal cord with the appearance of clinical symptoms in EAE [166]. cDNA microarray analysis of PLP transgenic mice, a model of remyelination failure in MS, showed up regulation of cathepsin B, L, and H expression [158] (Table 3).

## 2.4 Threonine and Aspartic Proteases

Proteosomes belong to the threonine class of proteases. The active site threonine residues are associated with three distinct cleavage preferences; that is, chymotryptic, tryptic and peptidylglutamyl. The proteosome is a proteolytic complex in which proteins are ubiquitin-tagged for selective destruction, although other proteins can be degraded within the proteosome without ubiquitination. Proteosome hydrolases are regulated by TMC-95s, endogenous proteasome inhibitors that bind to active site threonines. The ubiquitin proteosome process regulates levels and activity of numerous intracellular proteins including those involved in inflammation, regulation of the cell cycle, and gene expression. Proteosome inhibitors successfully alleviate symptoms in several inflammatory models [72, 202, 207]. The PS-519 proteasome inhibitor reduces clinical disease and results in fewer relapses in EAE [278], with inhibition of NF-kB activity thought to play a major role in disease attenuation. Ritonavir, which modulates proteasome function by inhibiting chymotrypsin-like and enhancing trypsin-like activity, also confers partial protection from EAE [110] (Table 3).

**Table 3** Summary of cysteine, threonine, and aspartic proteases implicated in MS pathogenesis or in the pathogenesis of animal models

| Pathogenesis | Protease Subfamily | Disease Association |
| --- | --- | --- |
| MS Sera | | |
| MS CSF | **Caspase** | |
| | Caspase-1 | Elevated acute MS [78] |
| | **Cathepsins** | |
| | Cathepsin B | Elevated [179] |
| MS PBMC | **Caspase** | |
| | Caspase-1 | Elevated [83, 112] |
| | **Cathepsins** | |
| | Cathepsin B | Elevated [22] |
| MS lesions | **Caspase** | |
| | Caspase-1 | Elevated microglia, inflammatory cells, and oligodendrocytes [173] |
| | **Calpain-1** | Elevated [62, 242] |
| | **Cathepsins** | |
| | Cathepsin B | Elevated [23] |
| | Cathepsin C | Elevated [39] |
| | **Aspartic** | |
| | Cathepsin D | Elevated [39] |
| Animal models | **Caspase** | |
| | Caspase-1 | Caspase-1$^{-/-}$ reduced incidence and severity of EAE [84] |
| | **Calapain-1** | Elevated EAE CNS, astrocytes, oligodendrocytes, inflammatory cells [241] |
| | | Calpain inhibitor reduces inflammation, demyelination, and clinical EAE [104] |
| | **Cathepsins** | |
| | Cathepsin B, L, H | Elevated PLP transgenic mice [158] |
| | Cathepsin A and C | Elevated with clinical symptoms [166] |
| | **Threonine** | PS-519 proteosome inhibitor reduces EAE clinical disease [278] |
| | **Aspartic** | |
| | Cathepsin D | Pepstain suppresses EAE [29] |

Far less is known regarding the role of aspartic proteases, cathepsins D and E, in MS. Cathepsin D degrades myelin basic protein (MBP) [15, 291], and at least one study has shown that pepstain, an inhibitor of cathepsin D, suppresses clinical and histological signs of EAE [29]. Of interest, cathepsin D was among the genes upregulated by more than 2.5-fold in a large-scale cDNA sequencing study of MS plaques [39].

# 3   Functional Roles of Proteases in MS

Regardless of the initiating event in MS, albeit tissue injury due to metabolic abnormality, infection, or autoimmune reaction, the host response designed to restore homeostasis is integrally dependent on the action of numerous extracellular and intracellular proteases. Partially overlapping proteolytic mechanisms govern blood clotting, fibrinolysis, complement activation, inflammation, and immunity, and these processes have co-evolved from common ancestral activation pathways [135]. Underscoring the importance of proteases in host defense, extracellular proteases often have multiple targets and are poised for rapid action and amplification. [300]. By virtue of their ability to release, activate, or inactivate bioactive molecules, proteolytic events are important post-translational control check points regulating hemostasis and immune function, and evidence suggests they play key roles in both the immune and neurodegenerative arms of MS (Fig. 1).

## 3.1   Proteolytic Modulation and Mediation of Immune Cell Effector Function

### 3.1.1   Regulation of Cytokine Activity

Proteolysis is critically involved in the activation of latent immunologic cytokines. Like proteases, cytokines are produced as precursor proteins necessitating cleavage of a pro-peptide for bioactivity. For example, plasmin activates such factors as latent transforming growth factor-$\beta$ [134], complement C3 [285], and the leukocyte chemoattractant CCL14 [274]. MMP-9 cleaves pro-IL-1$\beta$ [234], and pro-TNF-$\alpha$ [86]. TACE and possibly MMP-12 also cleave, thereby releasing membrane-bound pro-TNF-$\alpha$ [41]. Neutrophil proteinase 3 can activate pro-TNF-$\alpha$, pro-IL-1$\beta$, and pro-IL-18 [290]. Inflammatory caspases are also integrally involved in cytokine activation. Caspase-1 mediates maturation of pro-IL-1$\beta$ and pro-IL-18 to their biologically active forms [38, 263]. IL-18 in turn stimulates production of interferon-$\gamma$ and other pro-inflammatory cytokines, participates in T cell polarization, stimulates nitric oxide (NO) synthesis, activates natural killer cells, and upregulates adhesion molecules [65, 178]. IL-1$\beta$ initiates and amplifies a wide range of activities associated with innate immunity and host response to infection and tissue injury, including promotion of collagenase and metalloprotease synthesis [65]. In cuprizone-induced

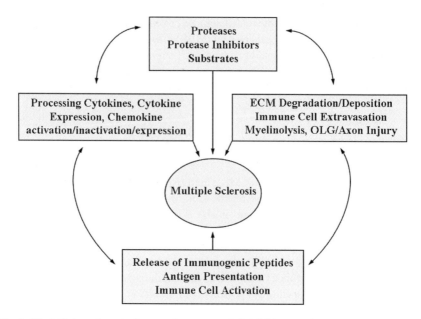

**Fig. 1** The MS degradome is that set of proteases, their inhibitors, and substrates that contribute to the development and progression of MS. Proteolysis plays a direct role in ECM turnover, immune cell extravasation, myelinolysis, and injury to oligodendrocytes (OLG) and axons. Limited proteolytic events also play key roles in regulating the activity and expression of cytokines, chemokines, and their receptors. Combined, these proteolytic activities promote the release of immunogenic peptides, antigen presentation, and immune cell activation. In turn, these events collectively affect the availability of proteases, their inhibitors, and substrates and, therefore, the development and progression of CNS inflammatory demyelinating disease

demyelination, IL-1β plays a critical role in remyelination [168]. Notably, underscoring overlap in hemostatic and immune pathways, IL-1β affects vessel wall elements promoting coagulation and thrombosis [260].

Mice deficient in caspase-1 have defective maturation of IL-1β and IL-18 and are resistant to endotoxicity [138, 148]. More recently, IL-33 has also been described as a possible substrate for caspase-1 [233]. Caspase-1 is activated in the inflammasome, an NALP (cryopyrin)-driven platform for caspase oligomerization. Mutation of the NALP3 gene results in defective control of inflammasome proteins, resulting in constitutively elevated IL-1β maturation and secretion, and this contributes to a clinical spectrum of autoinflammatory diseases such as Muckle Wells syndrome and familial cold urticaria, characterized by spontaneous systemic inflammation and episodes of fever [167]. Caspase-12 may inhibit caspase-1 activity, since caspase-12$^{-/-}$ mice secrete higher levels of IL-1β and IL-18 [226]. Caspase 12 polymorphisms in humans result in hyporesponsiveness to LPS-induced cytokine production [226]. Much remains to be learned regarding the substrates of inflammatory caspases and their role in MS.

Proteases not only activate pro-cytokines but, in turn, are regulated by cytokines. For example, MMP-9 is upregulated by Th1 cytokines, while Th2 cytokines, such as IL-4 and IL-10, have the opposite effect [1, 140]. MMP-12, which has a protective effect in EAE [140, 288], is elevated in macrophages after stimulation with cytokines IL-1β, TNF-α, macrophage colony stimulating factor, and growth factors, such as platelet derived growth factor and vascular endothelial growth factor. Transforming growth factor-β1 inhibits cytokine-mediated induction of MMP-12 [75]. Interestingly, vasoactive intestinal peptide promotes Th2 responses by suppressing upregulation of granzyme B in Th2 but not Th1 effector cells [240]. In Jurkat T cells, K2, K6, K10, and K11 are upregulated by IL-2, while K7 and K13 are simultaneously downregulated [230]. Notably, inhibition of K6 in EAE results in reduced sera levels of IFN-γ [27].

### 3.1.2  Regulation of Chemokine Activity

Ligands for many chemokine receptors undergo some level of proteolytic processing to enhance or inhibit local chemoattractant activity [300]. Carboxypeptidase modification is a common proteolytic regulatory mechanism for effector proteins of the innate immune response including the anaphylatoxins C5a, C3a, and C4a, for which cleavage results in partial inactivation. Chemerin is proteolytically activated by plasmin, mast cell tryptase, cathepsin G, and neutrophil elastase by carboxyl-terminal cleavage. CXCL12 (stromal-derived factor-1), a potent chemoattractant for leukocytes, is also proteolytically modified at the carboxy terminus, and this results in reduced activity [58]. CXCL10 (IP-10) is cleaved at the carboxy terminus by MMP-8, and CXCL9 (MIG) by MMP-9 [275], although the biological outcome is not defined. Carboxy terminus modification of CXCL7 (NAP2) by an unknown protease enhances receptor binding and triggers neutrophil degranulation [71]. CXCL7 itself is generated from CTAP-III by proteolytic cleavage and is a potent neutrophil chemoattractant acting at CXCR1 and CXCR2 [255].

Amino-terminal proteolysis is even more common among chemoattractant proteins than carboxyterminus modifications, likely due to the importance of this region in chemokine-receptor binding. Cathepsin G, elastase, and mast cell chymase cleave the amino-terminal of CCL15 and CCL23, promoting recruitment of CCR1+ and CCR3+ leukocytes to sites of neutrophil degranulation [20, 216]. Aside from neutrophil granule proteases, CD26/dipeptidyl-peptidase IV (DPP IV), a serine protease, has the largest number of chemoattractant targets removing dipeptides from their amino-terminus. CD26/DPP IV inactivates CXCL11, limiting chemotactic responses, and CXCL12, a chemokine essential for hematopoiesis [211, 212]. Other cell surface proteases, such as ADAM-17 and ADAM-10, promote ectodomain shedding of CX3CL1 [85, 113], and since both are expressed by inflamed vessels, they may play a role in the recruitment of monocytes from vasculature into tissues. CXCL16 is expressed by antigen-presenting cells and binds oxidized low-density lipoprotein and bacteria; however, upon ectodomain shedding mediated by ADAM-10, it is converted to a soluble chemoattractant for activated CD4+ and CD8+ lymphocytes acting through CXCR6 [91].

Using an exosite scanning approach, the Overall lab demonstrated that chemokines are substrates for MMP-2, pointing to novel roles for MMPs in the regulation of inflammation [170, 171]. For example, MMP-2 was shown to cleave monocyte chemoattractant protein-3 (MCP-3/CCL-7), resulting in loss of MCP-3 bioactivity [171]. Further, the cleavage product MCP-3 (amino acids 5–76) forms a receptor antagonist for native MCPs and for other chemokines such as macrophage inflammatory protein-1-alpha *in vitro* and *in vivo*. *In vivo*, MMP-2-cleaved MCP-3 reduces mononuclear infiltration in models of inflammation and, therefore, may serve as a natural anti-inflammatory agent [171]. Notably, other MMPs located in neutrophil granules also target chemoattractant proteins to enhance or inhibit activity. MMP-9 inactivates CXCL5, limiting neutrophil accumulation at sites of inflammation, while MMP-8 and MMP-9 inactivate CXCL6 [276]. Elastase released from neutrophils cleaves and inactivates CXCL12, blocking transendothelial cell migration of CD3+ T cells [215]. Conversely, certain MMPs activate chemoattractants serving to attract neutrophils. MMP-3 and mast cell chymase activate CXCL7 [137, 232].

### 3.1.3   Complement Activation

Components of the complement system are activated by serine proteases, such as C1r, C1s, the C3 convertases, and mannan-associated serine protease-1 and -2 [246]. Activation culminates in formation of C5b-9, the membrane attack complex (MAC) that damages membranes, induces release of proinflammatory mediators, controls entry into the cell cycle, and has apoptotic or anti-apoptotic effects [184]. Numerous studies link complement activation with MS [156] and its animal models [172]. MAC deposition occurs at the edge of active plaques [253] and in association with myelin in newly forming lesions [13]. While C5b-9 may be pro-inflammatory during the acute phase of disease and may promote demyelination, other studies point to a possible neuroprotective role in rescuing oligodendrocytes from apoptosis at sublytic concentrations *in vitro* [249]. Moreover, mice deficient in C5 show enhanced oligodendrocyte apoptosis in EAE [190, 224] and are more susceptible to kainic acid (KA)-induced neurotoxicity [264].

### 3.1.4   Direct Modulation of Immune Effector Function

A large body of experimental data indicates proteases with classic activities in the blood coagulation system also directly affect immune responses by binding to and cleaving PAR. Activation of these G-protein-linked receptors promotes production of cytokines, growth factors, reactive oxygen species (ROS), and MMPs, permitting rapid response to environmental stimuli. Proteolysis of PARs results in the formation of a tethered ligand that can bind and activate the receptor, resulting in activation of a wide range of signaling cascades [52]. Thrombin is known to activate PAR-1, -3, and -4, while trypsin, mast cell tryptase, mast cell granzymes, and factor Xa activate

PAR-2. PARs are widely expressed on endothelial cells, leukocytes, and in brain and therefore are poised to be mediators of pathogenesis of MS at multiple levels. PAR-1 activation promotes mast cell degranulation [46], mediates thrombin-induced macrophage production of IL-1, IL-6, and MMP-13, and inhibits IL-4 production [296] and thrombin-induced inflammation in crescentic glomerulonephritis [54]. Thrombin's effects on microglia appear to occur by a nonproteolytic mechanism as the effects are not diminished by hirudin. PAR-2 activation induces leukocyte rolling and adhesion and can trigger edema [52, 280] and allergic dermatitis [128]. Trypsin induces lymphocyte adhesion, production of ROS [150], and induction of dendritic cell maturation [53]. Tryptase activates peripheral mononuclear cells, inducing the synthesis and release of TNF-$\alpha$, IL-6, and IL-1$\beta$ but not IL-12, INF-$\gamma$, IL-4, or IL-10. Of particular interest, tryptase-induced cytokine secretion was greater in PBMC derived from secondary progressive and relapsing-remitting MS patients relative to healthy controls [163]. K14 activates PAR-1, -2, and -4, and K5 and K6 activate PAR-2 [196]. Notably, PAR-2-deficient mice are protected from CFA-induced arthritis [32] and are more resistant to EAE [191].

Immune homeostasis and maintenance of tolerance also depends heavily on apoptotic mechanisms and clearance of dead cells mediated, in part, by cell death caspases [244]. Autoimmune disease has been linked to defective apoptosis of autoreactive T or B cells, resulting in tissue destruction or defective clearance [143]. Removal of certain immune cell subsets, such as neutrophils, which contain proteolytic enzymes, ROS, and other bacteriocidal factors, is likewise induced by caspase-mediated apoptosis, since simple disintegration with release of inflammatory mediators would prolong inflammation [74]. Activation of caspase-3 is linked to release of $Ca^{2+}$-independent phospholipase A2, promoting attraction of macrophages and ensuring efficient removal of dying cells [143]. In addition to caspase-mediated apoptosis, granzyme B is involved in activation-induced apoptosis of T helper cells [240].

## 3.2 Proteases as Mediators of Immune Cell Extravasation

Inflammation in MS necessitates the recruitment of systemic leukocytes across the BBB into the brain parenchyma, a process mediated, in part, by secretion of proteases [106]. The BBB partially protects the CNS from abrupt changes in blood composition. The luminal endothelium of cerebral capillaries are joined by tight junctions and are separated from circumferential astrocyte end-feet by an intervening ECM, which cumulatively forms a unique barrier to the flow of blood proteins and cells. T cell transmigration involves both transient adhesion to vascular endothelium and focal degradation of endothelial basement membrane and surrounding ECM. BBB changes are deemed critical to pathogenesis of MS and imaging reveals dynamic and ongoing disruption.

MMPs may be one of the major players in the process of leukocyte transmigration into tissues. MMP-2 and MMP-9 degrade components of the capillary basal lamina, including collagen type IV, laminin, fibronectin, and gelatin, and therefore may play key roles in increasing BBB permeability and in T cell extravasation [89]. MMP-9 is produced by both endothelial cells and astrocytes, and upregulation may be a key event in breakdown of the BBB [219]. TNF-α induces expression of MMP-9 and, therefore likely contributes to opening of the BBB in inflammatory disease [219].

MMP-2 and MMP-3 also affect the integrity of the BBB. Like MMP-9, MMP-2 is constitutively expressed by astrocytes, including those astrocyte end-feet so critical to formation of the BBB. Pericytes are a type of macrophage embedded in the endothelial basal lamina and secrete both MMP-3 and MMP-9 in addition to other inflammatory mediators. MMPs arising from components of the BBB can therefore attack tight junction proteins. Intracerebral injection of MMP-2 opens the BBB [219]. MMP-3 knockout mice show reduced BBB damage in response to LPS [97]. TIMP-1 also inhibits transmigration of monocytes across an endothelial barrier *in vitro* [237]. Synthetic inhibitors of MMP activity also attenuate transmigration of T cells across basement membrane matrices *in vitro* [31, 293]. The most convincing evidence for the role of MMPs in leukocyte transmigration comes from studies demonstrating that IFN-β, used therapeutically for relapsing remitting MS, inhibits T cell MMP-9 production and restores BBB integrity [126, 146, 256].

Serine proteases such as tPA, thrombin, and plasmin, traditionally viewed as part of the blood homeostasis system, also contribute to BBB permeability. For example, thrombin stimulates release of prostaglandin $PGI_2$ from endothelial cells, increases vascular permeability, and promotes transendothelial migration by neutrophils [254]. Thrombin is characterized by its ability to cause retraction of astrocytic processes [98], a clear mechanism by which it may contribute to disruption of the BBB. Additionally, PAR-1 is associated with capillaries and may take part in response to influx of thrombin. Specialized receptors capable of binding tPA, annexin II tetramer (AIIt), and low-density lipoprotein receptor-related protein (LRP) are localized to BBB endothelial cells and surrounding microglia and therefore provide a mechanism to enhance localized proteolytic and nonproteolytic effects of tPA. A significant increase in AIIt and plasminogen is seen in MS lesions compared to NAWM [100]. As new proteases are identified and characterized, additional players in BBB permeabilization will be identified. For example, K6 is also capable of degrading all major extracellular components of the endothelial basal lamina, is produced by activated immune cells and astroglia, and inhibition of K6 activity reduces SDF-1-α-mediated immune cell invasion in a modified Boyden chamber assay [27].

Adhesion receptors expressed by cells of the cerebral microvasculature and astrocyte end-feet, including integrin and dystroglycan family members, also play key roles in maintaining BBB integrity in part by evoking changes in protease expression [59]. Engagement of T cell VLA-4 and endothelial cell VCAM-1 induces MMP-2 expression and activation, consistent with manifestation of an invasive phenotype in T cells and an activated phenotype in endothelial cells, resulting in proteolysis of basement membrane and interstitial matrix components, facilitating T cell extravasation toward the site of inflammation [161].

Proteases that mediate shedding also participate in migration of leukocytes from blood to inflamed tissues [116]. Limited proteolysis mediated by ADAMs at the level of both leukocytes and endothelial cells controls in part the activity of selectins, integrins, cell adhesion molecules, and transmembrane cytokines, that promote leukocyte extravasation [180, 247]. ADAM-10 and -17 are both expressed by endothelial cells and leukocytes and participate in shedding of L-selectin, CD44, transmembrane chemokines, and VCAM.

## 3.3    Neurodegenerative Activities

Neurodegenerative changes in the MS lesion include both acute and chronic demyelination, oligodendrocyte loss, axon injury, and neuronal degeneration. These changes encompass both white and gray matter and ultimately result in significant brain atrophy. Ample evidence suggests that alterations in both extracellular and intracellular proteolytic activity occurring in association with areas of inflammation and demyelination, and in areas of NAWM and normal-appearing gray matter (NAGM), play important roles in neurodegenerative events.

### 3.3.1    Myelinolysis

Proteases of multiple classes degrade myelin proteins. These include MMP-9 [40, 88, 210], MMP-2, MMP-3, MMP-7, MMP-12, interstitial collagenase [41, 94], thrombin [144], plasminogen activators [34, 193], plasmin [120], K6 [21, 26], calpain-1 [10, 11], and mast cell proteases, such as tryptase [63]. An important consideration is that two proteases known to degrade myelin, K6 and MMP-12, also appear critical to myelin formation [9, 142]. There is great interest in further understanding the regulation of myelinolytic proteases and their suitability as therapeutic targets.

All proteases shown to degrade myelin proteins are able to generate encephalitogenic epitopes triggering activation of autoreactive T cells, epitope spreading, and exacerbation of demyelination [88, 210]. This concept has been formalized as the Remnant Epitopes Generate Autoimmunity (REGA) model [197]. In this model, an external factor stimulates inflammatory processes resulting in production of cytokines and chemokines that, in turn, promote protease release. As described, depending on substrate specificity, proteases operate in cascades not only as extracellular matrix and myelin-degrading factors, but also as key modulators of cytokine and chemokine activity. While the brain is classically considered immunologically privileged, antigens drain from brain to cervical lymph nodes, and leukocyte recruitment takes place in postcapillary venules [228]. The net effect of extracellular proteolysis therefore alters the antigen repertoire qualitatively and quantitatively. This thesis holds that proteolytic events drive autoimmunity, such that inhibition of certain proteases may be beneficial to the treatment of autoimmune disease [197].

Extracellular proteolytic processing appears necessary for generation of encephalitogenic peptides. Both MMP-9 and MMP-7 degrade myelin proteins into immunogenic peptides [40, 210]. Proteolytic involvement continues through an intracellular pathway; most antigens enter antigen-presenting cells via an endocytic pathway, where endoproteases process antigens into appropriately sized peptides for MHC class II presentation. While the list of proteases likely to be involved in antigen processing in the endosomal/lysosome pathway may be incomplete, it includes cysteine proteases, such as cathepsin B, H, L, S, F, Z, V, O, C, and K, the aspartic proteases cathepsins D and E, and asparaginyl endopeptidase. IFN-γ regulation of several cathepsins may permit fine tuning of the antigen-processing machinery [17]. Moreover, the cysteine protease cathepsin S is necessary for degradation of invariant chain (Ii) from MHC class II-Ii complexes, allowing peptide binding in professional APCs [217]. Cathepsin S-null mice are associated with impaired invariant chain degradation, antigen presentation, and diminished collagen-induced arthritis [182].

Recent studies have also implicated heat shock protein αβ-crystallin as an important immunodominant protein in MS. αβ-crystallin is the most upregulated mRNA in MS lesions [39] and, like myelin peptides, is a candidate autoantigen in MS [277]. Notably, cleavage of αβ-crystallin by gelatinase B produces immunodominant T cell activating peptides in human [44] and a variety of mouse strains [251]. The identification of proteases converting self-proteins, such as myelin and αβ-crystallin, into class II MHC-peptide complexes that trigger autoimmune responses may point to new therapeutic targets whose activities could be inhibited to blunt the severity of the autoimmune attack.

### 3.3.2  Neurotoxicity

Axon damage occurs in both chronic and acute MS lesions, although the mechanisms involved at each stage and whether demyelination is a necessary prerequisite are far from clear [76]. Axonal loss appears to be associated with every newly formed lesion, and cumulative axon loss may be a major contributor to progressive and irreversible neurological disability [186]. While undoubtedly a variety of factors contribute to axon injury, likely culprits include a loss of trophic support and events mediated directly by resident and infiltrating inflammatory cells and the toxic factors they secrete, such as NO, oxygen radicals, glutamate, complement, cytokines, and proteases.

As in most other aspects of MS pathogenesis, MMPs are implicated in direct neurotoxicity, particularly since they are capable of damaging both myelin and axons [96, 123, 187]. MMP-2 [62], -7, and -9 [151] are expressed in both active plaques and adjacent NAWM, suggesting a role in axon damage. Microinjection of MMP -2, -7, or -9 into rodent subcortical white matter results in rapid and marked axon injury even in the absence of inflammation [187, 206]. TIMP-1 is rapidly upregulated in astrocytes by kainate-induced excitotoxic injury and is neuroprotective, although it does not prevent apoptosis [218, 257].

Serine proteases, their substrates, and cleavage products are also implicated in neuron/axon injury. Neuroserpin, an endogenous inhibitor of tPA and uPA, decreases cell death after carotid artery occlusion [297]. Importantly, tPA-deficient mice are more resistant to hippocampal degeneration in response to either

KA-induced excitotoxic injury or middle cerebral artery occlusion [268]. The ability of tPA to mediate direct neurotoxic effects has been linked to NO and peroxynitrite formation such that these compounds restore the toxic effects of KA in tPA$^{-/-}$ mice [203]. As a corollary, plasminogen-deficient mice are also resistant to hippocampal neurodegeneration mediated by excitotoxic events [269]. Paralleling this observation, exogenous application of α-2-antiplasmin, an endogenous inhibitor of plasmin, is neuroprotective in KA-induced hippocampal injury [268]. Also, direct injection of either plasminogen or plasmin into CNS promotes neuronal apoptosis and an increase in T cells, neutrophils, and macrophages/microglia [294]. Underscoring the concept of proteolytic cascades operating in parallel and serial pathways, tPA may increase tissue damage by activating MMP-9, while plasmin activates both MMP-2 and -9 [12, 149].

Highlighting the concept that the net effect of proteolytic activity depends heavily on its interactions with available substrates and inhibitors is growing evidence that reduced fibrinolytic activity contributes to axonal damage in MS. Opening of the BBB permits fibrin deposition in MS while at the same time fibrinolytic activity appears to be decreased due to increased PAI-1 inhibitor levels. Since fibrin localizes to demyelinated axons that stain for nonphosphorylated neurofilament, fibrin may contribute to axon damage [99]. Studies support the concept that fibrin accumulation in tPA-deficient mice exacerbates both axon damage and demyelination in response to sciatic nerve injury [2]. Notably, tPA-PAI-1 complexes increase in both NAWM and NAGM of MS lesions, indicating roles for reduced fibrinolysis in axon injury, even in apparently normal tissue. One suggested approach to axon damage reduction would be to remove inhibitors of the plasminogen activator system or otherwise stimulate local fibrinolytic activity.

Thrombin has both neuroprotective and pro-apoptotic effects *in vitro* [98]. At low concentrations, thrombin protects both hippocampal neurons and astrocytes from death [208]. However, at higher concentrations, thrombin inhibits neurite outgrowth [98]. Infusion of thrombin into CNS induces seizure [145], conduction block [43], tissue damage [294], inflammation, and gliosis [205]. Both thrombin and MMP-9 are toxic to cultured human fetal neurons, and these effects are enhanced in combination [295]. Glia-derived nexin-1 (PN-1), an endogenous inhibitor of thrombin, protects hippocampal neurons from injury [238]. PAR-1, -3, and -4, all activated by thrombin, are expressed in rodent CNS [121, 189, 289] and human brain [124] and likely mediate, in large part, thrombin's neurotoxic effects. PAR-1 overexpression in motor neurons promotes degeneration [77]. Also, PAR-1-deficient mice exhibit enhanced neuronal survival in optic nerve injury [81]. Of particular interest, the neuroprotective effect of autoimmune T cells in models of axon injury appears to relate to their production and secretion of ATIII [80].

Granzymes are a subfamily of serine proteases that includes granzyme A, B, H, K, and M. Granzymes A and B play important roles in destruction of target cells by cytotoxic lymphocytes. Granzyme B is stored in CD8$^+$, CD4$^+$, and gamma delta T cell granules along with other cytotoxic factors, including perforin [279]. Granzyme B is classically thought to cross the plasma membrane to activate caspases in a perforin, or manose-6-phosphate receptor-dependent manner. Perforin has been implicated in exacerbation of TMEV-induced disease with enhanced levels of demyelination, viral load, Th1 responses, and axon injury [111, 176]. Recently, activated T cells were shown to release soluble granzyme B, which had neurotoxic properties independent of perforin or mannose-6-phosphate receptor, although perforin enhanced the toxic effects [284]. In this case, soluble granzyme B-mediated neurotoxicity was found to involve a G-protein receptor and to activate caspase-3.

Calpains have an established role in axon damage in several models of axon injury such as stretch, crush, and ischemia [122, 225]. Suggesting a role in mediating axon injury in MS, an increasing gradient of calpain-1 expression appears in areas of no axon damage to areas of maximal damage [62]. Expression of MMP-2 and calpain-1 in periplaque white matter of acute MS lesions, prior to axon injury, suggests upregulation represents an early event in plaque evolution. Moreover, peak calpain-1 and MMP-2 expression parallel peak expression of β-amyloid precursor protein, at the border of all MS lesion subtypes, further supporting activities in axon injury [62].

Oligodendrocyte apoptosis is also an important component of pathogenesis in the MS lesion and can occur prior to manifestation of an inflammatory response [13]. Experimental evidence for a role of calpains in oligodendrocyte death in response to kainate- and NO-induced injury has been described [19]. Oligodendrocyte injury by TNF-α has also been described in experimental models [125, 301]. Caspases, particularly caspase-3, appears to be involved in TNF-induced apoptosis of embryonic mouse oligodendrocytes [95, 109], although mitochondrial-derived apoptosis-inducing factor (AIF) may mediate TNF-induced apoptosis of mature oligodendrocytes [125, 141]. K8-deficient mice exhibit both attenuated demyelination and delayed oligodendroglial death in EAE [262]. Interestingly, PAR-2 activation of macrophages results in release of an oligotoxic factor [191]. Oligodendrocytes also express MHC class I and are therefore susceptible to CD8+ T cell-mediated cytotoxicity [303].

# 4   Novel Hypothesis Regarding Role of Proteases in MS

Despite the dominant view that MS is a T-cell-dependent, macrophage-mediated disease that results in an autoimmune attack on the myelin sheath, growing MRI and pathological evidence indicates that alterations occur in normal-appearing myelin prior to the phagocytic attack [13]. T2-weighted MRI shows that NAWM and NAGM are always involved in MS, extending well beyond the plaque edge. Also, magnetic resonance spectroscopy points to metabolic changes in NAWM surrounding acute plaques, suggesting metabolic abnormalities precede inflammatory demyelination [56]. Magnetization transfer imaging, which probes proton pools, indicates that NAWM without inflammatory infiltrate, in addition to MS lesions, shows significant changes in MS patients relative to controls [245]. Taken together, these data support the emerging concept that changes in NAWM precede myelin degradation and inflammation. Disruption of the myelin sheath may initiate macrophage activity, which subsequently leads to amplification of an inflammatory response.

MBP is extensively post-translationally modified by deimination, phosphorylation, deamidation, methylation, and N-terminal acylation. One novel hypothesis, which may underlie biochemical changes in NAWM, relates to the degree of MBP cationicity as a result of peptidylarginine deiminase 2 (PAD2 EC 3.5.3.15) activity [175]. PAD2 converts arginyl residues to citrulline. The compaction of myelin relies, in part, on the ability of MBP to bind the cytoplasmic faces of the oligodendrocyte membrane, and this occurs by virtue of its net positive charge and through protein–lipid interactions. Therefore, alterations in the net charge of MBP represent an important regulatory mechanism for myelin turnover and assembly. Deimination gives rise to MBP charge variants referred to as C1 and C8, with C1 being the least modified and most cationic isomer and the most abundant form in the adult human CNS. The lesser cationic component, C8, has extensive deimination of arginyl residues. Each deiminated arginine results in loss of one positive charge. Deiminated MBP is structurally less ordered and more susceptible to vesiculation and proteolysis [15, 35, 209]. The C8, deiminated form of MBP, is elevated both in MS lesions and infants [175]. MS severity strongly correlates with the degree of arginine loss caused by deimination. In Marburg's syndrome, an aggressive fulminating type of MS, more than 80% of MBP is found as C8, compared to 45% in chronic MS, and 20% in normal adult brain [292]. MBP deimination may represent a primary defect preceding neurodegenerative events and autoimmune attack [177]. Deiminated C8 MBP is more susceptible to proteolytic digestion by MMP-3. C1 MBP isolated from MS patients is, interestingly, also more susceptible to MMP-3 cleavage relative to controls. Moreover, MMP-3 cleavage results in release of several peptides, including one containing an immunodominant epitope. Cathepsin D also digests the MBP C8 isomer 3-fold faster than C1 isomers [177]. Other post-translational modifications of MBP may also affect myelin stability. For example, phosphorylation of MBP C1 stabilizes $\beta$ structure [214] and is associated with enhanced resistance to calpain-1 proteolysis [271].

# 5  Proteases as Targets for Rationale Drug Design

The MS lesion is a complex cellular and molecular environment that can differ in early active, chronic active, inactive, and remyelinating lesions. Infiltrating inflammatory and resident CNS cells alter levels of cytokines, chemokines, growth factors and proteases, their substrates, and endogenous inhibitors, and therefore responsiveness of local cells. This reality offers both the promise of identification of new therapeutic targets, but clearly indicates that targeting any one factor is likely an inefficient strategy to promote repair. Since certain proteases have clear roles in either the inflammatory or neurodegenerative aspects of MS and several are easily detectable in serum and/or CSF, there is continuing interest in determining their utility as potential surrogate markers to aid in patient classification, treatment selection, and disease monitoring. Additionally, there is great interest in determining whether proteases may serve as unique therapeutic targets that could be used selectively to target different aspects of pathogenesis alone, in combination with each other, or with other existing therapeutic regimes.

As outlined, layered on the complex environment of the MS lesion, are secreted proteases of various families that directly impact not only cellular viability, myelin turnover, and the integrity of the extracellular matrix, but may also modify the activation state of key cellular mediators of MS, either directly or indirectly by processing cytokine precursor proteins and influencing the activation state of chemokines and their receptors. A single secreted protease, therefore, may drive pathogenesis along multiple pathways. Targeting certain secreted proteases therapeutically may therefore attenuate pathogenic activity in the MS lesion on multiple levels. An increased understanding of protease systems will be critical to the design of potential inhibitors either directed toward a single protease or capable of more broad-spectrum inhibitory activity.

Several therapies currently in use for MS or in clinical trials owe their efficacy, in part, to their effects on production of MMP. For example, IFN-βs have several proposed mechanisms of action including interaction with T cell receptors to decrease antigen presentation and Th1 activation, decreased expression of T cell adhesion molecules, and relevant to the present discussion, reduced production of MMPs. Suppression of MMP activity may also be part of the mechanism of action of statins as immune modulators [185]. Minocycline, a tetracycline antibiotic now shown to be of considerable benefit in several animal models of neurological injury or disease including MS, Parkinson's, Huntington's, amyotrophic lateral sclerosis, stroke, and spinal cord injury, also attenuates MMP production, resulting in decreased T cell proliferation and migration, reduced microglial activation, and inhibition of inflammatory cytokines [221].

The inflammatory caspase, caspase-1, is a suggested drug target for several inflammatory diseases. Pralnacasan, an orally bioavailable nonpeptidic inhibitor of caspase-1, inhibits serum cytokine levels in a murine osteoarthritis model [223] and Th1 activation in a murine model of colitis [153]. VX-765, a more recently identified caspase-1 inhibitor, also blocks IL-1β secretion from LPS stimulated PBMCs [250]. The role of caspase-1 in MS needs further exploration.

Other studies suggest therapeutic uses for oral proteases in inflammatory disease. Phlogenzym, consisting of the hydrolytic enzymes bromelain and trypsin as well as the antioxidant rutosid, is an oral therapeutic used in clinical trials in Western Europe to treat T cell-mediated inflammatory conditions including MS, type 1 diabetes, and rheumatoid arthritis [132, 199]. Oral phlogenzym confers complete protection from EAE. In these studies, T cell responses were shifted toward Th2 cytokines and showed increased activation thresholds. Notably, accessory molecules necessary for T cell co-stimulation, CD4, CD44, and B7-1 were hydrolyzed by Phlogenzym, while CD3 and MHC class II molecules, and LFA-1, were not affected, suggesting the neuroprotective effect may be due to cleavage of molecules necessary for T cell interactions with antigen-presenting cells [258]. Oral bromelain also decreased the incidence and severity of spontaneous colitis in IL-10-deficient mice [102]. Oral Phlogenzym lowered CD4+ cell number and IFN-γ production in splenocytes of endotoxemic mice [165]. Phlogenzym may also be an effective nonsteroidal anti-inflammatory agent for treatment of osteoarthritis [132]. A recent randomized, double-blind, placebo-controlled study of orally administered hydrolytic enzymes in MS, however, found no treatment effect on clinical or MRI parameters [16].

## Conclusion

Clearly, matrix metalloproteases are only one component of the MS degradome. Additional research regarding the activities of proteases of each major class and their likely activation/inactivation interactive cascades will be necessary to understand the full scope of action of proteases in MS pathogenesis and their potential therapeutic usefulness. It is also evident that proteases typically have multiple targets and that the consequence of their over- or underexpression in the MS lesion needs to be considered in terms of the full complement of other available proteases, substrates, and inhibitors. Given the identified roles of members of all major classes of protease in MS events, ongoing understanding of the physiologic consequences of alterations in the MS degradome will offer insight into novel therapeutic approaches.

**Acknowledgements** This work was supported in part by a grant from the National Multiple Sclerosis Society RG 3367-B-4 and the Craig H. Neilsen Foundation.

## References

1. Abraham M, Shapiro S, Lahat N, Miller A (2002) The role of IL-18 and IL-12 in the modulation of matrix metalloproteinases and their tissue inhibitors in monocytic cells. Int Immunol 14:1449–1457
2. Akassoglou K, Kombrinck KW, Degen JL, Strickland S (2000) Tissue plasminogen activator-mediated fibrinolysis protects against axonal degeneration and demyelination after sciatic nerve injury. J Cell Biol 149:1157–1166
3. Akassoglou K, Adams RA, Bauer J, Mercado P, Tseveleki V, Lassmann H, Probert L, Strickland S (2004) Fibrin depletion decreases inflammation and delays the onset of demyelination in a tumor necrosis factor transgenic mouse model for multiple sclerosis. Proc Natl Acad Sci USA 101:6698–6703
4. Akenami FO, Koskiniemi M, Farkkila M, Vaheri A (1997) Cerebrospinal fluid plasminogen activator inhibitor-1 in patients with neurological disease. J Clin Pathol 50:157–160
5. Angelo PF, Lima AR, Alves FM, Blaber SI, Scarisbrick IA, Blaber M, Juliano L, Juliano MA (2006) Substrate specificity of human kallikrein 6: salt and glycosaminoglycan activation effects. J Biol Chem 281:3116–3126
6. Anthony DC, Ferguson B, Matyzak MK, Miller KM, Esiri MM, Perry VH (1997) Differential matrix metalloproteinase expression in cases of multiple sclerosis and stroke. Neuropathol Appl Neurobiol 23:406–415
7. Balabanov R, Lisak D, Beaumont T, Lisak RP, Dore-Duffy P (2001) Expression of urokinase plasminogen activator receptor on monocytes from patients with relapsing-remitting multiple sclerosis: effect of glatiramer acetate (copolymer 1). Clin Diagn Lab Immunol 8:1196–1203
8. Balaji KN, Schaschke N, Machleidt W, Catalfamo M, Henkart PA (2002) Surface cathepsin B protects cytotoxic lymphocytes from self-destruction after degranulation. J Exp Med 196:493–503

9. Bando Y, Ito S, Nagai Y, Terayama R, Kishibe M, Jiang YP, Mitrovic B, Takahashi T, Yoshida S (2006) Implications of protease M/neurosin in myelination during experimental demyelination and remyelination. Neurosci Lett 405:175–180

10. Banik NL, McAlhaney WW, Hogan EL (1985) Calcium-stimulated proteolysis in myelin: evidence for a Ca2+-activated neutral proteinase associated with purified myelin of rat CNS. J Neurochem 45:581–588

11. Banik NL (1992) Pathogenesis of myelin breakdown in demyelinating diseases: role of proteolytic enzymes. Crit Rev Neurobiol 6:257–271

12. Baramova EN, Bajou K, Remacle A, L'Hoir C, Krell HW, Weidle UH, Noel A, Foidart JM (1997) Involvement of PA/plasmin system in the processing of pro-MMP-9 and in the second step of pro-MMP-2 activation. FEBS Lett 405:157–162

13. Barnett MH, Prineas JW (2004) Relapsing and remitting multiple sclerosis: pathology of the newly forming lesion. Ann Neurol 55:458–468

14. Bar-Or A, Nuttall RK, Duddy M, Alter A, Kim HJ, Ifergan I, Pennington C, Bourgoin P, Edwards DR, Yong VW (2003) Analyses of all matrix metalloproteinase members in leukocytes emphasize monocytes as major inflammatory mediators in multiple sclerosis. Brain 126:2738–2749

15. Bates IR, Boggs JM, Feix JB, Harauz G (2003) Membrane-anchoring and charge effects in the interaction of myelin basic protein with lipid bilayers studied by site-directed spin labeling. J Biol Chem 278:29041–29047

16. Baumhackl U, Kappos L, Radue EW, Freitag P, Guseo A, Daumer M, Mertin J (2005) A randomized, double-blind, placebo-controlled study of oral hydrolytic enzymes in relapsing multiple sclerosis. Mult Scler 11:166–168

17. Beers C, Honey K, Fink S, Forbush K, Rudensky A (2003) Differential regulation of cathepsin S and cathepsin L in interferon gamma-treated macrophages. J Exp Med 197:169–179

18. Beilin O, Karussis DM, Korczyn AD, Gurwitz D, Aronovich R, Hantai D, Grigoriadis N, Mizrachi-Kol R, Chapman J (2005) Increased thrombin inhibition in experimental autoimmune encephalomyelitis. J Neurosci Res 798:351–359

19. Benjamins JA, Nedelkoska L, George EB (2003) Protection of mature oligodendrocytes by inhibitors of caspases and calpains. Neurochem Res 28:143–152

20. Berahovich RD, Miao Z, Wang Y, Premack B, Howard MC, Schall TJ (2005) Proteolytic activation of alternative CCR1 ligands in inflammation. J Immunol 174:7341–7351

21. Bernett MJ, Blaber SI, Scarisbrick IA, Dhanarajan P, Thompson SM, Blaber M (2002) Crystal structure and biochemical characterization of human kallikrein 6 reveals a trypsin-like kallikrein is expressed in the central nervous system. J Biol Chem 277:24562–24570

22. Bever CT Jr, Panitch HS, Johnson KP (1994) Increased cathepsin B activity in peripheral blood mononuclear cells of multiple sclerosis patients. Neurology 44:745–748

23. Bever CT Jr, Garver DW (1995) Increased cathepsin B activity in multiple sclerosis brain. J Neurol Sci 131:71–73

24. Bjartmar C, Kinkel RP, Kidd G, Rudick RA, Trapp BD (2001) Axonal loss in normal-appearing white matter in a patient with acute MS. Neurology 57:1248–1252

25. Blaber S, Heysook Y, Scarisbrick IA, Juliani L, Blaber M (2007) The autolytic regulation of human kallkrein 6. Biochemistry, in press

26. Blaber SI, Scarisbrick IA, Bernett MJ, Dhanarajan P, Seavy MA, Jin Y, Schwartz MA, Rodriguez M, Blaber M (2002) Enzymatic properties of rat myelencephalon specific protease. Biochemistry 41:1165–1173

27. Blaber SI, Ciric B, Christophi GP, Bernett MJ, Blaber M, Rodriguez M, Scarisbrick IA (2004) Targeting kallikrein 6-proteolysis attenuates CNS inflammatory disease. FASEB J 19:920–922

28. Bo L, Vedeler CA, Nyland H, Trapp BD, Mork SJ (2003) Intracortical multiple sclerosis lesions are not associated with increased lymphocyte infiltration. Mult Scler 9:323–331

29. Boehme DH, Marks N (1979) Mitigation of experimental allergic encephalomyelitis by cathepsin D inhibition. Adv Exp Med Biol 121B:317–323

30. Borgono CA, Miacovos MP, Diamandis EP (2004) Human tissue kallikreins: physiologic roles and applications in cancer. Mol Cancer Res 2:257–280

31. Brundula V, Rewcastle NB, Metz LM, Bernard CC, Yong VW (2002) Targeting leukocyte MMPs and transmigration: minocycline as a potential therapy for multiple sclerosis. Brain 125:1297–1308
32. Busso N, Frasnelli M, Feifel R, Cenni B, Steinhoff M, Hamilton J, So A (2007) Evaluation of protease-activated receptor 2 in murine models of arthritis. Arthritis Rheum 56:101–107
33. Califano F, Giovanniello T, Pantone P, Campana E, Parlapiano C, Alegiani F, Vincentelli GM, Turchetti P (2000) Clinical importance of thrombomodulin serum levels. Eur Rev Med Pharmacol Sci 4:59–66
34. Cammer W, Bloom BR, Norton WT, Gordon S (1978) Degradation of basic protein in myelin by neutral proteases secreted by stimulated macrophages: a possible mechanism of inflammatory demyelination. Proc Natl Acad Sci USA 75:1554–1558
35. Cao L, Goodin R, Wood D, Moscarello MA, Whitaker JN (1999) Rapid release and unusual stability of immunodominant peptide 45–89 from citrullinated myelin basic protein. Biochemistry 38:6157–6163
36. Cassim B, Mody G, Bhoola KD (2002) Kallikrein cascade and cytokines in inflammed joints. Pharmacol Ther 94:1–34
37. Centonze D, Napolitano M, Saulle E, Gubellini P, Picconi B, Martorana A, Pisani A, Gulino A, Bernardi G, Calabresi P (2002) Tissue plasminogen activator is required for corticostriatal long-term potentiation. Eur J Neurosci 16:713–721
38. Cerretti DP, Kozlosky CJ, Mosley B, Nelson N, Van Ness K, Greenstreet TA, March CJ, Kronheim SR, Druck T, Cannizzaro LA et al (1992) Molecular cloning of the interleukin-1 beta converting enzyme. Science 256:97–100
39. Chabas D, Baranzini SE, Mitchell D, Bernard CC, Rittling SR, Denhardt DT, Sobel RA, Lock C, Karpuj M, Pedotti R, Heller R, Oksenberg JR, Steinman L (2001) The influence of the proinflammatory cytokine, osteopontin, on autoimmune demyelinating disease. Science 294:1731–1735
40. Chandler S, Coates R, Gearing A, Lury J, Wells G, Bone E (1995) Matrix metalloproteinases degrade myelin basic protein. Neurosci Lett 201:223–226
41. Chandler S, Cossins J, Lury J, Wells G (1996) Macrophage metalloelastase degrades matrix and myelin proteins and processes a tumour necrosis factor-alpha fusion protein. Biochem Biophys Res Commun 228:421–429
42. Chang C, Werb Z (2001) The many faces of metalloproteases: cell growth, invasion, angiogenesis and metastasis. Trends Cell Biol 11:S37–S43
43. Chapman J (2006) Thrombin in inflammatory brain diseases. Autoimmun Rev 5:528–531
44. Chou YK, Burrows GG, LaTocha D, Wang C, Subramanian S, Bourdette DN, Vandenbark AA (2004) CD4 T-cell epitopes of human alpha B-crystallin. J Neurosci Res 75:516–523
45. Christophi GP, Isackson PJ, Blaber SI, Blaber M, Rodriguez M, Scarisbrick IA (2004) Distinct promoters regulate tissue-specific and differential expression of kallikrein 6 in CNS demyelinating disease. J Neurochem 91:1439–1449
46. Cirino G, Cicala C, Bucci MR, Sorrentino L, Maraganore JM, Stone SR (1996) Thrombin functions as an inflammatory mediator through activation of its receptor. J Exp Med 183:821–827
47. Claudio L, Raine CS, Brosnan CF (1995) Evidence of persistent blood brain barrier abnormalities in chromic-progressive multiple sclerosis. Acta Neuropathol (Berl) 90:228–238
48. Clements JM, Cossins JA, Wells GM, Corkill DJ, Helfrich K, Wood LM, Pigott R, Stabler G, Ward GA, Gearing AJ, Miller KM (1997) Matrix metalloproteinase expression during experimental autoimmune encephalomyelitis and effects of a combined matrix metalloproteinase and tumour necrosis factor-alpha inhibitor. J Neuroimmunol 74:85–94
49. Colton CA, Keri JE, Chen WT, Monsky WL (1993) Protease production by cultured microglia: substrate gel analysis and immobilized matrix degradation. J Neurosci Res 35:297–304
50. Comabella M, Romera C, Camina M, Perkal H, Moro MA, Leza JC, Lizasoain I, Castillo M, Montalban X (2006) TNF-alpha converting enzyme (TACE) protein expression in different clinical subtypes of multiple sclerosis. J Neurol 253:701–706

51. Cossins JA, Clements JM, Ford J, Miller KM, Pigott R, Vos W, Van der Valk P, De Groot CJ (1997) Enhanced expression of MMP-7 and MMP-9 in demyelinating multiple sclerosis lesions. Acta Neuropathol (Berl) 94:590–598
52. Coughlin SR (2005) Protease-activated receptors in hemostasis, thrombosis and vascular biology. J Thromb Haemost 3:1800–1814
53. Csernok E, Ai M, Gross WL, Wicklein D, Petersen A, Lindner B, Lamprecht P, Holle JU, Hellmich B (2006) Wegener autoantigen induces maturation of dendritic cells and licenses them for Th1 priming via the protease-activated receptor-2 pathway. Blood 107:4440–4448
54. Cunningham MA, Rondeau E, Chen X, Coughlin SR, Holdsworth SR, Tipping PG (2000) Protease-activated receptor 1 mediates thrombin-dependent, cell-mediated renal inflammation in crescentic glomerulonephritis. J Exp Med 191:455–462
55. Cuzner ML, Gveric D, Strand C, Loughlin AJ, Paemen L, Opdenakker G, Newcombe J (1996) The expression of tissue-type plasminogen activator, matrix metalloproteases and endogenous inhibitors in the central nervous system in multiple sclerosis: comparison of stages in lesion evolution. J Neuropath Exp Neurol 55:1194–1204
56. Davie CA, Barker GJ, Thompson AJ, Tofts PS, McDonald WI, Miller DH (1997) 1H magnetic resonance spectroscopy of chronic cerebral white matter lesions and normal appearing white matter in multiple sclerosis. J Neurol Neurosurg Psychiatry 63:736–742
57. Davies B, Kearns IR, Ure J, Davies CH, Lathe R (2001) Loss of hippocampal serine protease BSP1/neuropsin predisposes to global seizure activity. J Neurosci 21:6993–7000
58. De La Luz Sierra M, Yang F, Narazaki M, Salvucci O, Davis D, Yarchoan R, Zhang HH, Fales H, Tosato G (2004) Differential processing of stromal-derived factor-1alpha and stromal-derived factor-1beta explains functional diversity. Blood 103:2452–2459
59. del Zoppo GJ, Milner R (2006) Integrin-matrix interactions in the cerebral microvasculature. Arterioscler Thromb Vasc Biol 26:1966–1975
60. Deshpande RV, Goust JM, Hogan EL, Banik NL (1995) Calpain secreted by activated human lymphoid cells degrades myelin. J Neurosci Res 42:259–265
61. Dhib-Jalbut S (2002) Mechanisms of action of interferons and glatiramer acetate in multiple sclerosis. Neurology 58:S3–S9.
62. Diaz-Sanchez M, Williams K, DeLuca GC, Esiri MM (2006) Protein co-expression with axonal injury in multiple sclerosis plaques. Acta Neuropathol (Berl) 111:289–299
63. Dietsch GN, Hinrichs DJ (1991) Mast cell proteases liberate stable encephalitogenic fragments from intact myelin. Cell Immunol 135:541–548
64. Dihanich M, Kaser M, Reinhard E, Cunningham D, Monard D (1991) Prothrombin mRNA is expressed by cells of the nervous system. Neuron 6:575–581
65. Dinarello CA, Fantuzzi G (2003) Interleukin-18 and host defense against infection. J Infect Dis 187 Suppl 2:S370–S384
66. Donovan FM, Cunningham DD (1998) Signaling pathways involved in thrombin-induced cell protection. J Biol Chem 273:12746–12752
67. D'Souza CA, Mak B, Moscarello MA (2002) The up-regulation of stromelysin-1 (MMP-3) in a spontaneously demyelinating transgenic mouse precedes onset of disease. J Biol Chem 277:13589–13596
68. Dubois B, Masure S, Hurtenbach U, Paemen L, Heremans H, van den Oord J, Sciot R, Meinhardt T, Hammerling G, Opdenakker G, Arnold B (1999) Resistance of young gelatinase B-deficient mice to experimental autoimmune encephalomyelitis and necrotizing tail lesions. J Clin Invest 104:1507–1515
69. Earnshaw WC (1999) Apoptosis. A cellular poison cupboard. Nature 397:387–389
70. East E, Baker D, Pryce G, Lijnen HR, Cuzner ML, Gveric D (2005) A role for the plasminogen activator system in inflammation and neurodegeneration in the central nervous system during experimental allergic encephalomyelitis. Am J Pathol 167:545–554
71. Ehlert JE, Gerdes J, Flad HD, Brandt E (1998) Novel C-terminally truncated isoforms of the CXC chemokine beta-thromboglobulin and their impact on neutrophil functions. J Immunol 161:4975–4982

72. Elliott PJ, Pien CS, McCormack TA, Chapman ID, Adams J (1999) Proteasome inhibition: A novel mechanism to combat asthma. J Allergy Clin Immunol 104:294–300
73. Esparza J, Kruse M, Lee J, Michaud M, Madri JA (2004) MMP-2 null mice exhibit an early onset and severe experimental autoimmune encephalomyelitis due to an increase in MMP-9 expression and activity. FASEB J 18:1682–1691
74. Fadeel B, Kagan VE (2003) Apoptosis and macrophage clearance of neutrophils: regulation by reactive oxygen species. Redox Rep 8:143–150
75. Feinberg MW, Jain MK, Werner F, Sibinga NE, Wiesel P, Wang H, Topper JN, Perrella MA, Lee ME (2000) Transforming growth factor-beta 1 inhibits cytokine-mediated induction of human metalloelastase in macrophages. J Biol Chem 275:25766–25773
76. Ferguson B, Matyszak MK, Esiri MM, Perry VH (1997) Axonal damage in acute multiple sclerosis lesions. Brain 120:393–399
77. Festoff BW, D'Andrea MR, Citron BA, Salcedo RM, Smirnova IV, Andrade-Gordon P (2000) Motor neuron cell death in wobbler mutant mice follows overexpression of the G-protein-coupled, protease-activated receptor for thrombin. Mol Med 6:410–429
78. Franciotta D, Martino G, Zardini E, Furlan R, Bergamaschi R, Gironi M, Bergami A, Angelini G, De Benedetti F, Pignatti P, Moscato G, Cosi V (2002) Caspase-1 levels in biological fluids from patients with multiple sclerosis and from patients with other neurological and non-neurological diseases. Eur Cytokine Netw 13:99–103
79. Fridman R, Toth M, Pena D, Mobashery S (1995) Activation of progelatinase B (MMP-9) by gelatinase A (MMP-2). Cancer Res 55:2548–2555
80. Friedmann I, Hauben E, Yoles E, Kardash L, Schwartz M (2001) T cell-mediated neuroprotection involves antithrombin activity. J Neuroimmunol 121:12–21
81. Friedmann I, Yoles E, Schwartz M (2001) Thrombin attenuation is neuroprotective in the injured rat optic nerve. J Neurochem 76:641–649
82. Frigerio S, Ariano C, Bernardi G, Ciusani E, Massa G, La Mantia L, Salmaggi A (1998) Cerebrospinal fluid thrombomodulin and sVCAM-1 in different clinical stages of multiple sclerosis patients. J Neuroimmunol 87:88–93
83. Furlan R, Filippi M, Bergami A, Rocca MA, Martinelli V, Poliani PL, Grimaldi LM, Desina G, Comi G, Martino G (1999) Peripheral levels of caspase-1 mRNA correlate with disease activity in patients with multiple sclerosis; a preliminary study. J Neurol Neurosurg Psychiatry 67:785–788
84. Furlan R, Martino G, Galbiati F, Poliani PL, Smiroldo S, Bergami A, Desina G, Comi G, Flavell R, Su MS, Adorini L (1999) Caspase-1 regulates the inflammatory process leading to autoimmune demyelination. J Immunol 163:2403–2409
85. Garton KJ, Gough PJ, Philalay J, Wille PT, Blobel CP, Whitehead RH, Dempsey PJ, Raines EW (2003) Stimulated shedding of vascular cell adhesion molecule 1 (VCAM-1) is mediated by tumor necrosis factor-alpha-converting enzyme (ADAM 17). J Biol Chem 278:37459–37464
86. Gearing AJ, Beckett P, Christodoulou M, Churchill M, Clements JM, Crimmin M, Davidson AH, Drummond AH, Galloway WA, Gilbert R et al (1995) Matrix metalloproteinases and processing of pro-TNF-alpha. J Leukoc Biol 57:774–777
87. Gijbels K, Masure S, Carton H, Opdenakker G (1992) Gelatinase in cerebrospinal fluid of patients with multiple sclerosis and other inflammatory neurological disorders. J Neuroimmunol 41:29–34
88. Gijbels K, Galardy RE, Steinman L (1994) Reversal of experimental allergic encephalomyelitis with a hydroxamate inhibitor of matrix metalloproteases. J Clin Invest 94:2177–2182
89. Goetzl EJ, Banda MJ, Leppert D (1996) Matrix metalloproteinases in immunity. J Immunol 156:1–4
90. Gottschall PE, Deb S (1996) Regulation of matrix metalloproteinase expressions in astrocytes, microglia and neurons. Neuroimmunomodulation 3:69–75
91. Gough PJ, Garton KJ, Wille PT, Rychlewski M, Dempsey PJ, Raines EW (2004) A disintegrin and metalloproteinase 10-mediated cleavage and shedding regulates the cell surface expression of CXC chemokine ligand 16. J Immunol 172:3678–3685

92. Gran B, Tabibzadeh N, Martin A, Ventura ES, Ware JH, Zhang G-X, Parr JL, Kennedy AR, Rostami AM (2006) The protease inhibitor, Bowman-Birk inhibitor, suppresses experimental autoimmune encephalomyelitis: a potential oral therapy for multiple sclerosis. Mult Scler 12:688–697

93. Greiner A, Lautwein A, Overkleeft HS, Weber E, Driessen C (2003) Activity and subcellular distribution of cathepsins in primary human monocytes. J Leukoc Biol 73:235–242

94. Gronski TJ Jr, Martin RL, Kobayashi DK, Walsh BC, Holman MC, Huber M, Van Wart HE, Shapiro SD (1997) Hydrolysis of a broad spectrum of extracellular matrix proteins by human macrophage elastase. J Biol Chem 272:12189–12194

95. Gu C, Casaccia-Bonnefil P, Srinivasan A, Chao MV (1999) Oligodendrocyte apoptosis mediated by caspase activation. J Neurosci 19:3043–3049

96. Gu Z, Kaul M, Yan B, Kridel SJ, Cui J, Strongin A, Smith JW, Liddington RC, Lipton SA (2002) S-nitrosylation of matrix metalloproteinases: signaling pathway to neuronal cell death. Science 297:1186–1190

97. Gurney KJ, Estrada EY, Rosenberg GA (2006) Blood-brain barrier disruption by stromelysin-1 facilitates neutrophil infiltration in neuroinflammation. Neurobiol Dis 23:87–96

98. Gurwitz D, Cunningham DD (1990) Neurite outgrowth activity of protease nexin-1 on neuroblastoma cells requires thrombin inhibition. J Cell Physiol 142:155–162

99. Gveric D, Hanemaaijer R, Newcombe J, van Lent NA, Sier CF, Cuzner ML (2001) Plasminogen activators in multiple sclerosis lesions: implications for the inflammatory response and axonal damage. Brain 124:1978–1988

100. Gveric D, Herrera BM, Cuzner ML (2005) tPA receptors and the fibrinolytic response in multiple sclerosis lesions. Am J Pathol 166:1143–1151

101. Halangk W, Lerch MM, Brandt-Nedelev B, Roth W, Ruthenbuerger M, Reinheckel T, Domschke W, Lippert H, Peters C, Deussing J (2000) Role of cathepsin B in intracellular trypsinogen activation and the onset of acute pancreatitis. J Clin Invest 106:773–781

102. Hale LP, Greer PK, Trinh CT, Gottfried MR (2005) Treatment with oral bromelain decreases colonic inflammation in the IL-10-deficient murine model of inflammatory bowel disease. Clin Immunol 116:135–142

103. Harkness KA, Adamson P, Sussman JD, Davies-Jones GA, Greenwood J, Woodroofe MN (2000) Dexamethasone regulation of matrix metalloproteinase expression in CNS vascular endothelium. Brain 123:698–709

104. Hassen GW, Feliberti J, Kesner L, Stracher A, Mokhtarian F (2006) A novel calpain inhibitor for the treatment of acute experimental autoimmune encephalomyelitis. J Neuroimmunol 180:135–146

105. Helfer B, Boswell BC, Finlay D, Cipres A, Vuori K, Bong Kang T, Wallach D, Dorfleutner A, Lahti JM, Flynn DC, Frisch SM (2006) Caspase-8 promotes cell motility and calpain activity under nonapoptotic conditions. Cancer Res 66:4273–4278

106. Hemmer B, Archelos JJ, Hartung H-P (2002) New concepts in the immunopathogenesis of multiple sclerosis. Nat Rev 3:291–301

107. Hewson AK, Smith T, Leonard JP, Cuzner ML (1995) Suppression of experimental allergic encephalomyelitis in the Lewis rat by the matrix metalloproteinase inhibitor Ro31–9790. Inflammation Res 44:345–349

108. Hibbs MS, Hasty KA, Seyer JM, Kang AH, Mainardi CL (1985) Biochemical and immunological characterization of the secreted forms of human neutrophil gelatinase. J Biol Chem 260:2493–2500

109. Hisahara S, Shoji S, Okano H, Miura M (1997) ICE/CED-3 family executes oligodendrocyte apoptosis by tumor necrosis factor. J Neurochem 69:10–20

110. Hosseini H, Andre P, Lefevre N, Viala L, Walzer T, Peschanski M, Lotteau V (2001) Protection against experimental autoimmune encephalomyelitis by a proteasome modulator. J Neuroimmunol 118:233–244

111. Howe CL, Adelson JD, Rodriguez M (2007) Absence of perforin expression confers axonal protection despite demyelination. Neurobiol Dis 25:354–359

112. Huang WX, Huang P, Hillert J (2004) Increased expression of caspase-1 and interleukin-18 in peripheral blood mononuclear cells in patients with multiple sclerosis. Mult Scler 10:482–487
113. Hundhausen C, Misztela D, Berkhout TA, Broadway N, Saftig P, Reiss K, Hartmann D, Fahrenholz F, Postina R, Matthews V, Kallen KJ, Rose-John S, Ludwig A (2003) The disintegrin-like metalloproteinase ADAM10 is involved in constitutive cleavage of CX3CL1 (fractalkine) and regulates CX3CL1-mediated cell-cell adhesion. Blood 102:1186–1195
114. Huovila AP, Turner AJ, Pelto-Huikko M, Karkkainen I, Ortiz RM (2005) Shedding light on ADAM metalloproteinases. Trends Biochem Sci 30:413–422
115. Ibrahim MZ, Reder AT, Lawand R, Takash W, Sallouh-Khatib S (1996) The mast cells of the multiple sclerosis brain. J Neuroimmunol 70:131–138
116. Imai C, Okamura A, Peng JF, Kitamura Y, Printz MP (2005) Interleukin-1beta enhanced action of kinins on extracellular matrix of spontaneous hypertensive rat cardiac fibroblasts. Clin Exp Hypertens 27:59–69
117. Inaba Y, Ichikawa M, Inoue A, Itoh M, Kyogashima M, Sekiguchi Y, Nakamura S, Komiyama A, Koh C (2001) Plasma thrombin-antithrombin III complex is associated with the severity of experimental autoimmune encephalomyelitis. J Neurol Sci 185:89–93
118. Inoue A, Koh CS, Shimada K, Yanagisawa N, Yoshimura K (1996) Suppression of cell-transferred experimental autoimmune encephalomyelitis in defibrinated Lewis rats. J Neuroimmunol 71:131–137
119. Inoue A, Koh CS, Yamazaki M, Yanagisawa N, Ishihara Y, Kim BS (1997) Fibrin deposition in the central nervous system correlates with the degree of Theiler's murine encephalomyelitis virus-induced demyelinating disease. J Neuroimmunol 77:185–194
120. Inuzuka T, Sato S, McIntyre LJ, Quarles RH (1984) Effects of trypsin and plasmin treatment of myelin on the myelin-associated glycoprotein and basic protein. J Neurochem 43:582–585
121. Ishihara H, Connolly AJ, Zeng D, Kahn ML, Zheng YW, Timmons C, Tram T, Coughlin SR (1997) Protease-activated receptor 3 is a second thrombin receptor in humans. Nature 386:502–506
122. Iwata A, Stys PK, Wolf JA, Chen XH, Taylor AG, Meaney DF, Smith DH (2004) Traumatic axonal injury induces proteolytic cleavage of the voltage-gated sodium channels modulated by tetrodotoxin and protease inhibitors. J Neurosci 24:4605–4613
123. Johnston JB, Zhang K, Silva C, Shalinsky DR, Conant K, Ni W, Corbett D, Yong VW, Power C (2001) HIV-1 Tat neurotoxicity is prevented by matrix metalloproteinase inhibitors. Ann Neurol 49:230–241
124. Junge CE, Lee CJ, Hubbard KB, Ahoabin A, Olson JJ, Hepler JR, Brat DJ, Traynelis SF (2004) Protease-activated receptor-1 in human brain: localization and functional expression in astrocytes. Exp Neurol 1888:94–103
125. Jurewicz A, Matysiak M, Tybor K, Kilianek L, Raine CS, Selmaj K (2005) Tumour necrosis factor-induced death of adult human oligodendrocytes is mediated by apoptosis inducing factor. Brain 128:2675–2688
126. Karabudak R, Kurne A, Guc D, Sengelen M, Canpinar H, Kansu E (2004) Effect of interferon beta-1a on serum matrix metalloproteinase-9 (MMP-9) and tissue inhibitor of matrix metalloproteinase (TIMP-1) in relapsing remitting multiple sclerosis patients. One year follow-up results. J Neurol 251:279–283
127. Kastenbauer S, Koedel U, Wick M, Kieseier BC, Hartung HP, Pfister HW (2003) CSF and serum levels of soluble fractalkine (CX3CL1) in inflammatory diseases of the nervous system. J Neuroimmunol 137:210–217
128. Kawagoe J, Takizawa T, Matsumoto J, Tamiya M, Meek SE, Smith AJ, Hunter GD, Plevin R, Saito N, Kanke T, Fujii M, Wada Y (2002) Effect of protease-activated receptor-2 deficiency on allergic dermatitis in the mouse ear. Jpn J Pharmacol 88:77–84
129. Kermode AG, Thompson AJ, Tofts P, MacManus DG, Kendall BE, Kingsley DP, Moseley IF, Rudge P, McDonald WI (1990) Breakdown of the blood–brain barrier precedes symptoms and other MRI signs of new lesions in multiple sclerosis. Pathogenetic and clinical implications. Brain 113:1477–1489

130. Kieseier BC, Kiefer R, Clements JM, Miller K, Wells GM, Schweitzer T, Gearing AJ, Hartung HP (1998) Matrix metalloproteinase-9 and -7 are regulated in experimental autoimmune encephalomyelitis. Brain 121:159–166
131. Kieseier BC, Pischel H, Neuen-Jacob E, Tourtellotte WW, Hartung HP (2003) ADAM-10 and ADAM-17 in the inflamed human CNS. Glia 42:398–405
132. Klein G, Kullich W, Schnitker J, Schwann H (2006) Efficacy and tolerance of an oral enzyme combination in painful osteoarthritis of the hip. A double-blind, randomised study comparing oral enzymes with non-steroidal anti-inflammatory drugs. Clin Exp Rheumatol 24:25–30
133. Koh CS, Gausas J, Paterson PY (1993) Neurovascular permeability and fibrin deposition in the central neuraxis of Lewis rats with cell-transferred experimental allergic encephalomyelitis in relationship to clinical and histopathological features of the disease. J Neuroimmunol 47:141–145
134. Koli K, Saharinen J, Hyytiainen M, Penttinen C, Keski-Oja J (2001) Latency, activation, and binding proteins of TGF-beta. Microsc Res Tech 52:354–362
135. Krem MM, Di Cera E (2002) Evolution of enzyme cascades from embryonic development to blood coagulation. Trends Biochem Sci 27:67–74
136. Kruger PG (2001) Mast cells and multiple sclerosis: a quantitative analysis. Neuropathol Appl Neurobiol 27:275–280
137. Kruidenier L, MacDonald TT, Collins JE, Pender SL, Sanderson IR (2006) Myofibroblast matrix metalloproteinases activate the neutrophil chemoattractant CXCL7 from intestinal epithelial cells. Gastroenterology 130:127–136
138. Kuida K, Lippke JA, Ku G, Harding MW, Livingston DJ, Su MS, Flavell RA (1995) Altered cytokine export and apoptosis in mice deficient in interleukin-1 beta converting enzyme. Science 267:2000–2003
139. Kwon EE, Prineas JW (1994) Blood-brain barrier abnormalities in longstanding multiple sclerosis lesions. An immunohistochemical study. J Neuropathol Exp Neurol 53:625–636
140. Lacraz S, Nicod L, Galve-de Rochemonteix B, Baumberger C, Dayer JM, Welgus HG (1992) Suppression of metalloproteinase biosynthesis in human alveolar macrophages by interleukin-4. J Clin Invest 90:382–388
141. Ladiwala U, Lachance C, Simoneau SJ, Bhakar A, Barker PA, Antel JP (1998) p75 neurotrophin receptor expression on adult human oligodendrocytes: signaling without cell death in response to NGF. J Neurosci 18:1297–1304
142. Larsen PH, DaSilva AG, Conant K, Yong VW (2006) Myelin formation during development of the CNS is delayed in matrix metalloproteinase-9 and -12 null mice. J Neurosci 26:2207–2214
143. Lauber K, Bohn E, Krober SM, Xiao YJ, Blumenthal SG, Lindemann RK, Marini P, Wiedig C, Zobywalski A, Baksh S, Xu Y, Autenrieth IB, Schulze-Osthoff K, Belka C, Stuhler G, Wesselborg S (2003) Apoptotic cells induce migration of phagocytes via caspase-3-mediated release of a lipid attraction signal. Cell 113:717–730
144. Law MJ, Martenson RE, Deibler GE (1984) Cleavage of rabbit myelin basic protein by thrombin. J Neurochem 42:559–568
145. Lee KR, Drury I, Vitarbo E, Hoff JT (1997) Seizures induced by intracerebral injection of thrombin: a model of intracerebral hemorrhage. J Neurosurg 87:73–78
146. Leppert D, Waubant E, Burk MR, Oksenberg JR, Hauser SL (1996) Interferon beta-1b inhibits gelatinase secretion and in vitro migration of human T cells: a possible mechanism for treatment efficacy in MS. Ann Neurol 40:846–852
147. Lerch MM, Halangk W, Kruger B (2000) The role of cysteine proteases in intracellular pancreatic serine protease activation. Adv Exp Med Biol 477:403–411
148. Li P, Allen H, Banerjee S, Franklin S, Herzog L, Johnston C, McDowell J, Paskind M, Rodman L, Salfeld J et al (1995) Mice deficient in IL-1 beta-converting enzyme are defective in production of mature IL-1 beta and resistant to endotoxic shock. Cell 80:401–411
149. Lijnen HR, Silence J, Lemmens G, Frederix L, Collen D (1998) Regulation of gelatinase activity in mice with targeted inactivation of components of the plasminogen/plasmin system. Thromb Haemost 79:1171–1176

150. Lim SY, Tennant GM, Kennedy S, Wainwright CL, Kane KA (2006) Activation of mouse protease-activated receptor-2 induces lymphocyte adhesion and generation of reactive oxygen species. Br J Pharmacol 149:591–599

151. Lindberg RLP, De Groot CJA, Montagne L, Freitag P, van der Valk P, Kappos L, Leppert D (2001) The expression profile of matrix metalloproteinases (MMPs) and their inhibitors (TIMPs) in lesions and normal appearing white matter of multiple sclerosis. Brain 124:1743–1753

152. Liu Z, Zhou X, Shapiro SD, Shipley JM, Twining SS, Diaz LA, Senior RM, Werb Z (2000) The serpin alpha1-proteinase inhibitor is a critical substrate for gelatinase B/MMP-9 in vivo. Cell 102:647–655

153. Loher F, Bauer C, Landauer N, Schmall K, Siegmund B, Lehr HA, Dauer M, Schoenharting M, Endres S, Eigler A (2004) The interleukin-1 beta-converting enzyme inhibitor pralnacasan reduces dextran sulfate sodium-induced murine colitis and T helper 1 T-cell activation. J Pharmacol Exp Ther 308:583–590

154. Lopez-Otin C, Overall CM (2002) Protease degradomics: a new challenge for proteomics. Nat Rev Mol Cell Biol 3:509–519

155. Lu W, Bhasin M, Tsirka SE (2002) Involvement of tissue plasminogen activator in onset and effector phases of experimental allergic encephalomyelitis. J Neurosci 22:10781–10789

156. Lucchinetti C, Bruck W, Parisi J, Scheithauer B, Rodriguez M, Lassmann H (2000) Heterogeneity of multiple sclerosis lesions: implications for the pathogenesis of demyelination. Ann Neurol 47:707–717

157. Luo LY, Jiang W (2006) Inhibition profiles of human tissue kallikreins by serine protease inhibitors. Biol Chem 387:813–816

158. Ma J, Tanaka KF, Yamada G, Ikenaka K (2006) Induced expression of cathepsins and cystatin C in a murine model of demyelination. Neurochem Res 32:311–320

159. Macfelda K, Weiss TW, Kaun C, Breuss JM, Zorn G, Oberndorfer U, Voegele-Kadletz M, Huber-Beckmann R, Ullrich R, Binder BR, Losert UM, Maurer G, Pacher R, Huber K, Wojta J (2002) Plasminogen activator inhibitor 1 expression is regulated by the inflammatory mediators interleukin-1alpha, tumor necrosis factor-alpha, transforming growth factor-beta and oncostatin M in human cardiac myocytes. J Mol Cell Cardiol 34:1681–1691

160. Maciejewski-Lenoir D, Chen S, Feng L, Maki R, Bacon KB (1999) Characterization of fractalkine in rat brain cells: migratory and activation signals for CX3CR-1-expressing microglia. J Immunol 163:1628–1635

161. Madri JA, Graesser D, Haas T (1996) The roles of adhesion molecules and proteinases in lymphocyte transendothelial migration. Biochem Cell Biol 74:749–757

162. Maeda A, Sobel RA (1996) Matrix metalloproteinases in the normal human central nervous system, microglia nodules, and multiple sclerosis lesions. J Neuropathol Exp Neurol 55:300–309

163. Malamud V, Vaaknin A, Abramsky O, Mor M, Burgess LE, Ben-Yehudah A, Lorberboum-Galski H (2003) Tryptase activates peripheral blood mononuclear cells causing synthesis and release of TNF-a, IL-6 and IL-1B: possible relevance to multiple sclerosis. J Neuroimmunology 138:115–122

164. Mandler RN, Dencoff JD, Midani F, Ford CC, Ahmed W, Rosenberg GA (2001) Matrix metalloproteinases and tissue inhibitors of metalloproteinases in cerebrospinal fluid differ in multiple sclerosis and Devic's neuromyelitis optica. Brain 124:493–498

165. Manhart N, Akomeah R, Bergmeister H, Spittler A, Ploner M, Roth E (2002) Administration of proteolytic enzymes bromelain and trypsin diminish the number of CD4+ cells and the interferon-gamma response in Peyer's patches and spleen in endotoxemic balb/c mice. Cell Immunol 215:113–119

166. Marks N, Grynbaum A, Levine S (1977) Proteolytic enzymes in ordinary, hyperacute, monocytic and passive transfer forms of experimental allergic encephalomyelitis. Brain Res 123:147–157

167. Martinon F, Tschopp J (2007) Inflammatory caspases and inflammasomes: master switches of inflammation. Cell Death Differ 14:10–22

168. Mason JL, Suzuki K, Chaplin DD, Matsushima GK (2001) Interleukin-1beta promotes repair of the CNS. J Neurosci 21:7046–7052

169. McCawley LJ, Matrisian LM (2001) Matrix metalloproteinases: they're not just for matrix anymore! Curr Opin Cell Biol 13:534–540

170. McQuibban GA, Butler GS, Gong JH, Bendall L, Power C, Clark-Lewis I, Overall CM (2001) Matrix metalloproteinase activity inactivates the CXC chemokine stromal cell-derived factor-1. J Biol Chem 276:43503–43508

171. McQuibban GA, Gong JH, Wong JP, Wallace JL, Clark-Lewis I, Overall CM (2002) Matrix metalloproteinase processing of monocyte chemoattractant proteins generates CC chemokine receptor antagonists with anti-inflammatory properties in vivo. Blood 100:1160–1167

172. Mead RJ, Singhrao SK, Neal JW, Lassmann H, Morgan BP (2002) The membrane attack complex of complement causes severe demyelination associated with acute axonal injury. J Immunol 168:458–465

173. Ming X, Li W, Maeda Y, Blumberg B, Raval S, Cook SD, Dowling PC (2002) Caspase-1 expression in multiple sclerosis plaques and cultured glial cells. J Neurol Sci 197:9–18

174. Mitsui S, Okui A, Uemura H, Mizuno T, Yamada T, Yamamura Y, Yamaguchi N (2002) Decreased cerebrospinal fluid levels of neurosin (KLK6), an aging-related protease, as a possible new risk factor for Alzheimer's disease. Ann NY Acad Sci 977:216–223

175. Moscarello MA, Mastronardi FG, Wood DD (2006) The role of citrullinated proteins suggests a novel mechanism in the pathogenesis of multiple sclerosis. Neurochem Res 32:251–256

176. Murray PD, McGavern DB, Lin X, Njenga MK, Leibowitz J, Pease LR, Rodriguez M (1998) Perforin-dependent neurologic injury in a viral model of multiple sclerosis. J Neurosci 18:7306–7314

177. Musse AA, Boggs JM, Harauz G (2006) Deimination of membrane-bound myelin basic protein in multiple sclerosis exposes an immunodominant epitope. Proc Natl Acad Sci USA 103:4422–4427

178. Nadiri A, Wolinski MK, Saleh M (2006) The inflammatory caspases: key players in the host response to pathogenic invasion and sepsis. J Immunol 177:4239–4245

179. Nagai A, Terashima M, Harada T, Shimode K, Takeuchi H, Murakawa Y, Nagasaki M, Nakano A, Kobayashi S (2003) Cathepsin B and H activities and cystatin C concentrations in cerebrospinal fluid from patients with leptomeningeal metastasis. Clin Chim Acta 329:53–60

180. Nagano O, Murakami D, Hartmann D, De Strooper B, Saftig P, Iwatsubo T, Nakajima M, Shinohara M, Saya H (2004) Cell-matrix interaction via CD44 is independently regulated by different metalloproteinases activated in response to extracellular Ca(2+) influx and PKC activation. J Cell Biol 165:893–902

181. Nagase H, Woessner JF Jr (1999) Matrix metalloproteinases. J Biol Chem 274:21491–1494

182. Nakagawa TY, Brissette WH, Lira PD, Griffiths RJ, Petrushova N, Stock J, McNeish JD, Eastman SE, Howard ED, Clarke SR, Rosloniec EF, Elliott EA, Rudensky AY (1999) Impaired invariant chain degradation and antigen presentation and diminished collagen-induced arthritis in cathepsin S null mice. Immunity 10:207–217

183. Nam RK, Diamandis EP, Toi A, Trachtenberg J, Magklara A, Scorilas A, Papnastasiou PA, Jewett MA, Narod SA (2000) Serum human glandular kallikrein-2 protease levels predict the presence of prostate cancer among men with elevated prostate-specific antigen. J Clin Oncol 18:1036–1042

184. Nauta AJ, Daha MR, Tijsma O, van de Water B, Tedesco F, Roos A (2002) The membrane attack complex of complement induces caspase activation and apoptosis. Eur J Immunol 32:783–792

185. Neuhaus O, Strasser-Fuchs S, Fazekas F, Kieseier BC, Niederwieser G, Hartung HP, Archelos JJ (2002) Statins as immunomodulators: comparison with interferon-beta 1b in MS. Neurology 59:990–997

186. Neumann H (2003) Molecular mechanisms of axonal damage in inflammatory central nervous system diseases. Curr Opin Neurol 16:267–273

187. Newman TA, Woolley ST, Hughes PM, Sibson NR, Anthony DC, Perry VH (2001) T-cell- and macrophage-mediated axon damage in the absence of a CNS-specific immune response: involvement of metalloproteinases. Brain 124:2203–214

188. Nicholson DW (1999) Caspase structure, proteolytic substrates, and function during apoptotic cell death. Cell Death Differ 6:1028–1042

189. Niclou SP, Suidan HS, Pavlik A, Vejsada R, Monard D (1998) Changes in the expression of protease-activated receptor 1 and protease nexin-1 mRNA during rat nervous system development and after nerve lesion. Eur J Neurosci 10:1590–1607

190. Niculescu T, Weerth S, Niculescu F, Cudrici C, Rus V, Raine CS, Shin ML, Rus H (2004) Effects of complement C5 on apoptosis in experimental autoimmune encephalomyelitis. J Immunol 172:5702–5706

191. Noorbakhsh F, Tsutsui S, Vergnolle N, Boven LA, Shariat N, Vodjgani M, Warren KG, Andrade-Gordon P, Hollenberg MD, Power C (2006) Proteinase-activated receptor 2 modulates neuroinflammation in experimental autoimmune encephalomyelitis and multiple sclerosis. J Exp Med 203:425–435

192. Norga K, Paemen L, Masure S, Dillen C, Heremans H, Billiau A, Carton H, Cuzner L, Olsson T, Van Damme J, Opdenakker G (1995) Prevention of acute autoimmune encephalomyelitis and abrogation of relapses in murine models of multiple sclerosis by the protease inhibitor D-penicillamine. Inflammation Res 44:529–534

193. Norton WT, Cammer W, Bloom BR, Gordon S (1978) Neutral proteinases secreted by macrophages degrade basic protein: a possible mechanism of inflammatory demyelination. Adv Exp Med Biol 100:365–381

194. Nygardas PT, Hinkkanen AE (2002) Up-regulation of MMP-8 and MMP-9 activity in the BALB/c mouse spinal cord correlates with the severity of experimental autoimmune encephalomyelitis. Clin Exp Immunol 128:245–254

195. Ogata Y, Enghild JJ, Nagase H (1992) Matrix metalloproteinase 3 (stromelysin) activates the precursor for the human matrix metalloproteinase 9. J Biol Chem 267:3581–3584

196. Oikonomopoulou K, Hansen KK, Saifeddine M, Tea I, Blaber M, Blaber SI, Scarisbrick I, Andrade-Gordone P, Cottrellf GS, Bunnett NW, Diamandis EP, Hollenberg MD (2006) Proteinase-activated receptors (PARs): Targets for kallikrein signalling. J Biol Chem 281:32095–32112

197. Opdenakker G, Dillen C, Fiten P, Martens E, Van Aelst I, Van den Steen PE, Nelissen I, Starckx S, Descamps FJ, Hu J, Piccard H, Van Damme J, Wormald MR, Rudd PM, Dwek RA (2006) Remnant epitopes, autoimmunity and glycosylation. Biochim Biophys Acta 1760:610–615

198. Overall CM, Kleifeld O (2006) Towards third generation matrix metalloproteinase inhibitors for cancer therapy. Br J Cancer 94:941–946

199. Paczek L, Kropiewnicka EH, Bartlomiejczyk I, Gradowska L, Heidland A, Wood G (2000) Systemic proteolytic enzyme treatment diminishes urinary interleukin 6 in diabetic patients. Nephron 84:194–195

200. Paemen L, Olsson T, Soderstron M, Damme JV, Openakker G (1994) Evaluation of gelatinases and IL-6 in the cerebrospinal fluid of patients with optic neuritis, multiple sclerosis and other inflammatory neurological diseases. Eur J Neurosci 1:55–63

201. Pagenstecher A, Stalder AK, Kincaid CL, Shapiro SD, Campbell IL (1998) Differential expression of matrix metalloproteinase and tissue inhibitor of matrix metalloproteinase genes in the mouse central nervous system in normal and inflammatory states. Am J Pathol 152:729–741

202. Palombella VJ, Conner EM, Fuseler JW, Destree A, Davis JM, Laroux FS, Wolf RE, Huang J, Brand S, Elliott PJ, Lazarus D, McCormack T, Parent L, Stein R, Adams J, Grisham MB (1998) Role of the proteasome and NF-kappaB in streptococcal cell wall-induced polyarthritis. Proc Natl Acad Sci USA 95:15671–15676

203. Parathath SR, Parathath S, Tsirka SE (2006) Nitric oxide mediates neurodegeneration and breakdown of the blood-brain barrier in tPA-dependent excitotoxic injury in mice. J Cell Sci 119:339–349

204. Paterson PY (1976) Experimental allergic encephalomyelitis: role of fibrin deposition in immunopathogenesis of inflammation in rats. Fed Proc 35:2428–2434

205. Perraud F, Besnard F, Sensenbrenner M, Labourdette G (1987) Thrombin is a potent mitogen for rat astroblasts but not for oligodendroblasts and neuroblasts in primary culture. Int J Dev Neurosci 5:181–188

206. Peterson JW, Bo L, Mork S, Chang A, Trapp BD (2001) Transected neurites, apoptotic neurons, and reduced inflammation in cortical multiple sclerosis lesions. Ann Neurol 50:389–400

207. Phillips JB, Williams AJ, Adams J, Elliott PJ, Tortella FC (2000) Proteasome inhibitor PS519 reduces infarction and attenuates leukocyte infiltration in a rat model of focal cerebral ischemia. Stroke 31:1686–1693

208. Pike CJ, Vaughan PJ, Cunningham DD, Cotman CW (1996) Thrombin attenuates neuronal cell death and modulates astrocyte reactivity induced by beta-amyloid in vitro. J Neurochem 66:1374–1382

209. Pritzker LB, Joshi S, Gowan JJ, Harauz G, Moscarello MA (2000) Deimination of myelin basic protein. 1. Effect of deimination of arginyl residues of myelin basic protein on its structure and susceptibility to digestion by cathepsin D. Biochemistry 39:5374–5381

210. Proost P, Van Damme J, Opdenakker G (1993) Leukocyte gelatinase B cleavage releases encephalitogens from human myelin basic protein. Biochem Biophys Res Comm 192:1175–1781

211. Proost P, Struyf S, Schols D, Durinx C, Wuyts A, Lenaerts JP, De Clercq E, De Meester I, Van Damme J (1998) Processing by CD26/dipeptidyl-peptidase IV reduces the chemotactic and anti-HIV-1 activity of stromal-cell-derived factor-1alpha. FEBS Lett 432:73–76

212. Proost P, Schutyser E, Menten P, Struyf S, Wuyts A, Opdenakker G, Detheux M, Parmentier M, Durinx C, Lambeir AM, Neyts J, Liekens S, Maudgal PC, Billiau A, Van Damme J (2001) Amino-terminal truncation of CXCR3 agonists impairs receptor signaling and lymphocyte chemotaxis, while preserving antiangiogenic properties. Blood 98:3554–3561

213. Puente SS, Sanchez LM, Overall CM, Lopez-Otin C (2003) Human and mouse proteases: a comparative genomic approach. Nat Rev Genet 4:544–558

214. Ramwani JJ, Epand RM, Moscarello MA (1989) Secondary structure of charge isomers of myelin basic protein before and after phosphorylation. Biochemistry 28:6538–6543

215. Rao RM, Betz TV, Lamont DJ, Kim MB, Shaw SK, Froio RM, Baleux F, Arenzana-Seisdedos F, Alon R, Luscinskas FW (2004) Elastase release by transmigrating neutrophils deactivates endothelial-bound SDF-1alpha and attenuates subsequent T lymphocyte transendothelial migration. J Exp Med 200:713–724

216. Richter R, Bistrian R, Escher S, Forssmann WG, Vakili J, Henschler R, Spodsberg N, Frimpong-Boateng A, Forssmann U (2005) Quantum proteolytic activation of chemokine CCL15 by neutrophil granulocytes modulates mononuclear cell adhesiveness. J Immunol 175:1599–1608

217. Riese RJ, Mitchell RN, Villadangos JA, Shi GP, Palmer JT, Karp ER, De Sanctis GT, Ploegh HL, Chapman HA (1998) Cathepsin S activity regulates antigen presentation and immunity. J Clin Invest 101:2351–2363

218. Rivera S, Tremblay E, Timsit S, Canals O, Ben-Ari Y, Khrestchatisky M (1997) Tissue inhibitor of metalloproteinases-1 (TIMP-1) is differentially induced in neurons and astrocytes after seizures: evidence for developmental, immediate early gene, and lesion response. J Neurosci 17:4223–4235

219. Rosenberg GA, Estrada EY, Dencoff JE, Stetler-Stevenson WG (1995) TNF-alpha-induced gelatinase beta causes delayed opening of the blood–brain barrier: an expanded therapeutic window. Brain Res 703:151–155

220. Rosenberg GA, Dencoff JE, Correa NJ, Reiners M, Ford CC (1996) Effect of steroids on CSF matrix metalloproteinases in multiple sclerosis: relation to blood–brain barrier injury. Neurology 46:1626–1632

221. Rosenberg GA, Estrada EY, Mobashery S (2007) Effect of synthetic matrix metalloproteinase inhibitors on lipopolysaccharide-induced blood–brain barrier opening in rodents: Differences in response based on strains and solvents. Brain Res 1133:186–192

222. Rozniecki JJ, Hauser SL, Stein M, Lincoln R, Theoharides TC (1995) Elevated mast cell tryptase in cerebrospinal fluid of multiple sclerosis patients. Ann Neurol 37:63–66

223. Rudolphi K, Gerwin N, Verzijl N, van der Kraan P, van den Berg W (2003) Pralnacasan, an inhibitor of interleukin-1beta converting enzyme, reduces joint damage in two murine models of osteoarthritis. Osteoarthritis Cartilage 11:738–746

224. Rus H, Cudrici C, Niculescu F (2006) C5b-9 complement complex in autoimmune demyelination: dual role in neuroinflammation and neuroprotection. Adv Exp Med Biol 586:139–151

225. Saatman KE, Abai B, Grosvenor A, Vorwerk CK, Smith DH, Meaney DF (2003) Traumatic axonal injury results in biphasic calpain activation and retrograde transport impairment in mice. J Cereb Blood Flow Metab 23:34–42

226. Saleh M, Vaillancourt JP, Graham RK, Huyck M, Srinivasula SM, Alnemri ES, Steinberg MH, Nolan V, Baldwin CT, Hotchkiss RS, Buchman TG, Zehnbauer BA, Hayden MR, Farrer LA, Roy S, Nicholson DW (2004) Differential modulation of endotoxin responsiveness by human caspase-12 polymorphisms. Nature 429:75–79

227. Salmena L, Lemmers B, Hakem A, Matysiak-Zablocki E, Murakami K, Au PY, Berry DM, Tamblyn L, Shehabeldin A, Migon E, Wakeham A, Bouchard D, Yeh WC, McGlade JC, Ohashi PS, Hakem R (2003) Essential role for caspase 8 in T-cell homeostasis and T-cell-mediated immunity. Genes Dev 17:883–895

228. Sanz MJ, Hickey MJ, Johnston B, McCafferty DM, Raharjo E, Huang PL, Kubes P (2001) Neuronal nitric oxide synthase (NOS) regulates leukocyte-endothelial cell interactions in endothelial NOS deficient mice. Br J Pharmacol 134:305–312

229. Scarisbrick IA, Blaber SI, Lucchinetti CF, Genain CP, Blaber M, Rodriguez M (2002) Activity of a newly identified serine protease in CNS demyelination. Brain 125:1283–1296

230. Scarisbrick IA, Blaber SI, Tingling JT, Rodriguez M, Blaber M, Christophi GP (2006) Potential scope of action of tissue kallikreins in CNS immune-mediated disease. J Neuroimmunology 178: 167–176

231. Schaecher K, Rocchini A, Dinkins J, Matzelle DD, Banik NL (2002) Calpain expression and infiltration of activated T cells in experimental allergic encephalomyelitis over time: increased calpain activity begins with onset of disease. J Neuroimmunol 129:1–9

232. Schiemann F, Grimm TA, Hoch J, Gross R, Lindner B, Petersen F, Bulfone-Paus S, Brandt E (2006) Mast cells and neutrophils proteolytically activate chemokine precursor CTAP-III and are subject to counterregulation by PF-4 through inhibition of chymase and cathepsin G. Blood 107:2234–2242

233. Schmitz J, Owyang A, Oldham E, Song Y, Murphy E, McClanahan TK, Zurawski G, Moshrefi M, Qin J, Li X, Gorman DM, Bazan JF, Kastelein RA (2005) IL-33, an interleukin-1-like cytokine that signals via the IL-1 receptor-related protein ST2 and induces T helper type 2-associated cytokines. Immunity 23:479–490

234. Schonbeck U, Mach F, Libby P (1998) Generation of biologically active IL-1 beta by matrix metalloproteinases: a novel caspase-1-independent pathway of IL-1 beta processing. J Immunol 161:3340–3346

235. Secor VH, Secor WE, Gutekunst CA, Brown MA (2000) Mast cells are essential for early onset and severe disease in a murine model of multiple sclerosis. J Exp Med 191:813–822

236. Seeds NW, Williams BL, Bickford PC (1995) Tissue plasminogen activator induction in Purkinje neurons after cerebellar motor learning. Science 270:1992–1994

237. Seguin R, Biernacki K, Rotondo RL, Prat A, Antel JP (2003) Regulation and functional effects of monocyte migration across human brain-derived endothelial cells. J Neuropathol Exp Neurol 62:412–419

238. Seidel B, Keilhoff G, Reinheckel T, Wolf G (1998) Differentially expressed genes in hippocampal cell cultures in response to an excitotoxic insult by quinolinic acid. Brain Res Mol Brain Res 60:296–300

239. Seifert T, Kieseier BC, Ropele S, Strasser-Fuchs S, Quehenberger F, Fazekas F, Hartung HP (2002) TACE mRNA expression in peripheral mononuclear cells precedes new lesions on MRI in multiple sclerosis. Mult Scler 8:447–451

240. Sharma V, Delgado M, Ganea D (2006) VIP protects Th2 cells by downregulating granzyme B expression. Ann N Y Acad Sci 1070:540–544

241. Shields DC, Banik NL (1998) Upregulation of calpain activity and expression in experimental allergic encephalomyelitis: a putative role for calpain in demyelination. Brain Res 794:68–74

242. Shields DC, Schaecher KE, Saido TC, Banik NL (1999) A putative mechanism of demyelination in multiple sclerosis by a proteolytic enzyme, calpain. Proc Natl Acad Sci USA 96:11486–11491

243. Shipley JM, Wesselschmidt RL, Kobayashi DK, Ley TJ, Shapiro SD (1996) Metalloelastase is required for macrophage-mediated proteolysis and matrix invasion in mice. Proc Natl Acad Sci U S A 93:3942–3946

244. Siegel RM, Chan FK, Chun HJ, Lenardo MJ (2000) The multifaceted role of Fas signaling in immune cell homeostasis and autoimmunity. Nat Immunol 1:469–474

245. Siger-Zajdel M, Selmaj K (2001) Magnetisation transfer ratio analysis of normal appearing white matter in patients with familial and sporadic multiple sclerosis. J Neurol Neurosurg Psychiatry 71:752–756

246. Sim RB, Tsiftsoglou SA (2004) Proteases of the complement system. Biochem Soc Trans 32:21–27

247. Smalley DM, Ley K (2005) L-selectin: mechanisms and physiological significance of ecto-domain cleavage. J Cell Mol Med 9:255–266

248. Smith ME, van der Maesen K, Somera FP (1998) Macrophage and microglial responses to cytokines in vitro: phagocytic activity, proteolytic enzyme release, and free radical production. J Neurosci Res 54:68–78

249. Soane L, Cho HJ, Niculescu F, Rus H, Shin ML (2001) C5b-9 terminal complement complex protects oligodendrocytes from death by regulating Bad through phosphatidylinositol 3-kinase/Akt pathway. J Immunol 167:2305–2311

250. Stack JH, Beaumont K, Larsen PD, Straley KS, Henkel GW, Randle JC, Hoffman HM (2005) IL-converting enzyme/caspase-1 inhibitor VX-765 blocks the hypersensitive response to an inflammatory stimulus in monocytes from familial cold autoinflammatory syndrome patients. J Immunol 175:2630–2634

251. Starckx S, Van den Steen PE, Verbeek R, van Noort JM, Opdenakker G (2003) A novel rationale for inhibition of gelatinase B in multiple sclerosis: MMP-9 destroys alpha B-crystallin and generates a promiscuous T cell epitope. J Neuroimmunol 141:47–57

252. Sternlicht MD, Werb Z (2001) How matrix metalloproteinases regulate cell behavior. Annu Rev Cell Dev Biol 17:463–516

253. Storch MK, Stefferl A, Brehm U, Weissert R, Wallstrom E, Kerschensteiner M, Olsson T, Linington C, Lassmann H (1998) Autoimmunity to myelin oligodendrocyte glycoprotein in rats mimics the spectrum of multiple sclerosis pathology. Brain Pathol 8:681–694

254. Strukova SM (2001) Thrombin as a regulator of inflammation and reparative processes in tissues. Biochemistry (Mosc) 66:8–18

255. Struyf S, Schutyser E, Gouwy M, Gijsbers K, Proost P, Benoit Y, Opdenakker G, Van Damme J, Laureys G (2003) PARC/CCL18 is a plasma CC chemokine with increased levels in childhood acute lymphoblastic leukemia. Am J Pathol 163:2065–2075

256. Stuve O, Dooley NP, Uhm JH, Antel JP, Francis GS, Williams G, Yong VW (1996) Interferon beta-1b decreases the migration of T lymphocytes in vitro: effects on matrix metalloproteinase-9. Ann Neurol 40:853–863

257. Tan HK, Heywood D, Ralph GS, Bienemann A, Baker AH, Uney JB (2003) Tissue inhibitor of metalloproteinase 1 inhibits excitotoxic cell death in neurons. Mol Cell Neurosci 22:98–106

258. Targoni OS, Tary-Lehmann M, Lehmann PV (1999) Prevention of murine EAE by oral hydrolytic enzyme treatment. J Autoimmun 12:191–198

259. Tarui T, Mazar AP, Cines DB, Takada Y (2001) Urokinase-type plasminogen activator receptor (CD87) is a ligand for integrins and mediates cell–cell interaction. J Biol Chem 276:3983–3990

260. Tedgui A, Mallat Z (2006) Cytokines in atherosclerosis: pathogenic and regulatory pathways. Physiol Rev 86:515–581

261. Teesalu T, Hinkkanen AE, Vaheri A (2001) Coordinated induction of extracellular proteolysis systems during experimental autoimmune encephalomyelitis in mice. Am J Pathol 159:2227–2237

262. Terayama R, Bando Y, Yamada M, Yoshida S (2005) Involvement of neuropsin in the pathogenesis of experimental autoimmune encephalomyelits. Glia 52:108–118

263. Thornberry NA, Bull HG, Calaycay JR, Chapman KT, Howard AD, Kostura MJ, Miller DK, Molineaux SM, Weidner JR, Aunins J et al (1992) A novel heterodimeric cysteine protease is required for interleukin-1 beta processing in monocytes. Nature 356:768–774

264. Tocco G, Musleh W, Sakhi S, Schreiber SS, Baudry M, Pasinetti GM (1997) Complement and glutamate neurotoxicity. Genotypic influences of C5 in a mouse model of hippocampal neurodegeneration. Mol Chem Neuropathol 31:289–300

265. Toft-Hansen H, Nuttall RK, Edwards DR, Owens T (2004) Key metalloproteinases are expressed by specific cell types in experimental autoimmune encephalomyelitis. J Immunol 173:5209–5218

266. Trapp BD, Peterson J, Ransohoff RM, Rudick R, Mork S, Bo L (1998) Axonal transection in the lesions of multiple sclerosis. N Engl J Med 338:278–285

267. Trojano M, Avolio C, Liuzzi GM, Ruggieri M, Defazio G, Liguori M, Santacroce MP, Paolicelli D, Giuliani F, Riccio P, Livrea P (1999) Changes of serum ICAM-1 and MMP-9 induced by IFNbeta-1b treatment in relapsing-remitting MS. Neurology 153:1402–1408

268. Tsirka SE, Gualandris A, Amaral DG, Strickland S (1995) Excitotoxin-induced neuronal degeneration and seizure are mediated by tissue plasminogen activator. Nature 377:340–344

269. Tsirka SE, Bugge TH, Degen JL, Strickland S (1997) Neuronal death in the central nervous system demonstrates a non-fibrin substrate for plasmin. Proc Natl Acad Sci USA 94:9779–9781

270. Tsirka SE, Rogove AD, Bugge TH, Degan JL, Strickland S (1997) An extracellular proteolytic cascade promotes neuronal degeneration in the mouse hippocampus. J Neurosci 15:543–552

271. Tsubata T, Takahashi K (1989) Limited proteolysis of bovine myelin basic protein by calcium-dependent proteinase from bovine spinal cord. J Biochem (Tokyo) 105:23–28

272. Uchida A, Oka Y, Aoyama M, Suzukim S, Yokoi T, Katano H, Mase M, Tada T, Asai K, Yamada K (2004) Expression of myelencephalon-specific protease in transient middle cerebral artery occlusion model of rat brain. Mol Brain Res 126:129–136

273. Ulrich R, Baumgartner W, Gerhauser I, Seeliger F, Haist V, Deschl U, Alldinger S (2006) MMP-12, MMP-3, and TIMP-1 are markedly upregulated in chronic demyelinating Theiler murine encephalomyelitis. J Neuropath Exp Neurol 65:783–793

274. Vakili J, Standker L, Detheux M, Vassart G, Forssmann WG, Parmentier M (2001) Urokinase plasminogen activator and plasmin efficiently convert hemofiltrate CC chemokine 1 into its active. J Immunol 167:3406–3413

275. Van den Steen PE, Husson SJ, Proost P, Van Damme J, Opdenakker G (2003) Carboxyterminal cleavage of the chemokines MIG and IP-10 by gelatinase B and neutrophil collagenase. Biochem Biophys Res Commun 310:889–896

276. Van Den Steen PE, Wuyts A, Husson SJ, Proost P, Van Damme J, Opdenakker G (2003) Gelatinase B/MMP-9 and neutrophil collagenase/MMP-8 process the chemokines human GCP-2/CXCL6, ENA-78/CXCL5 and mouse GCP-2/LIX and modulate their physiological activities. Eur J Biochem 270:3739–3749

277. van Noort JM, van Sechel AC, Bajramovic JJ, el Ouagmiri M, Polman CH, Lassmann H, Ravid R (1995) The small heat-shock protein alpha B-crystallin as candidate autoantigen in multiple sclerosis. Nature 375:798–801

278. Vanderlugt CL, Rahbe SM, Elliott PJ, Dal Canto MC, Miller SD (2000) Treatment of established relapsing experimental autoimmune encephalomyelitis with the proteasome inhibitor PS-519. J Autoimmun 14:205–211.

279. Vergelli M, Hemmer B, Muraro PA, Tranquill L, Biddison WE, Sarin A, McFarland HF, Martin R (1997) Human autoreactive CD4+ T cell clones use perforin- or Fas/Fas ligand-mediated pathways for target cell lysis. J Immunol 158:2756–2761

280. Vergnolle N, Wallace JL, Bunnett NW, Hollenberg MD (2001) Protease-activated receptors in inflammation, neuronal signaling and pain. Trends Pharmacol Sci 22:146–152

281. Vos CM, van Haastert ES, de Groot CJ, van der Valk P, de Vries HE (2003) Matrix metalloproteinase-12 is expressed in phagocytotic macrophages in active multiple sclerosis lesions. J Neuroimmunol 138:106–114

282. Wakefield AJ, More LJ, Difford J, McLaughlin JE (1994) Immunohistochemical study of vascular injury in acute multiple sclerosis. J Clin Pathol 47:129–133
283. Waltz DA, Natkin LR, Fujita RM, Wei Y, Chapman HA (1997) Plasmin and plasminogen activator inhibitor type 1 promote cellular motility by regulating the interaction between the urokinase receptor and vitronectin. J Clin Invest 100:58–67
284. Wang T, Allie R, Conant K, Haughey N, Turchan-Chelowo J, Hahn K, Rosen A, Steiner J, Keswani S, Jones M, Calabresi PA, Nath A (2006) Granzyme B mediates neurotoxicity through a G-protein-coupled receptor. FASEB J 20:1209–1211
285. Ward PA (1967) A plasmin-split fragment of C'3 as a new chemotactic factor. J Exp Med 126:189–206
286. Waubant E, Goodkin DE, Gee L, Bacchetti P, Sloan R, Stewart T, Andersson P-B, Stabler G, Miller K (1999) Serum MMP-9 and TIMP-1 levels are related to MRI activity in relapsing multiple sclerosis. Neurolology 53:1397–1401
287. Waubant E, Goodkin D, Bostrom A, Bacchetti P, Hietpas J, Lindberg R, Leppert D (2003) IFNbeta lowers MMP-9/TIMP-1 ratio, which predicts new enhancing lesions in patients with SPMS. Neurology 60:52–57
288. Weaver A, Goncalves da Silva A, Nuttall RK, Edwards DR, Shapiro SD, Rivest S, Yong VW (2005) An elevated matrix metalloproteinase (MMP) in an animal model of multiple sclerosis is protective by affecting Th1/Th2 polarization. FASEB J 19:1668–1670
289. Weinstein JR, Gold SJ, Cunningham DD, Gall CM (1995) Cellular localization of thrombin receptor mRNA in rat brain: expression by mesencephalic dopaminergic neurons and codistribution with prothrombin mRNA. J Neurosci 15:2906–2919
290. Wiedow O, Meyer-Hoffert U (2005) Neutrophil serine proteases: potential key regulators of cell signalling during inflammation. J Intern Med 257:319–328
291. Williams KR, Williams ND, Konigsberg W, Yu RK (1986) Acidic lipids enhance cathepsin D cleavage of the myelin basic protein. J Neurosci Res 15:137–145
292. Wood DD, Bilbao JM, O'Connors P, Moscarello MA (1996) Acute multiple sclerosis (Marburg type) is associated with developmentally immature myelin basic protein. Ann Neurol 40:18–24
293. Xia M, Leppert D, Hauser SL, Sreedharan SP, Nelson PJ, Krensky AM, Goetzl EJ (1996) Stimulus specificity of matrix metalloproteinase dependence of human T cell migration through a model basement membrane. J Immunol 156:160–167
294. Xue M, Del Bigio MR (2001) Acute tissue damage after injections of thrombin and plasmin into rat striatum. Stroke 32:2164–2169
295. Xue M, Hollenberg MD, Yong VW (2006) Combination of thrombin and matrix metalloproteinase-9 exacerbates neurotoxicity in cell culture and intracerebral hemorrhage in mice. J Neurosci 26:10281–10291
296. Yang YH, Hall P, Little CB, Fosang AJ, Milenkovski G, Santos L, Xue J, Tipping P, Morand EF (2005) Reduction of arthritis severity in protease-activated receptor-deficient mice. Arthritis Rheum 52:1325–1332
297. Yepes M, Sandkvist M, Wong MK, Coleman TA, Smith E, Cohan SL, Lawrence DA (2000) Neuroserpin reduces cerebral infarct volume and protects neurons from ischemia-induced apoptosis. Blood 96:569–776
298. Yong VW (2005) Metalloproteinases: mediators of pathology and regeneration in the CNS. Nat Rev Neurosci 6:931–944
299. Yushchenko M, Mader M, Elitok E, Bitsch A, Dressel A, Tumani H, Bogumil T, Kitze B, Poser S, Weber F (2003) Interferon-beta-1 b decreased matrix metalloproteinase-9 serum levels in primary progressive multiple sclerosis. J Neurol 250:1224–1228
300. Zabel BA, Zuniga L, Ohyama T, Allen SJ, Cichy J, Handel TM, Butcher EC (2006) Chemoattractants, extracellular proteases, and the integrated host defense response. Exp Hematol 34:1021–1032
301. Zajicek JP, Wing M, Scolding NJ, Compston DA (1992) Interactions between oligodendrocytes and microglia. A major role for complement and tumour necrosis factor in oligodendrocyte adherence and killing. Brain 115:1611–1631

302. Zarghooni M, Soosaipillai A, Grass L, Scorilas A, Mirazimi N, Diamandis EP (2002) Decreased concentration of human kallikrein 6 in brain extracts of Alzheimer's disease patients. Clin Biochem 35:225–231
303. Zeine R, Pon R, Ladiwala U, Antel JP, Filion LG, Freedman MS (1998) Mechanism of gammadelta T cell-induced human oligodendrocyte cytotoxicity: relevance to multiple sclerosis. J Neuroimmunol 87:49–61
304. Zhang WH, Wang X, Narayanan M, Zhang Y, Huo C, Reed JC, Friedlander RM (2003) Fundamental role of the Rip2/caspase-1 pathway in hypoxia and ischemia-induced neuronal cell death. Proc Natl Acad Sci USA 100:16012–16017

# Genetic Analysis of CNS Remyelination

A.J. Bieber

**Abstract** Myelin repair (remyelination) following the demyelination of central nervous system (CNS) axons in diseases such as multiple sclerosis plays a critical role in determining the level of accompanying neurologic disability. While remyelination can be quite robust, in multiple sclerosis it often fails. Understanding and stimulating the remyelination process are therefore important goals in MS research. Remyelination is a complex cellular process that involves an intimate interplay between the myelin-producing cells of the CNS (oligodendrocytes), the axons to be myelinated, as well as CNS-infiltrating immune cells. Genetic analysis can be a powerful tool for the functional analysis of complex cellular processes and has recently been applied to the problem of remyelination failure during disease. This chapter reviews the recent use of genetic approaches for the study of CNS remyelination in mouse models of demyelinating disease.

A.J. Bieber

Department of Neurology, Mayo Clinic College of Medicine, 200 First Street SW, Rochester, MN 55905, USA

e-mail: bieber.allan@mayo.edu

M. Rodriguez (ed.), *Advances in Multiple Sclerosis and Experimental Demyelinating Diseases. Current Topics in Microbiology and Immunology 318.*
© Springer-Verlag Berlin Heidelberg 2008

# 1  Introduction

Human multiple sclerosis (MS) is a complex disease with a multifaceted etiology and heterogeneous pathology. Demyelinated central nervous system (CNS) lesions are the pathologic hallmark of MS and are accompanied by varying degrees of inflammation, reactive gliosis, oligodendrocyte death, axonal loss, complement activation, and antibody deposition [13, 30].

Remyelination can occur in MS lesions. Prineas and colleagues described remyelination in several patients with chronic MS lesions [41]. Nerve fibers with abnormally thin sheaths and shorter than normal myelin internodes were observed at the margins of many chronic plaques that were examined but the extent of the observed remyelination was extremely limited. In contrast, remyelination in acute lesions is often more substantial. Remyelination exceeding 10% of total lesion area was found in many lesions from 15 patients with early-stage MS [40]. Numerous shadow plaques were also observed that contained large numbers of thinly myelinated nerve fibers, suggesting remyelination of entire lesions.

The strong remyelination in acute MS lesions is similar to that observed following toxin-induced demyelination in animals. Demyelination resulting from the injection of lysolecithin into the CNS is rapidly and completely remyelinated with myelin sheaths that are uniformly thinner than normal and with characteristically shorter myelin internodes [12, 25]. A strong remyelination response is also observed following recovery from murine hepatitis virus (MHV)-induced demyelination in mice. Demyelination follows initial virus infection and is accompanied by the development of ataxia and paralysis. Recovery of neurologic function is mediated by nearly complete remyelination that begins as early as 14 days after infection [34, 47], concomitant with viral clearance; if virus persists, remyelination does not occur. The significant remyelination observed during early stages of MS in humans, as well as the strong remyelination observed in noninflammatory animal models of demyelination and in murine hepatitis virus (MHV)-infected mice, suggest that complete myelin repair is possible.

While demyelination is a defining pathologic characteristic of the disease, axonal injury and degeneration have been identified as the primary determinants of permanent neurologic deficits in patients with MS [13, 14]. Axonal injury probably begins early in the disease during active myelin breakdown but the damage continues in chronic demyelinated lesions in which exposed axons are highly vulnerable to secondary injury. While protective therapies that act directly at the demyelinated axon have not yet been established, remyelination can potentially protect vulnerable axons from secondary injury. Strategies to promote remyelination are therefore an important goal for the treatment of MS and a better understanding of the molecular and genetic mechanisms of remyelination is central to this goal.

Much of what we know about the development of demyelinated lesions and their potential for remyelination comes from histologic, immunochemical, and gene expression studies of lesioned tissue from human MS and from animal models of demyelinating disease. The application of genetic analysis to mouse models of demyelinating disease is an increasingly powerful tool for understanding the functions of particular gene products in the disease process and in repair. The following sections will introduce the various mouse models of demyelinating disease, describe the various genetic approaches used in mice for the study of disease and repair, and describe some of the recent applications of genetic analysis to the study of CNS remyelination.

## 2 Mouse Models of Demyelinating Disease

Human MS is a complex disease and no single mouse model exactly reproduces the clinical and pathological patterns observed in this disease. Three distinctly different approaches are available for the induction of demyelination in mice: exposure to toxins, autoimmunity, and virus-induced demyelination. Each approach results in demyelinating conditions with uniquely different features; taken together, these experimental systems have provided a useful set of animal models for the study of CNS repair following demyelinating disease.

Injection of ethidium bromide or lysolecithin into the white matter tracts of the brain or spinal cord, or administration of cuprizone in the diet, results in the rapid induction of focal demyelinated lesions due to toxic effects on the myelin sheath or oligodendrocytes [18, 22, 33]. The demyelination observed following toxin-induced demyelination is not immune-mediated and occurs even in mice with genetically deficient immune responses. However, following injury, there is frequently a strong immune infiltration of T cells, B cells, and hematogenous macrophages at lesion sites. This infiltration is usually short-lived but several studies have suggested its importance in CNS repair [9, 45, 46]. Remyelination following focal demyelination in these models is usually quite robust which suggests that in the absence of inhibiting factors significant remyelination may be the default physiologic response to myelin injury.

One of the most commonly used models of CNS demyelination is experimental autoimmune encephalitis (EAE) [21]. EAE is induced by sensitizing animals to myelin components either by direct immunization or by adoptive transfer of myelin reactive T cells. Crude homogenates of myelin can be used as an immunogen to induce encephalitis, but more commonly, specific myelin proteins are used such as myelin-basic protein (MBP), proteolipid protein (PLP), myelin oligodendrocyte glycoprotein (MOG), myelin-associated glycoprotein (MAG) or S-100. Sensitivity to myelin antigens results in CNS inflammation and frequently also CD4+ T cell-mediated demyelination. Depending upon the method of induction both acute and chronic forms of EAE can be induced. Remyelination is common in the acute forms but less so in the chronic forms of the disease.

Demyelinating disease also results following CNS infection with several mouse viruses, in particular, murine hepatitis virus (MHV) and Theiler's murine encephalomyelitis virus (TMEV) [10, 34]. Intracerebral infection with certain strains of these viruses results in an acute encephalitis that is characterized by an influx of many types of immune effector cells including CD4+ and CD8+ T cells, B cells, macrophages, and natural killer cells. In susceptible strains of mice, resolution of the acute inflammatory response is followed by development of viral persistence and chronic immune-mediated demyelinating disease. Remyelination following TMEV-mediated demyelination can be significant but is strongly dependent upon the strain of mouse that is infected [11]. This strain dependence of the remyelination response is discussed more fully below.

## 3  Cellular Events in Remyelination

Demyelination occurs as the result of damage to the myelin sheath and to oligodendrocytes. Following myelin damage, several lines of evidence suggest that surviving oligodendrocytes at the site of the lesion are unable to contribute to the remyelination process. Instead, new myelin-producing oligodendrocytes are generated from CNS resident multi-potent glial progenitor cells which are commonly referred to as oligodendrocyte progenitor cells (OPCs). These cells are relatively abundant and may comprise as much as 5%–8% of all CNS glia [27].

The first step in the remyelination process is the population of the lesion site with sufficient OPCs to mediate complete myelin repair. This initial recruitment phase involves both OPC proliferation and the migration of these new cells into the lesion. Once recruited to the lesion site, OPCs differentiate into premyelinating oligodendrocytes that establish an association with demyelinated axons and then become mature oligodendrocytes as they extend the membranous sheets that wrap the axon and eventually form mature myelin. Several excellent reviews on remyelination and OPC biology have recently been published [19, 27].

Remyelination is therefore a multi-step process involving OPC proliferation and migration, OPC differentiation and axonal recognition, and finally the generation of new myelin. One can easily imagine failure to remyelinate as the result of perturbation of any of these steps. Demyelination and remyelination most often occur following CNS injury and are therefore often accompanied by CNS inflammation. The quality of the inflammatory response may play an important role in determining whether OPC proliferation and differentiation proceeds normally and is probably also an important determinant of axonal survival. The quality of the immune response and the health of surviving axons must therefore also be considered as important components of the remyelination process.

## 4  Genetic Analysis in the Mouse

Despite having diverged evolutionarily over 75 million years ago, laboratory mice and humans share a high degree of genomic and physiologic similarity, making mice an excellent experimental model for the study of complex cellular processes with relevance to human disease. Mice are small, have a short generation time, and are easily bred and maintained. Perhaps more importantly, a large number of well-characterized inbred strains exist which allows investigators to carry out experiments on controlled genetic backgrounds, greatly minimizing the effects of genetic variation that are present in out-bred populations. Finally, technologies have been developed for the production of transgenic mice and for targeted gene knock-outs. These technologies have been invaluable for testing hypotheses about the function of particular gene products in many different biological processes.

There are two general approaches for genetic analysis in mice. Forward genetics utilizes naturally occurring or induced mutations to identify genes important for a biological process of interest [1, 26]. Mutations in these genes are detected based on the presence of a predetermined phenotype that is known to occur when the process is disrupted. Linkage analysis is used to identify genetic loci that contain likely candidate genes and these genes are then tested to determine whether alteration in their function induces the observed mutant phenotype. Once candidate genes are identified and confirmed, the full range of biochemical, molecular, genetic, and cell biological techniques can be applied to study their biological function.

Reverse genetics relies on the selection of candidate gene whose function in a particular biological process is suspected, often not based on phenotypic evidence, but on other experimental observations such as its expression in a specific tissue or cell type [1, 44]. The expression of this candidate gene is then altered and the effects of this alteration on the process of interest are assessed. Gene function can be altered in several ways. Technologies for the production of transgenic mice have made it possible to insert any fragment of DNA into the mouse genome. The power of this approach is that the coding sequence for any protein of interest can be linked with inducible or tissue-specific promoters to allow the overexpression or misexpression of that protein. The integration of DNA is not targeted to a specific site and therefore does not result in the insertional mutation of any specific gene. The endogenous gene that is homologous to the inserted transgene is therefore present in the genetic background and only dominant phenotypic effects of transgene expression are observed.

Homologous recombination allows the generation of insertional mutations in specific genes that knock out the function of the gene and allow an assessment of the effects of a loss of function mutation for that gene. Knock-out mice of this type have been a mainstay of reverse genetics for many years. However, if the gene to be mutated plays a critical role in development or general physiology, a knock-out may be lethal and therefore not useful for the study of cellular function in the adult animal. To circumvent this problem, the cre-*loxP* system has become an increasingly important tool for creating conditional gene deletions in which a gene of interest is deleted but only from specific cell types [8, 42, 48]. Cre recombinase is a type I topoisomerase that catalyzes site-specific recombination between *loxP* recognition elements; this results in deletion of the DNA sequences that lie between those sites. In this system, two lines of mice are created. In one line, the cre recombinase coding sequence is linked to a tissue-specific promoter, for example, the myelin-basic protein (MBP) promoter which is specifically expressed in oligodendrocytes. A second line is created in which homologous recombination is used to insert *loxP* elements into genomic DNA (frequently in introns) at sites flanking the coding sequence of a particular gene of interest; such genes are frequently referred to as floxed genes. When these two lines are crossed together, expression of the cre protein from the tissue-specific promoter catalyzes recombination at the *loxP* sites. This deletes the floxed gene but only in the tissues that express cre. In our example, expression of the cre protein from the MBP promoter deletes the floxed gene in oligodendrocytes. Using this system, delayed deletion of the gene of interest until adulthood avoids lethal phenotypes.

As mentioned previously, several mouse models of demyelinating disease are used to study the mechanisms of demyelination and the process of remyelination, and to serve as experimental systems for the development of MS therapeutics. The following sections summarize how both forward and reverse genetic approaches have been used to elucidate the roles of specific genes in the process of remyelination in there models.

# 5   Reverse Genetic Analysis of CNS Remyelination

The cellular and molecular biology of myelin and myelination have been studied intensively for many years. While the remyelination process is probably similar to myelination that occurs during normal development, remyelination appears to differ in many ways and probably needs to be studied as a unique and distinct process. At present, genetic analysis of the roles of specific genes in remyelination has only been applied to a small collection of genes. In the following sections, the genetic analysis of several of these genes is presented as a case study in how genetics can be used to understand the molecular biology of remyelination.

## 5.1   *Interferon-γ Is an Inhibitor of CNS Remyelination*

Interferon gamma (IFN-γ) is a pleiotropic cytokine produced by activated T cells and natural killer cells. While not normally present in large numbers in the nervous system, these cells enter the CNS following injury where the secretion of IFN-γ results in the activation of macrophages and microglia, and in the upregulation of class I and class II major histocompatibility molecules on many different cell types. The aggregate result of these changes is an enhanced immune response at the site of injury.

Some of the earliest indications that IFN-γ may be deleterious to CNS repair came from studies on the use of interferons for the treatment of human MS. While interferons alpha and beta (IFN-α and IFN-β) decrease MS exacerbations and are currently standard therapeutic treatments for multiple sclerosis, IFN-γ exacerbates the disease [37, 38].

Experiments in mice support the idea that IFN-γ plays a deleterious role in remyelination and recovery from demyelinating disease. The IFN-γ coding sequence was linked to the myelin-basic protein promoter region and this construct was used to create transgenic mice that specifically expressed IFN-γ in oligodendrocytes [17, 24]. This expression resulted in hypomyelination, oligodendrocyte cell death, and a tremoring phenotype. However, IFN-γ expression in these models begins during the first few weeks of postnatal development and it is difficult to rigorously apply results on the effects of IFN-γ on myelin development to an understanding of the role that IFN-γ plays in remyelination later in life.

To address these concerns and to specifically assess the effects of IFN-γ on remyelination, transgenic mice that express IFN-γ in a temporally controlled manner have been created [28, 29]. In these animals, the glial fibrillary acidic protein (GFAP) promoter, which directs gene expression in mature astrocytes, is linked to the coding sequence for the tetracycline-controlled transactivator protein (tTA). The mice also contain a second transgene in which the IFN-γ coding sequence is linked to the tetracycline regulatory element (TRE). In these GFAP/tTA;TRE/IFN-γ double transgenic mice, the tTA protein is expressed in astrocytes. However, in the presence of doxycycline, a tetracycline analog, the tTA protein is inactive, does not bind the TRE sequence, and, therefore, does not induce IFN-γ expression. When these mice are raised in the presence of dietary doxycycline, they develop normally and show no CNS IFN-γ expression. When doxycycline is removed from the diet, IFN-γ expression is induced in CNS astrocytes and reaches a maximal level of expression after about 2 weeks.

To examine the role of IFN-γ on remyelination, demyelinating disease was induced in double transgenic animals either by dietary administration of cuprizone or by immunization with myelin oligodendrocyte glycoprotein (MOG) to induce EAE. Once demyelinating disease was established, doxycycline was removed from the diet to induce the secretion of IFN-γ by astrocytes. IFN-γ expression suppressed remyelination in both experimental systems. In cuprizone-treated animals, remyelination in the corpus callosum was reduced from 48.4% to 26.9% of demyelinated axons following 8 weeks of doxycycline withdrawal [29]. Myelin-specific gene expression was also much reduced, consistent with a general inhibition of myelination.

Following cuprizone-induced demyelination, OPCs repopulate demyelinated lesions and then differentiate into mature oligodendrocytes responsible for remyelination. NG2 staining to detect OPCs revealed similar numbers of progenitors in GFAP/tTA;TRE/IFN-γ double transgenic mice with continued doxycycline treatment compared to doxycycline withdrawal. Despite similar OPC numbers, there was a significant reduction of mature oligodendrocytes in mice with induced IFN-γ expression in the CNS [29]. These observations are consistent with in vitro studies demonstrating that mature myelinating oligodendrocytes are more sensitive to IFN-γ than are OPCs. IFN-γ expression may therefore inhibit remyelination at the stage following OPC recruitment when oligodendrocytes begin to differentiate.

Similar observations were made in double transgenic mice with MOG-induced EAE [29]. IFN-γ expression induced following establishment of the disease resulted in reduced expression of myelin-specific proteins, reduced numbers of mature oligodendrocytes at demyelinated lesions, and reduced remyelination. Furthermore, IFN-γ expression significantly delayed clinical recovery. Axonal integrity did not appear to be affected, suggesting that the delay in recovery may be a consequence of remyelination failure.

While the inhibition of remyelination by IFN-γ may result from direct effects on oligodendrocytes, the global effects of IFN-γ on CNS tissue make it difficult to exclude indirect effects mediated by other cells such as activated microglia. To address this question another transgenic system has been employed. Suppressors of cytokine signaling (SOCS) are a family of proteins that inhibit the JAK/STAT signaling pathways. As such, they are key regulators of cytokine-mediated events. Of particular interest is SOCS1, which functions as a cellular regulator of IFN-γ responsiveness. Transgenic mice were created in which SOCS1 expression was driven specifically in oligodendrocytes by the proteolipid protein promoter; expression of SOCS1 in these mice protects them against the damaging effects of IFN-γ expression [6]. In culture, oligodendrocytes are normally quite sensitive to IFN-γ and die by necrosis within a few days after treatment [5]. Oligodendrocytes from PLP/SOCS1 transgenic mice were cultured and treated with IFN-γ and the nuclear translocation of the IFN-γ signaling molecule STAT1 was used as an assay for IFN-γ responsiveness [6]. In oligodendrocytes that express SOCS1, STAT1 remains in the cytoplasm while wild type cells respond with STAT1 nuclear translocation. In vivo, IFN-γ expression in oligodendrocytes from a MBP/IFN-γ transgene causes the upregulation of MHC class I on oligodendrocytes and myelin. In MBP/IFN-γ, PLP/SOCS1 double transgenic mice, oligodendrocytes and myelin do not express detectable levels of MHC class I. The results, both in culture and in vivo, indicate that SOCS1 expression in oligodendrocytes diminishes their responsiveness to IFN-γ and that the deleterious effects of IFN-γ are a direct effect on oligodendrocytes.

In addition to the cellular effects of SOCS1 protection, PLP/SOCS1 transgenic mice are also protected from the neurologic abnormalities that accompany IFN-γ overexpression during myelin development [6]. As mentioned previously, transgenic expression of IFN-γ in developing mice results in hypomyelination and a tremoring phenotype. When the PLP/SOCS1 transgene is crossed into transgenic lines that overexpress IFN-γ during myelination, the expression of SOCS1 significantly decreases the incidence of tremor. These results demonstrate that the expression of SOCS1 not only diminishes the responsiveness of oligodendrocytes to the deleterious effects of IFN-γ but that this protection may also affect neurologic function.

While these experiments demonstrate that IFN-γ has a direct effect on oligodendrocytes which reduces oligodendrocyte numbers and inhibits remyelination, they do not address the cellular basis for this inhibition. Recent studies strongly suggest that this effect is the result of endoplasmic reticulum stress. The endoplasmic reticulum is the site of synthesis for secreted and membrane-bound proteins. As these proteins are synthesized, they are folded properly with the help of ER chaperone proteins and only correctly folded proteins are transported on the Golgi apparatus. Abnormally folded proteins are retained in the ER, translocated into the cytoplasm and degraded by the proteosome. Under certain conditions, unfolded proteins accumulate in the ER forming toxic aggregates, a condition called ER stress [51]. When this happens, eukaryotic cells activate an ER stress response that attenuates protein synthesis, upregulates the transcription of ER chaperone proteins and the proteins involved in the clearance of misfolded proteins, and eventually induces apoptosis to remove the damaged cell.

The endoplasmic reticulum kinase, *PERK*, plays an important role in the response to ER stress by phosphorylating eIF2α to attenuate translation. *PERK* also phosphorylates the ATF4 transcription factor to enhance the production of other proteins involved in the ER stress response. Mice that are homozygous for a targeted knock-out of the *PERK* gene die soon after birth due to a variety of developmental and metabolic defects [23, 52]. While *PERK* heterozygotes are viable, their levels of *PERK* are half those observed in wild type animals and they exhibit mild deficiencies in some physiologic functions such as the ability to clear glucose from the serum, which suggests that reduced levels of *PERK* are physiologically relevant [23]. *PERK* heterozygotes were used to test whether ER stress might be responsible for the deleterious effects of IFN-γ on oligodendrocytes and remyelination [28]. In the corpus callosum of GFAP/tTA;TRE/IFN-γ double transgenic mice with cuprizone-induced demyelination, IFN-γ expression following doxycycline withdrawal is accompanied by the upregulation of several genes associated with the ER stress response. In addition, increased phosphorylation of eIF2α was observed in oligodendrocytes, demonstrating a link between IFN-γ effects on oligodendrocytes and ER stress. When these double transgenic mice are crossed onto a *PERK* $^{+/-}$ genetic background, very few oligodendrocytes were detected in the corpus callosum and the number of remyelinated axons was greatly reduced. Of the oligodendrocytes present in the corpus callosum, a significant number were caspase 3-positive, suggesting that they were undergoing apoptosis. Taken together, these observations strongly support the idea that IFN-γ expression in the CNS results in ER stress, causing oligodendrocyte loss and remyelination failure.

## 5.2 Efficient CNS Remyelination Requires T Cells

Examining the extent of remyelination in mice with genetic deficiencies in immune function demonstrates a positive role for immune function in the remyelination process [9]. Mice deficient in recombination-activating gene 1 (*RAG-1*) lack both B cells and T cells. Following lysolecthin-induced demyelination in the spinal cord, *RAG-1* mutant mice show a 65% reduction in remyelination compared to control mice. Mice lacking either CD4[+] or CD8[+] T cells show a similar inhibition of remyelination. These experiments demonstrate that both CD4[+] and CD8[+] CNS-infiltrating T cells provide functions necessary for efficient remyelination. A neuroprotective role for T cells following CNS injury has previously been proposed [45, 46], although the exact mechanism of this effect is still not fully understood.

## 5.3 Growth Factors Play Diverse Roles During CNS Remyelination

Cultured oligodendrocytes respond to a variety of growth factors in culture and reverse genetics has been used to study several of these in vivo for their roles in myelination and remyelination. Fibroblast growth factor 2 (FGF2) is a potent mitogen for OPCs, especially in combination with platelet-derived growth factor (PDGF). FGF2 expression is strongly upregulated at the sites of demyelinated lesions and is likely to play a role in remyelination.

FGF2 knock-out mice have been studied using several systems of demyelinating disease to determine the role of FGF in remyelination. Following both cuprizone- and MHV-induced demyelination, oligodendrocyte repopulation of demyelinated lesions increases in FGF2 knock-out mice [4, 36]. In the cuprizone model, increased remyelination accompanies this enhanced oligodendroglial regeneration [3]. Treatment of spinal cord glia in culture with FGF2 or with function-neutralizing FGF2 antibodies demonstrates that elevated FGF2 favors OPC proliferation, while FGF2 depletion promotes the differentiation of OPCs into mature oligodendrocytes [4]. Therefore, while FGF2 acts as a mitogen for OPCs in culture and probably also in vivo, it apparently inhibits oligodendrocytre differentiation and, thus, remyelination.

PDGF also acts as a mitogen for OPCs in vitro. PDGF overexpression in astrocytes under the control of the glial fibrillar acidic protein promoter (GFAP/PDGF), results in increased OPC density in adult mice. This suggests a role for PDGF expression levels in determining the number of OPCs that develop in the adult CNS [49]. However, when demyelination was induced in GFAP/PDGF transgenic mice with dietary cuprizone or by lysolecithin injection into the spinal cord, no differences are observed in the extent or rate of remyelination despite significantly increased OPC density in lesions [49]. These data demonstrate a key role for PDGF levels in establishing the density of the OPC population but also show that remyelination is generally not limited by the number of available OPCs.

A third growth factor, insulin-like growth factor 1 (IGF-1), appears to protect mature oligodendrocytes from death following demyelinating insults. IGF-1 promotes the long-term survival of oligodendrocytes in culture and protects them from undergoing apoptosis. Overexpression of IGF-1 in the brain during development, under the control of the metallothionein-I promoter (IGF-1 Tg mice), results in increased numbers of myelinated axons with thicker myelin sheaths, increased numbers of oligodendrocytes and increased levels of PLP and MBP mRNA in the CNS. These data indicate that IGF-1 stimulates both oligodendrocyte growth and myelination [50]. Cuprizone-induced demyelination in wild type mice results in oligodendrocyte apoptosis and the depletion of oligodendrocytes in the corpus callosum with concomitant demyelination. In IGF-1 Tg mice, acute demyelination is observed following cuprizone treatment but oligodendrocyte apoptosis is greatly reduced. As a consequence, mature oligodendrocytes survive the initial demyelinating insult and demyelinated lesions are rapidly remyelinated [32]. These observations suggest a role for IGF-1 in preventing the depletion of mature oligodendrocytes during demyelination and thereby enhancing the rate of myelin repair.

Subsequent studies on the role of interleukin-1$\beta$ (IL-1$\beta$) in remyelination support the notion that IGF-1 enhances myelin repair [31]. IL-1$\beta$ is a proinflammatory cytokine expressed in MS lesions [15] and associated with blood–brain barrier breakdown [2] and with cytotoxic effects on oligodendrocytes in culture [35]. All of these observations suggest a role for IL-1$\beta$ in the MS pathology. However, IL-1$\beta$ knock-out mice show a reduced capacity for myelin repair following cuprizone-induced demyelination [31]. This failure to remyelinate correlates with reduced IGF-1 production by macrophages, microglia and astrocytes and with delayed OPC differentiation in demyelinated lesions. The promotion of myelin repair by IL-1β therefore appears to be the result of IL-1β-induced secretion of IGF-1 at the lesion.

## 5.4   The Extracellular Matrix Receptor, β 1-Integrin, Is Not Essential for Remyelination

Integrins are an important class of receptors for extracellular matrix molecules. Oligodendrocytes express β1-integrin which appears to play a role in the elaboration of myelin sheets on laminin in culture [43] and in oligodendrocyte survival in vivo [20]. However, deletion of the β1-integrin gene results in perinatal death preventing a detailed genetic analysis of the role of β1-integrin in myelination or remyelination [16].

Investigators used the cre-lox system to generate a conditional deletion of the β1-integrin gene after the completion of early development to avoid the problem of early lethality [7, 39]. The cyclic nucleotide phosphodiesterase (CNP) promoter, which is expressed in mature oligodendrocytes, was used to drive cre recombinase expression in mice carrying a floxed allele of β1-integrin on a β1-integrin-deficient background. The floxed allele provides β1-integrin expression during embryonic development but the gene is deleted in oligodendrocytes when CNP expression begins during myelin development. While β1-integrin deletion results in increased apoptosis in premyelinating oligodendrocytes, this increase in cell death during development does not appear to significantly affect myelination. Remyelination proceeds normally when lysolecithin-induced demyelination occurs in the spinal cords of adult mice with a conditional deletion of the β1-integrin. These results demonstrate that β1-integrin does not play an essential role in either myelination or remyelination.

The experiments described above demonstrate the creative use of transgenic mice and mice with targeted gene knock-outs to identify the likely functions of a specific gene product. The eventual development of a complete understanding of the remyelination process will undoubtedly rely heavily on this type of genetic analysis.

## 6   Forward Genetic Analysis of CNS Remyelination

The studies described above illustrate the power of reverse genetics in studying the role of a particular gene in remyelination. The disadvantage of this approach is that it requires the identification of candidate genes prior to experimentation and is therefore biased towards our previously existing knowledge of the remyelination process.

Forward genetic analysis provides a less biased alternative but requires a phenotype that can serve as a biological readout for mutations in genes that affect remyelination. Forward genetics approaches might utilize either naturally occurring allelic variation or induced mutations to identify genes that are important for remyelination. Recently, naturally occurring variation in the ability of different inbred mouse strains to remyelinate following Theiler's virus-induced demyelination has been reported [11] and this variation may have potential as a phenotypic readout for genes involved in myelin repair.

Persistent TMEV infection results in chronic progressive demyelinating disease. Disease progression has been characterized in four susceptible inbred strains: SJL, B10.D1-H2$^q$ (B10.Q), FVB, and SWR. In SJL and B10.Q mice, demyelination begins 2–3 weeks after infection and progresses over the next several months. Demyelination persists throughout the life of the animal with very little remyelination. Chronic demyelination is accompanied by a progressive accumulation of neurological deficits. In contrast, FVB and SWR mice develop extensive CNS remyelination between 3.5 months and 11 months after infection. By 1 year after infection, many lesions in FVB and SWR mice are completely remyelinated postinfection. The late onset and the thoroughness of the repair after relatively severe prior demyelination are noteworthy.

All four strains show similar functional phenotypes in the first 3 months after infection. Approximately 1 week after infection they became transiently lethargic due to acute encephalitis in response to viral infection. This stage of disease lasts for 1–2 weeks after which the mice recover. Mice retain normal activity and appearance until 3–4 months after infection, beyond which SJL and B10.Q mice develop progressive neurologic dysfunction. In contrast, few signs of neurologic disease are observed in FVB or SWR mice at any time up to 1 year after infection. Neurologic ability was quantified for SJL and FVB mice using an accelerated rotarod assay, comparing performance at several time points during disease to preinfection baseline performance. Motor function declines slightly during the first 30–120 days in both strains. SJL performance continues to decline beyond 120 days after infection while FVB performance is maintained out to 325 days after infection. Thus, FVB mice, in which remyelination progresses rapidly, show little obvious clinical presentation of disease, and motor function stabilizes concomitant with remyelination.

The inheritance of this myelin repair phenotype can be examined by crossing FVB mice with SJL and B10.Q to generate FVB/SJL and FVB/B10.Q F1 hybrid mice. Infected mice from these crosses develop demyelinated lesions followed by extensive remyelination with a time course similar to that observed in FVB mice (Fig. 1). F1 hybrids are clinically normal up to 1 year after infection. Both lesion repair and preservation of neurological function are inherited as dominant traits in the F1 generation. When (FVB/B10.Q)F1 mice are backcrossed to the B10.Q parent strain to produce (FVB/B10.Q x B10.Q)N2 progeny, the extent of remyelination in the N2 generation is distributed continuously between mice with very little remyelination 300 days after infection and mice that show complete remyelination

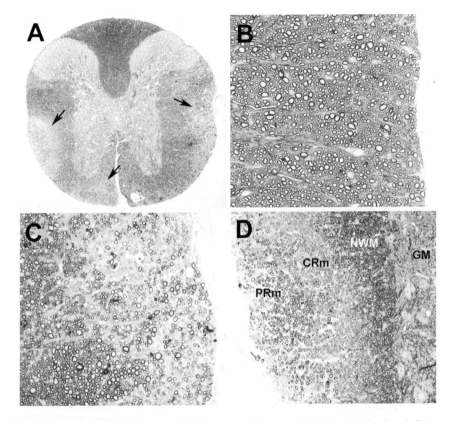

**Fig. 1** Demyelination and remyelination in the spinal cord of TMEV infected mice. **A** Cross-section of a mouse spinal cord 350 days after infection, stained with ρ-phenylenediamine to show myelin. Normal myelin picks up the stain evenly; several lightly stained areas (*arrow*) indicate demyelinated lesions. The lesion on the left also contains significant remyelination. **B** Normal-appearing white matter. **C** Sites of demyelination show significant myelin loss but a few intact myelin sheaths remain **D** Remyelination is frequently oligodendrocyte-mediated with varying amounts of Schwann cell remyelination. *CRm*, central (oligodendrocyte) remyelination; *PRm*, peripheral (Schwann cell) remyelination; *NWM*, normal white matter; *GM*, grey matter. The mice presented here are FVB/B10.Q hybrid mice which show significant potential for spontaneous CNS repair following TMEV-induced demyelination.

(A.J. Bieber, unpublished observations). The reparative phenotype therefore behaves as a quantitative trait in the N2 generation.

The appearance in the N2 generation of both mice with a strong remyelination phenotype and those that do not repair opens up possibilities for a forward genetic analysis of the potential for remyelination. Classic Mendelian inheritance is characterized by the dichotomous appearance of discrete phenotypes, often based on the inheritance of alternative alleles of a single gene. A quantitative trait is one that shows measurable phenotypic variation based on the multifactorial inheritance of alleles from several genetic loci that differ between strains and are called quantitative trait loci (or QTLs) for that phenotype. In the past, DNA microsatellites were routinely used to map QTLs but mapping with SNPs (single nucleotide polymorphisms). To map the genetic loci involved in remyelination, N2 animals scored for remyelination at 300 days after infection, and their genomic DNA would then be typed for a large collection of SNP markers that are polymorphic between the FVB and B10.Q strains. The preferential segregation of the strong remyelination phenotype with any particular SNP would indicate recombinational linkage between them, thereby identifying the chromosomal position of the SNP as a genetic locus containing a gene involved in remyelination. Such a screen will allow the unbiased identification of genes involved in CNS repair.

The technical aspects of mouse genetics, both forward and reverse, are now at a point where rapid progress should occur in the identification and functional analysis of the genes and pathways involved in remyelination and CNS repair. Ultimately, such analysis will lead to better understanding of the pathophysiology of human demyelinating disease and, hopefully, to the development of novel treatment strategies.

# References

1. Allayee H, Andalibi A, Mehrabian M (2006) Using inbred mouse strains to identify genes for complex diseases. Front Biosci 11:1216–1226
2. Argaw AT, Zhang Y, Snyder BJ, Zhao ML, Kopp N, Lee SC, Raine CS, Brosnan CF, John GR (2006) IL-1beta regulates blood–brain barrier permeability via reactivation of the hypoxia-angiogenesis program. J Immunol 177:5574–5584
3. Armstrong RC, Le TQ, Flint NC, Vana AC, Zhou YX (2006) Endogenous cell repair of chronic demyelination. J Neuropathol Exp Neurol 65:245–256
4. Armstrong RC, Le TQ, Frost EE, Borke RC, Vana AC (2002) Absence of fibroblast growth factor 2 promotes oligodendroglial repopulation of demyelinated white matter. J Neurosci 22:8574–8585
5. Baerwald KD, Popko B (1998) Developing and mature oligodendrocytes respond differently to the immune cytokine interferon-gamma. J Neurosci Res 52:230–239
6. Balabanov R, Strand K, Kemper A, Lee JY, Popko B (2006) Suppressor of cytokine signaling 1 expression protects oligodendrocytes from the deleterious effects of interferon-gamma. J Neurosci 26:5143–5152
7. Benninger Y, Colognato H, Thurnherr T, Franklin RJ, Leone DP, Atanasoski S, Nave KA, Ffrench-Constant C, Suter U, Relvas JB (2006) Beta1-integrin signaling mediates premyelinating oligodendrocyte survival but is not required for CNS myelination and remyelination. J Neurosci 26:7665–7673
8. Betz UA, Vosshenrich CA, Rajewsky K, Muller W (1996) Bypass of lethality with mosaic mice generated by cre-loxP-mediated recombination. Curr Biol 6:1307–1316
9. Bieber AJ, Kerr S, Rodriguez M (2003) Efficient central nervous system remyelination requires T cells. Ann Neurol 53:680–684
10. Bieber AJ, Rodriguez M (2003) Experimental models of virus-induced demyelination. In: Griffin J, Lassmann H, Nave K-A, Trapp B, Lazzarini R, Miller R (eds) Myelin and Its Diseases. Academic Press, New York, pp. 1073–1100.
11. Bieber AJ, Ure DR, Rodriguez M (2005) Genetically dominant spinal cord repair in a murine model of chronic progressive multiple sclerosis. J Neuropathol Exp Neurol 64:46–57

12. Bieber AJ, Warrington A, Asakura K, Ciric B, Kaveri SV, Pease LR, Rodriguez M (2002) Human antibodies accelerate the rate of remyelination following lysolecithin-induced demyelination in mice. Glia 37:241–249
13. Bjartmar C, Trapp BD (2001) Axonal and neuronal degeneration in multiple sclerosis: Mechanisms and functional consequences. Curr Opin Neurol 14:271–278
14. Bjartmar C, Trapp BD (2003) Axonal degeneration and progressive neurologic disability in multiple sclerosis. Neurotox Res 5:157–164
15. Brosnan CF, Cannella B, Battistini L, Raine CS (1995) Cytokine localization in multiple sclerosis lesions: Correlation with adhesion molecule expression and reactive nitrogen species. Neurology 45:S16–S21
16. Colognato H, Baron W, Avellana-Adalid V, Relvas JB, Baron-Van Evercooren A, Georges-Labouesse E, Ffrench-Constant C (2002) CNS integrins switch growth factor signalling to promote target-dependent survival. Nat Cell Biol 4:833–841
17. Corbin JG, Kelly D, Rath EM, Baerwald KD, Suzuki K,Popko B (1996) Targeted CNS expression of interferon-gamma in transgenic mice leads to hypomyelination, reactive gliosis, and abnormal cerebellar development. Mol Cell Neurosci 7:354–370
18. Crang AJ, Blakemore WF (1991) Remyelination of demyelinated rat axons by transplanted mouse oligodendrocytes. Glia 4:305–313
19. Franklin RJ (2002) Why does remyelination fail in multiple sclerosis? Nat Rev Neurosci 3:705–714
20. Frost EE, Buttery PC, Milner R, ffrench-Constant C (1999) Integrins mediate a neuronal survival signal for oligodendrocytes. Curr Biol 9:1251–1254
21. Gold R, Hartung HP, Toyka KV (2000) Animal models for autoimmune demyelinating disorders of the nervous system. Mol Med Today 6:88–91
22. Hall SM (1972) The effect of injections of lysophosphatidyl choline into white matter of the adult mouse spinal cord. J Cell Sci 10:535–546
23. Harding HP, Zeng H, Zhang Y, Jungries R, Chung P, Plesken H, Sabatini DD, Ron D (2001) Diabetes mellitus and exocrine pancreatic dysfunction in *PERK*-/- mice reveals a role for translational control in secretory cell survival. Mol Cell 7:1153–1163
24. Horwitz MS, Evans CF, McGavern DB, Rodriguez M, Oldstone MB (1997) Primary demyelination in transgenic mice expressing interferon-gamma. Nat Med 3:1037–1041
25. Jeffery ND, Blakemore WF (1995) Remyelination of mouse spinal cord axons demyelinated by local injection of lysolecithin. J Neurocytol 24:775–781
26. Kile BT, Hilton DJ (2005) The art and design of genetic screens: Mouse. Nat Rev Genet 6:557–567
27. Levine JM, Reynolds R, Fawcett JW (2001) The oligodendrocyte precursor cell in health and disease. Trends Neurosci 24:39–47
28. Lin W, Harding HP, Ron D, Popko B (2005) Endoplasmic reticulum stress modulates the response of myelinating oligodendrocytes to the immune cytokine interferon-gamma. J Cell Biol 169:603–612
29. Lin W, Kemper A, Dupree JL, Harding HP, Ron D, Popko B (2006) Interferon-gamma inhibits central nervous system remyelination through a process modulated by endoplasmic reticulum stress. Brain 129:1306–1318
30. Lucchinetti C, Bruck W, Parisi J, Scheithauer B, Rodriguez M, Lassmann H (2000) Heterogeneity of multiple sclerosis lesions: Implications for the pathogenesis of demyelination. Ann Neurol 47:707–717
31. Mason JL, Suzuki K, Chaplin DD, Matsushima GK (2001) Interleukin-1beta promotes repair of the CNS. J Neurosci 21:7046–7052
32. Mason JL, Ye P, Suzuki K, D'Ercole AJ, Matsushima GK (2000) Insulin-like growth factor-1 inhibits mature oligodendrocyte apoptosis during primary demyelination. J Neurosci 20:5703–5708
33. Matsushima GK, Morell P (2001) The neurotoxicant, cuprizone, as a model to study demyelination and remyelination in the central nervous system. Brain Pathol 11:107–116

34. Matthews AE, Weiss SR, Paterson Y (2002) Murine hepatitis virus – A model for virus-induced CNS demyelination. J Neurovirol 8:76–85
35. Merrill JE (1991) Effects of interleukin-1 and tumor necrosis factor-alpha on astrocytes, microglia, oligodendrocytes, and glial precursors in vitro. Dev Neurosci 13:130–137
36. Murtie JC, Zhou YX, Le TQ, Vana AC, Armstrong RC (2005) PDGF and FGF2 pathways regulate distinct oligodendrocyte lineage responses in experimental demyelination with spontaneous remyelination. Neurobiol Dis 19:171–182
37. Panitch HS (1992) Interferons in multiple sclerosis. A review of the evidence. Drugs 44:946–962
38. Panitch HS, Hirsch RL, Schindler J, Johnson KP (1987) Treatment of multiple sclerosis with gamma interferon: Exacerbations associated with activation of the immune system. Neurology 37:1097–1102
39. Potocnik AJ, Brakebusch C, Fassler R (2000) Fetal and adult hematopoietic stem cells require beta1 integrin function for colonizing fetal liver, spleen, and bone marrow. Immunity 12:653–663
40. Prineas JW, Barnard RO, Kwon EE, Sharer LR, Cho ES (1993) Multiple sclerosis: remyelination of nascent lesions. Ann Neurol 33:137–151
41. Prineas JW, Connell F (1979) Remyelination in multiple sclerosis. Ann Neurol 5:22–31
42. Rajewsky K, Gu H, Kuhn R, Betz UA, Muller W, Roes J, Schwenk F (1996) Conditional gene targeting. J Clin Invest 98:600–603
43. Relvas JB, Setzu A, Baron W, Buttery PC, LaFlamme SE, Franklin RJ, Ffrench-Constant C (2001) Expression of dominant-negative and chimeric subunits reveals an essential role for beta1 integrin during myelination. Curr Biol 11:1039–1043
44. Ristevski S (2005) Making better transgenic models: Conditional, temporal, and spatial approaches. Mol Biotechnol 29:153–163
45. Schwartz M (2000) Beneficial autoimmune T cells and posttraumatic neuroprotection. Ann N Y Acad Sci 917:341–347
46. Schwartz M, Moalem G, Leibowitz-Amit R, Cohen IR (1999) Innate and adaptive immune responses can be beneficial for CNS repair. Trends Neurosci 22:295–299
47. Stohlman SA, Hinton DR (2001) Viral induced demyelination. Brain Pathol 11:92–106
48. Van der Neut R (1997) Targeted gene disruption: Applications in neurobiology. J Neurosci Methods 71:19–27
49. Woodruff RH, Fruttiger M, Richardson WD, Franklin RJ (2004) Platelet-derived growth factor regulates oligodendrocyte progenitor numbers in adult CNS and their response following CNS demyelination. Mol Cell Neurosci 25:252–262
50. Ye P, Carson J, D'Ercole AJ (1995) In vivo actions of insulin-like growth factor-1 (IGF-1) on brain myelination: Studies of IGF-1 and IGF binding protein-1 (IGFBP-1) transgenic mice. J Neurosci 15:7344–7356
51. Yoshida H (2007) ER stress and diseases. FEBS J 274:630–658
52. Zhang P, McGrath B, Li S, Frank A, Zambito F, Reinert J, Gannon M, Ma K, McNaughton K, Cavener DR (2002) The *PERK* eukaryotic initiation factor 2 alpha kinase is required for the development of the skeletal system, postnatal growth, and the function and viability of the pancreas. Mol Cell Biol 22:3864–3874

# Remyelination in Experimental Models of Toxin-Induced Demyelination

**W.F. Blakemore(✉) and R.J.M. Franklin**

**Abstract**  Remyelination is the regenerative process by which demyelinated axons are reinvested with new myelin sheaths. It is associated with functional recovery and maintenance of axonal health. It occurs as a spontaneous regenerative response following demyelination in a range of pathologies including traumatic injury as well as primary demyelinating disease such as multiple sclerosis (MS). Experimental models of demyelination based on the use of toxins, while not attempting to accurately mimic a disease with complex etiology and pathogenesis such as MS, have nevertheless proven extremely useful for studying the biology of remyelination. In this chapter, we review the main toxin models of demyelination, drawing attention to their differences and how they can be used to study different aspects of remyelination. We also describe the optimal use of these models, highlighting potential pitfalls in interpretation, and how remyelination can be unequivocally recognized. Finally, we discuss the role of toxin models alongside viral and immune-mediated models of demyelination.

W.F. Blakemore
Department of Veterinary Medicine and Cambridge Centre for Brain Repair,
University of Cambridge, Madingley Road, Cambridge, CB3 OES, UK
e-mail: wfb1000@cam.ac.uk

M. Rodriguez (ed.), *Advances in Multiple Sclerosis and Experimental*
*Demyelinating Diseases. Current Topics in Microbiology and Immunology 318.*
© Springer-Verlag Berlin Heidelberg 2008

# 1   Introduction

A number of toxins create demyelinating lesions that allow investigators to explore the biology of remyelination. These have proved invaluable for gaining insights into the cellular and the molecular mechanism underlying the process. These models have also been used to understand remyelination failure in MS and the prospects for remyelination-enhancing therapies, but in this context, it must be remembered that nearly all demyelinating lesions in experimental animals are small compared to demyelinating lesions in humans and most will undergo spontaneous remyelination, albeit in an age- and sex-dependent manner. This chapter will not review the extensive knowledge of the biology of remyelination gleaned from these models (reviewed elsewhere [38] but instead will describe their principal features drawing attention to the several potential pitfalls that may lead to misinterpretation of data.

## 1.1   Identification of Remyelination

Although early studies on MS speculated that thin myelin sheaths might represent remyelination, it was not until the late 1960s and early 1970s that studies using experimental models of demyelination [23] and, in particular, cuprizone intoxication in mice [10, 11] and focal demyelinating lesions in the spinal cord of cats [41, 76] firmly established the morphological features of remyelinated myelin sheaths. These studies showed that remyelinated myelin sheaths are too thin for the axons they surround and that internodes are shorter than normal. However, this definition needs qualification; with the exception of the earliest stages of remyelination, the reduction in myelin sheath thickness is only apparent when large-diameter axons are remyelinated. With axons up to 1.5 μm in diameter and particularly in situations where there are no larger-diameter axons in the same white matter tract, it is very difficult to distinguish remyelinated fibers from normal fibers on the basis of myelin sheath thickness [10, 77], an issue especially pertinent to the now widely used model of corpus callosum demyelination in mice induced by low-dose cuprizone intoxication [90]. Remyelination is associated with a decrease in internodal length, and this will result in an increase in nodal density. With the availability of antibodies to nodal and paranodal proteins such as casper and neurofascin, it should now be possible to document remyelination by demonstrating an increase in nodal density.

The change in myelin sheath thickness associated with remyelination is best detected using 1-μm resin embedded sections or by electron microscopy (Fig. 1), ideally using tissue perfusion–fixed with gluteraldehyde to preserve myelin sheath structure and axon circularity. Many investigators use luxol fast blue staining of paraffin-embedded tissue to document remyelination. However, this stain lacks the resolution to separate unequivocally, remyelination from normal myelination and particularly to separate myelin loss due to axon degeneration from myelin loss due to primary demyelination. The extent of myelination shown following luxol fast blue staining can also be affected by factors entirely independent of whether axons

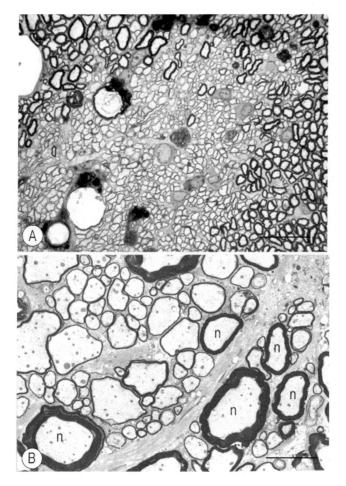

**Fig. 1** Light (**A**) and electron (**B**) micrographs of oligodendrocyte remyelination 2 months after lysolecithin injection into the spinal cord of an adult rat. The remyelinated axons can be distinguished from the normally myelinated axons because myelin sheaths of remyelinated axons are too thin for the axons they surround. In resin sections, they stain less intensely with toluidine blue (**A**). Bar in **A**=12 μm; **B**=3 μm

are myelinated, such as the presence of edema or cellular infiltrates, which change the density of myelinated fibers and, hence, the extent of luxol fast blue staining. The use of this stain, without the concurrent use of another one preferably to demonstrate axons [101], may lead to the mistaken conclusion that certain treatments enhance remyelination when they are actually just enhancing axon survival, which allows remyelination to occur and be visualized. Also, when considering treatments for stimulating remyelination, it is essential to ensure a similar extent of demyelination between groups of animals, since treatments may be protective for oligodendrocytes either by a direct effect on the oligodendrocyte, for example, LIF [24], or indirectly by interfering with the demyelinating mechanism such as systemic IGF-I treatment in EAE (see discussion in [78]).

# 2  Demyelinating Toxins

## 2.1  Focal Toxins

A number of fundamental studies can be conducted by injecting chemicals into white matter tracts that specifically destroy glial cells and/or their myelin while leaving the axons mostly intact. This approach demonstrates the physiological properties of demyelinated and remyelinated CNS axons [87], the recovery of function following remyelination [51] and the importance of axon degeneration for failure of recovery of behavioral function following demyelinating lesions [52]. To show a direct relationship between demyelination, remyelination and electrophysiological function, it is necessary to produce a single demyelinated area in a specific location so that animals can be implanted with stimulating electrodes above and below the lesion site to allow repeated evaluation of the conduction properties of the axons in the area of demyelination [88]. Then, following injection of the demyelinating toxin records of axonal conduction through the area of, demyelination and subsequent remyelination can be obtained from the saphenous nerve following stimulation above and below the lesion. Studies using this approach showed there was a close correlation between return of conduction and remyelination and that the speed of nerve conduction returns to normal following remyelination. However, these studies (and also the subsequent locomotor function studies of Jeffery and Blakemore using focal area of demyelination in the cervical spinal cord of rats to investigate functional consequences of demyelination and remyelination [51, 52]) also showed that, even with complete remyelination of a previously demyelinated area, full functional recovery does not occur if there is significant axon loss. In addition, in establishing the model system used for the electrophysiological studies, it was found that multiple focal areas of demyelination on the same axon resulted in increased axon degeneration.

The demyelinating agents used so far are lysolecithin, ethidium bromide, 6-aminonicotinamide, antibodies to oligodendrocyte-related molecules and bacterial endotoxin. The locations used include the dorsal and ventrolateral funiculi of the spinal cord (usually at the thoracolumbar level), the caudal cerebellar peduncle, the corpus callosum, the optic nerve and subcortical white matter. Usually, increasing the volume or concentration of the injected toxin enhances axon degeneration, and hemorrhage occurs with some toxins. Of note with all toxins, axon degeneration in the corpus callosum can be extensive due to the small size of the axons. Although it has been possible to induce focal demyelinating lesions in the optic nerves of cats [25, 53] and monkeys [61], attempts to induce such lesions in rodent have resulted in extensive axon degeneration. A major difference in the pathology induced by the different toxins is the extent of astrocyte loss induced and the speed of myelin sheath breakdown (Table 1). In the case of the injected toxins, demyelination is synchronized, and the initial tissue response to demyelination occurs in the absence of the toxin. However, with a systemic toxin such as cuprizone, demyelination is progressive, and initially the tissue response to

**Table 1** Following injection of different toxins into white matter tracts of the central nervous system to induce demyelination, the nature of subsequent remyelination is influenced by which glial cells are killed, and in general, astrocyte loss is associated with Schwann cell remyelination. In addition, the choice of toxin influences the speed of post-exposure demyelination and its synchronicity

| Toxin | Time of demyelination relative to exposure | Synchronous | Type of cell killed | | | Nature of remyelination | |
|---|---|---|---|---|---|---|---|
| | | | Oligodendrocytes | Astrocytes | OPCs | Oligodendrocyte | Schwann cell |
| Ethidium bromide | Slight delay | Small variation | Yes | Yes | Yes | Yes | Yes Major in spinal cord Minor in rostral cerebellar peduncle |
| Lysolecithin | Rapid | Yes | Some survive | Minor loss | ? | Yes | Minor |
| 6-Aminonicotinamide | Rapid | Yes | Yes | Yes | ? | Occasional | Yes |
| Endotoxin | ? | ? | Yes | Yes | ? | Occasional | Yes |
| Anti-galactocerebroside antibodies plus complement | Rapid | Yes | Yes | No | ? | Yes | Rare |
| Cuprizone | Prolonged exposure | No | Yes | No | No | Yes | Very occasional |

demyelination occurs in the presence of the toxin. Such differences have implications when analysing molecular changes associated with demyelination and remyelination. By comparing lysolecithin with ethidium bromide-induced lesions, it is possible to observe the influences astrocytes have on remyelination [17].

### 2.1.1   Lysolecithin (Lysophosphatidyl Choline)

Hall [45] was the first to use this membrane-dissolving agent as a demyelinating agent. It has since been used in numerous studies in mouse, rat, rabbit and cat. It is normally used as a 1% saline solution. At this strength, 1 µl injected into the white matter of the spinal cord of a rat or mouse produces an ellipsoid-shaped area of demyelination that extends over 3–8 mm (depending on the speed of injection and bore of the injecting needle). It has a particular toxicity for myelin and spares some but not the majority of oligodendrocytes [5, 73], which can be distinguished from newly generated oligodendrocytes by the myelin lamellae that surround them [56, 73]. There may also be some survival of progenitors. There is some loss of axons and astrocytes around the injection site. The majority of the demyelinated axons are remyelinated by oligodendrocytes (Fig. 1). However, some axons, particularly those in the center of the area of demyelination, are remyelinated by Schwann cells. If lesions are large, or poor technique causes excessive axon degeneration, Schwann cell remyelination can be extensive. In young animals, lysolecithin lesions in the spinal cord of all species remyelinate rapidly. However, remyelination in older animals occurs more slowly [84]. Following lysolecithin-induced demyelination in the rabbit, remyelination is incomplete even after 6 months [13]. In the caudal cerebellar peduncle, remyelination is faster after demyelination with lysolecithin than with ethidium bromide or Gal-C antibodies [98]. When injected into the optic nerve of monkeys, remyelination is poor in contrast to lesions made in the spinal cord [61]. Lysolecithin lesions have been induced in the shiverer mouse spinal cord to examine remyelination following cell transplant into and at a distance from the area of demyelination [42]. Injection of the calcium ionophore ionomycin has been used to induce demyelination in the spinal cord of rats and produces changes not unlike those caused by lysolecithin [89], after which axons are mainly remyelinated by oligodendrocytes.

### 2.1.2   Ethidium Bromide

Ethidium bromide was first used as an infusion into the cisterna magna of rats [82, 100] but is now most commonly injected directly into white matter tracts, either as a 0.05% or 0.1% saline solution depending on the tract targeted. One microliter injected into the dorsal funiculus of the rat spinal cord results in a much larger area of demyelination than can be induced with lysolecithin. Lesions can involve almost all of the dorsal funiculus and extend 4–8 mm longitudinally. This DNA-intercalating agent kills both astrocytes and oligodendrocytes [15] as well as oligodendrocyte progenitors

[86] throughout the demyelinated area. In young animals (<3 months), remyelination is rapid and undertaken mainly by oligodendrocytes (60%–80% of demyelinated axons); in older animals (>5 months), remyelination is slower, and an increased percentage (up to 80%) are remyelinated by Schwann cells (Fig. 2). Ethidium bromide also produces demyelinating lesions in the caudal cerebellar peduncles (CCP) of rats, where the lesions have a cross-sectional area of 0.6 mm$^2$ when 4 μl of 0.01% ethidium bromide is injected [98] (Fig. 3). The extent of Schwann cell

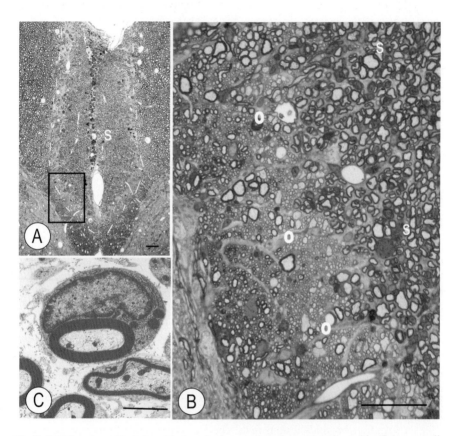

**Fig. 2** Ethidium bromide-induced lesions in the spinal cord are remyelinated by Schwann cells and oligodendrocytes. Schwann cell remyelination predominates in the center of the area of remyelination in the spinal cord of rats. **A** Low-power toluidine blue-stained 1-μm resin section of a remyelinated area in the spinal cord of a 5-month-old rat 1 month after its induction. The area of remyelination is outlined by the *broken white line*, and the *box* indicates the area shown in higher magnification **B**. The resolution offered by well-fixed resin-embedded tissue allows oligodendrocyte (*o*) and Schwann cell (*s*) remyelination to be distinguished from normally myelinated white matter. **C** Schwann cell myelin has a greater periodicity than oligodendrocyte myelin, and the myelinating cell is surrounded by a basal lamina and separated from adjacent myelinated axons by a larger-than-normal extracellular space in which collagen fibers are present. Bar in **A**=150 μm, **B**=15 μm and **C**=3 μm

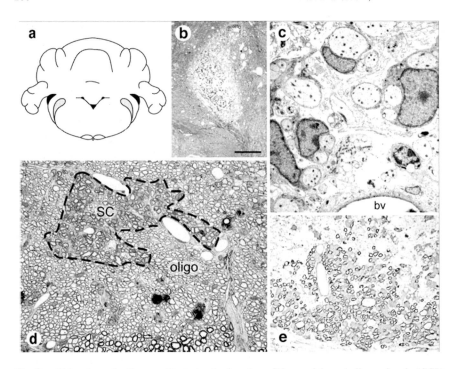

**Fig. 3 a** This schematic diagram illustrates the location of the caudal cerebellar peduncle (CCP) (*pale-shaded areas*) in adult rats. **b** Following stereotactic injection of ethidium bromide into the CCP, the demyelinated lesion can be identified on resin sections stained with toluidine blue (14-day lesion in an old rat). **c** At the lesion core, especially in the vicinity of blood vessels (BV), large numbers of premyelinating Schwann cells are seen engaging demyelinated axons 14 days after lesion induction (dpl). **d** At 66 dpl, the process of remyelination is largely completed in both young and old animals. Areas of Schwann cell remyelination, in the vicinity of blood vessels, are identified on morphological criteria within dotted region (**d**) and by expression of the peripheral myelin protein $P_0$ (**e**). Scale bar in **b** = 250 μm, **c** = 3.5 μm, **d** = 25 μm, **e** = 20 μm. (From [85], with permission)

remyelination in lesions made at this site is considerably less than in spinal cord lesions and even in old animals constitutes less than 15% of total remyelination (Fig. 3). Ethidium bromide lesions in the cervical spinal cord of rats have been used for functional studies [51], while the CCP lesion has been used in remyelination biology studies including analysis of the effects of repeat lesioning at the same site [79] and the effects of growth factors, steroids, age and the presence of myelin debris on remyelination [48, 58, 80]. The toxin also produces demyelinating lesions in the spinal cords of cats [15] and pigs (W.F. Blakemore, unpublished observations), and in both species, the predominant remyelinating cells are Schwann cells.

It is now clearer why ethidium bromide lesions in the spinal cord show extensive Schwann cell remyelination. Initially, it was thought that these cells were generated from the spinal nerve roots or peripheral nerves associated with blood vessels or present in the pia mater, since Schwann cells were always seen adjacent to these structures [37]. However, several lines of evidence provide a strong case that most remyelinating Schwann cells are generated from endogenous CNS precursors [16]. Whether all Schwann cells present in astrocyte-free areas of demyelination come from this source is currently unclear. Injection of ethidium bromide results in demyelinated axons lying in an astrocyte-free environment, and OPCs are rapidly recruited into the area of demyelination soon after lesion induction [86, 93]. This results in OPC exposure to an environment rich in bone morphogenic proteins (BMPs) produced by infiltrating macrophages and low in Noggin because of the absence of astrocytes [40, 91]. Such an environment in vitro inhibits oligodendrocyte differentiation from OPCs [44] and induces neural crest lineage differentiation from glial precursors during development [75]. Moreover, by using EB lesions exposed to X-irradiation to deplete endogenous precursors and hence prevent their contribution to remyelination, transplanted neonatal and adult OPCs can be shown to give rise to both oligodendrocytes and Schwann cells [33, 55]. Exposure of adult OPCs in vitro to BMPs also results in Schwann cell differentiation [33].

A further, frequently seen feature of EB lesions, especially in older animals, is the prolonged presence of myelin debris in the extracellular space and its association with delayed remyelination [43, 48, 84]. Recent studies have shown that myelin debris impairs remyelination by inhibiting OPC differentiation into oligodendrocytes rather than by influencing OPC recruitment [58].

### 2.1.3  Anti-galactocerebroside Antibodies and Complement

Galactocerebroside is a major sphingolipid constituent of myelin, and antibodies to these molecules identify oligodendrocytes in tissue culture. Large volumes (4 μl) are required to induce demyelination with this preparation [56]. It is very axon-sparing, and the areas of demyelination are shorter in length but involve a greater area of the dorsal funiculus than those induced by lysolecithin. Oligodendrocytes usually undertake remyelination unless the lesions are large, in which case Schwann cells remyelinate axons in the center of the lesions. Some oligodendrocytes survive within the area of demyelination. The main advantage of antibody-mediated `demyelination over lysolecithin is that it is more axon sparing. The same approach has also been used to induce demyelination in the adult rat caudal cerebellar peduncle, creating a lesion predominantly remyelinated by oligodendrocytes [98]. Anatomically targeted oligodendrocyte death can also be induced by recombination in transgenic mice carrying a floxed diptheria toxin (fragment A) gene under the CNP promoter following stereotactic injection of a Cre-expressing virus [22].

### 2.1.4  X-Irradiation

Although X-irradiation does not result in demyelination, it provides a valuable tool for creating demyelinating lesions devoid of endogenous remyelinating capacity.

These lesions are useful in investigating the remyelinating potential of transplanted glial cell preparations or exploring the reasons for remyelination failure in MS. X-irradiating the rat spinal cord with a single dose of 40 Gy of X-irradiation inhibits remyelination by depleting tissue of its endogenous oligodendrocyte progenitor cell (OPC) population [21, 46]. When demyelinating lesions are made in tissue exposed to 40 Gy of X-irradiation, the host cells do not remyelinate if the length of tissue irradiated is sufficiently long (usually 4 cm) to preclude OPC repopulation of tissue from nonirradiated tissue. This takes place at a rate determined by the animals' age [30], and provided the length of X-irradiation takes this into account any cell observed in the post-transplant demyelinated area can be judged to be transplant-derived. In addition to its use in evaluating the remyelinating potential of different progenitors, this approach has also been used to illustrate the inhibitory effect of astrocytes on remyelination [20] and the limited remyelinating potential of mature oligodendrocytes [32, 56, 94]. The use of X-irradiation to deplete endogenous OPCs also provides a system to compare the relative remyelinating capacity of endogenous adult and transplanted neonatal OPCs [19] and, by further manipulation, to model large areas of OPC-depleted demyelination. This is done by creating an OPC depletion zone between a source of transplanted or endogenous OPCs and a demyelinated area that must be repopulated before OPCs can interact with demyelinated axons (Fig. 4). Since repopulation takes time, this delays the interaction of OPCs with demyelinated axons and thus allows examination of the consequences of dissociating the process of remyelination from that of demyelination [17]. These studies form the basis for the proposed temporal mismatch hypothesis to explain failed remyelination in MS [29]. According to this hypothesis, non-remyelinated MS lesions arise because OPCs are destroyed along with oligodendrocytes during the destructive phase of lesion generation. Then because areas of demyelination in MS are larger than those induced in experimental animals and repopulation of OPC-depleted tissue is slow in older individuals, the repopulating OPCs arrive amongst the demyelinated axons after the disappearance of the inflammatory response associated with demyelination and necessary for activation of OPCs and generation of replacement oligodendrocytes. This hypothesis provides an explanation why OPCs and premyelinating oligodendrocytes can reside adjacent to demyelinated axons without remyelination occurring [27, 28, 36, 96, 97].

### 2.1.5  X-Irradiated Ethidium Bromide Lesions and Transplantation

The X-irradiated ethidium bromide model has been extensively used to examine the myelin-generating potential of different cell preparations. In general, there has been a close relationship between the ability of a cell preparation to generate oligodendrocytes in vitro and its ability to generate oligodendrocytes following introduction into lesions 3 days after their induction [90]. CNS preparations lacking the ability to generate significant numbers of oligodendrocytes in vitro, notably human embryonic spinal cord [26] and human adult neural precursor cells [2], as well as certain peripheral stem cell preparations such as bone marrow mesenchymal

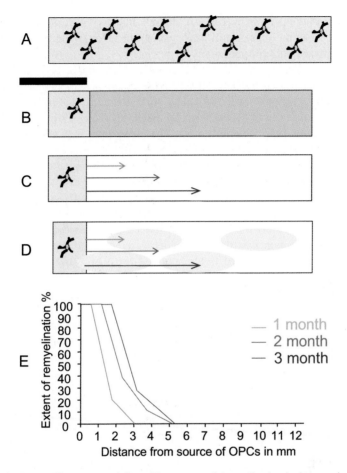

**Fig. 4** This diagram illustrates modeling of large areas of demyelination in the rat spinal cord by placing areas of demyelination at a distance from a source of oligodendrocyte progenitor cells (OPCs). The normal CNS contains oligodendrocyte progenitor cells (**A**), which, in the rat, can be almost completely depleted by exposing tissue to 40 Gy of X-irradiation (**B**). Depleted tissue is then progressively repopulated by OPCs from adjacent nonirradiated tissue at an age-dependent rate (0.5 mm/week in 4- to 6-month-old rats) (**C**). Placing focal areas of demyelination within the X-irradiated tissue means OPCs have to repopulate the OPC-depleted tissue before they can inter-act with the demyelinated axons (**D**) a situation that mimics what would exist in a large area of OPC-depleted demyelination. This approach makes it possible to show a delayed interaction between OPCs and demyelinated axons results in impaired remyelination as can be seen when the extent of remyelination at different distance from the source of OPCs is plotted for different sur-vival times (**E**). From this graph it is apparent that less myelination occurs during the 2nd month than in the first and is further reduced during the 3rd month

stromal cells [3, 4, 83], have generated Schwann cells within X-EB lesions. However, these data do not imply that this form of remyelination would necessarily happen following the therapeutic use of such cells in MS. Mesenchymal stem cells may well have therapeutic value in multiple sclerosis through their ability to modulate

the immune system [62]. However, it is unlikely that they would generate remyelinating cells, since the presence of astrocytes in the areas of demyelination would
preclude Schwann cell differentiation.

An issue that remains to be fully explored, which cannot be examined using
immune-mediated models of demyelination, is the requirement for haplotype matching
of host and donor tissue in order to achieve sustained transplant-mediated remyelination. So far only one publication has addressed this issue in adult animals, and it
used X-EB lesions [95]. This lesion was chosen because it would be possible to
monitor survival of transplant-generated tissue without using immunogenic trans-
plant-markers such as GFP and Lac-Z. By transplanting a mixed glial cell prepared
from a donor mismatched for MHC-1 and MHC-2 to the host, this study showed
that in vivo OPCs and oligodendrocytes do not express MHC-1 or -2 but could be
induced to express MHC-1 in the presence of pro-inflammatory cytokines such as
IFN-γ. Transplanted cells were rejected within 1 month; however, when the transplanted cell preparation was depleted of its astrocytes and thereby enriched for
OPCs, the transplant-generated tissue survived for over 2 months. When this is
taken with unpublished studies showing that transplanted cells are more readily
rejected when injected into X-irradiated host tissue than when introduced into normal
tissue, these preliminary studies would indicate that with its anti-inflammatory
environment, close tissue-matching may not be required if CNS precursors are to be
used in a clinical context. In addition, it also has to be appreciated that should areas
of transplant-mediated remyelination be rejected this would likely be followed by
remyelination by host-derived cells [18].

## 2.2   Systemic Toxins

There are a number of models of toxin-induced demyelination in which demyelination is more widespread. These include demyelination induced by intrathecal
injection of Cholera toxin B-subunit conjugated to saporin [50] and cuprizone
intoxication in mice.

### 2.2.1   Cuprizone

Cuprizone intoxication in mice results in demyelination of the corpus callosum,
internal capsule, white matter in the thalamus, anterior commissure and cerebellar
peduncles [8]. The early studies of Blakemore and Ludwin used much higher
doses of cuprizone (0.5%–0.6%) than are currently used (0.2%) and evaluated
remyelination in the rostral (superior) cerebellar peduncle [9–12, 54, 65–69].
Today the corpus callosum is the site used for analysis [72, 74], and this, together
with the lower dose of cuprizone, has led to a less reproducible model of demyelination [91]. Moreover, the change in the mouse strain used has resulted in a significant incidence of axon degeneration [49, 91], which increases when using aged

**Table 2** The early cuprizone intoxication studies of Ludwin and Blakemore used outbred Swiss mice. Little evidence of axon degeneration was reported or detected when sections of the corpus callosum from these experiments were re-examined; however, recent studies using lower doses of cuprizone in C57Bl/6 mice have found significant evidence of axon degeneration, and interestingly, the incidence of axonal degeneration increases with age. The table shows the incidence of axonal spheroids in one micron plastic section taken from the corpus callosum of young and old Swiss and C57Bl/6 mice (From [49]. Used with permission)

| | YNG Swiss | YNG C57Bl/6 | OLD Swiss | OLD C57Bl/6 |
|---|---|---|---|---|
| Dose | 0.5% | 0.2% | 0.75% | 0.4% |
| 5 Weeks of feeding | 8 (n=2) | NA | NA | NA |
| 6 Weeks of feeding | 4 (n=2) | 48 (n=3) | NA | NA |
| 7 Weeks of feeding | 7 (n=2) | NA | 3 (n=2) | 99 (n=4) |
| 8 Weeks of feeding | 8 (n =2) | NA | NA | NA |
| 10 Weeks of feeding | NA | NA | 32 (n=2) | NA |
| Mean±SE | 8±0.3[a] | 48±2.0 | 18±9.0[b] | 99±5.0 |

[a] $p=<0.05$ vs young C57Bl/6
[b] $p=<0.05$ vs old C57Bl/6

adult mice (6–7 months old) rather than the more usual 8- to 12-week-old animals [49] (Table 2).

Early cuprizone studies identified the morphological features of remyelinated axons and also established some fundamental aspects of remyelination. They established that remyelinating cells were recruited in association with demyelination [9, 66], and they confirmed in vitro observations [81] that remyelination consisted of two phases: a recruitment phase and a differentiation phase that could be blocked by continued toxin exposure [9, 14]. They also indicated that the inflammatory response stimulated by myelin sheath breakdown was important for remyelination [54, 67]. More recent studies have confirmed the importance of inflammation in this and other model systems [31, 36, 59, 60, 64] by highlighting the role of IL-1β [70] and TNF-α [6] for successful remyelination. They have also confirmed that prolonged cuprizone feeding results in remyelination failure [67] and that transplanted cells can remyelinate chronically demyelinated axons [71].

# 3 What is the Place of Toxin Models in the Study of CNS Demyelination and Remyelination?

Experimental models in neuropathology fall into two groups: those that attempt to replicate a disease process as accurately as possible and those that provide a more reductionist approach with which to study a specific aspect of a complex pathology; these have been described as disease and mechanism models, respectively [34]. Experimental autoimmune encephalomyelitis (EAE) and some viral models are examples of disease models for MS, while the toxin-induced models offer a more

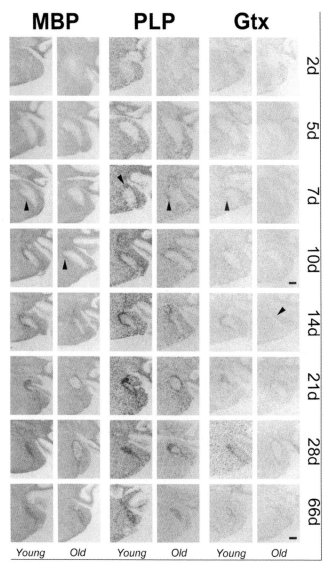

**Fig. 5** An alternative method for analysing remyelination is to document the re-expression of myelination-associated transcripts. In this figure, this has been done by in situ hybridization of ethidium bromide-induced lesions in the caudal cerebellar peduncle. Expression patterns of mRNAs of two major myelin proteins, MBP and PLP, and the mRNA of an oligodendrocyte-specific transcription factor Gtx during remyelination are illustrated in a way that clearly reveals the differences in the tempo of remyelination in young and old adult animals. Sections were hybridized with [35]S-labelled oligonucleotide probes and visualized by autoradiography. *Arrowheads* indicate the initial point at which re-expression of each mRNA could be detected. Scale bar=50 μm. (From [85], with permission)

reductionist system for studying myelin sheath regeneration, since the processes of demyelination and remyelination have a clear temporal dissociation. That said, even this straightforward distinction may be less clear than previously thought, since some forms of MS may have more in common with toxin-induced demyelination [7], while the immune system (T cells) has a significant involvement in some toxin-induced demyelination (specifically that following lysolecithin injection) [39].

The focal toxin-induced demyelinating lesions were first introduced for secondary procedures requiring lesions in specific sites. Thus, lysolecithin lesions were made in cat and, subsequently, the rat dorsal funiculus to examine the electrophysiological properties of demyelinated and remyelinated CNS axons [35, 88], while the caudal cerebellar lesions were developed to allow the placement of secure in-dwelling cannula for infusion [80, 98]. In contrast, lesions associated with immune-mediated and virus-induced demyelination are multifocal, and thus it is difficult to correlate demyelinated areas with observed loss of function. Moreover, lesions of different ages can occur within a single animal, which makes it difficult to study the temporal progression of cellular and molecular changes. The development of a new model of focal immune-mediated injury, which is based on systemic exposure to myelin antigen and focal injection of a cytokine combination in Lewis rats, partially addresses these problems [57]. However, the extent to which this model represents primary demyelination rather than primary axonal injury in white matter is still unclear.

A further advantage of focal toxin-induced lesions is that, unlike many viral and immune-mediated models of demyelination, they are not dependent on age, stain or species. Instead, the two most widely used demyelinating toxins, lysolecithin and ethidium bromide, make lesions in any white matter tract of any species, of any sex and of any age. (The possible exception is rodent optic nerve, where it is difficult to inject solutions into the tight confines of this tissue without inducing axon injury.) Only cuprizone, a systemic toxin, has constraints on white matter tracts affected and the species in which it can be used (mouse only, although a recent study suggests that it may also demyelinate the corpus callosum of adult rats [1]). The differences imposed by these variables predominantly relate to the regenerative process. Remyelination rates progressively decrease with age (Fig. 5) due to a decline in the efficiency of precursor recruitment and especially their differentiation [86, 99] resulting from intrinsic changes in aging precursors [30] and extrinsic changes in the signaling environment [47, 102]. Aging also reveals a divergence between the sexes because males remyelinate more slowly than females as they age [63]. Studying the causes of both the age- and gender-associated declines in remyelination efficiency allows us to identify factors critical for efficient remyelination and hence, in theory, identify pro-remyelination strategies. In this regard, the focal toxin models are especially useful, since the acute process of demyelination has a clear temporal separation from the subsequent repair process, allowing study of the specific reparative roles played by individual molecules. In contrast, the two processes occur simultaneously in EAE, making it difficult to separate an effect that renders the environment less hostile to remyelination from an effect that truly makes remyelination more effective.

# References

1. Adamo AM, Paez PM, Escobar Cabrera OE, Wolfson M, Franco PG, Pasquini JM, Soto EF (2006) Remyelination after cuprizone-induced demyelination in the rat is stimulated by apotransferrin. Exp Neurol 198:519–529
2. Akiyama Y, Honmou O, Kato T, Uede T, Hashi K, Kocsis JD (2001) Transplantation of clonal neural precursor cells derived from adult human brain establishes functional peripheral myelin in the rat spinal cord. Exp Neurol 167:27–39
3. Akiyama Y, Radtke C, Honmou O, Kocsis JD (2002) Remyelination of the spinal cord following intravenous delivery of bone marrow cells. Glia 39:229–236
4. Akiyama Y, Radtke C, Kocsis JD (2002) Remyelination of the rat spinal cord by transplantation of identified bone marrow stromal cells. J Neurosci 22:6623–6630
5. Arnett HA, Fancy SP, Alberta JA, Zhao C, Plant SR, Kaing S, Raine CS, Rowitch DH, Franklin RJ, Stiles CD (2004) Bhlh transcription factor olig1 is required to repair demyelinated lesions in the CNS. Science 306:2111–2115
6. Arnett HA, Mason J, Marino M, Suzuki K, Matsushima GK, Ting JP (2001) TNF-alpha promotes proliferation of oligodendrocyte progenitors and remyelination. Nat Neurosci 4:1116–1122
7. Barnett MH, Prineas JW (2004) Relapsing and remitting multiple sclerosis: Pathology of the newly forming lesion. Ann Neurol 55:458–468
8. Blakemore WF (1972) Observations on oligodendrocyte degeneration, the resolution of status spongiosus and remyelination in cuprizone intoxication in mice. J Neurocytol 1:413–426
9. Blakemore WF (1973) Demyelination of the superior cerebellar peduncle in the mouse induced by cuprizone. J Neurol Sci 20:63–72
10. Blakemore WF (1973) Remyelination of the superior cerebellar peduncle in the mouse following demyelination induced by feeding cuprizone. J Neurol Sci 20:73–83
11. Blakemore WF (1974) Pattern of remyelination in the CNS. Nature 249:577–578
12. Blakemore WF (1974) Remyelination of the superior cerebellar peduncle in old mice following demyelination induced by cuprizone. J Neurol Sci 22:121–126
13. Blakemore WF (1978) Observations on remyelination in the rabbit spinal cord following demyelination induced by lysolecithin. Neuropathol Appl Neurobiol 4:47–59
14. Blakemore WF (1981) Observations on myelination and remyelination in central nervous system. In: Development in the nervous system. Gerrod DR, Feldman JD (eds) Cambridge University Press, Cambridge, pp 289–308.
15. Blakemore WF (1982) Ethidium bromide induced demyelination in the spinal cord of the cat. Neuropathol Appl Neurobiol 8:365–375
16. Blakemore WF (2005) The case for a central nervous system (CNS) origin for the Schwann cells that remyelinate CNS axons following concurrent loss of oligodendrocytes and astrocytes. Neuropathol Appl Neurobiol 31:1–10
17. Blakemore WF, Chari DM, Gilson JM, Crang AJ (2002) Modelling large areas of demyelination in the rat reveals the potential and possible limitations of transplanted glial cells for remyelination in the CNS. Glia 38:155–168
18. Blakemore WF, Crang AJ, Franklin RJ, Tang K, Ryder S (1995) Glial cell transplants that are subsequently rejected can be used to influence regeneration of glial cell environments in the CNS. Glia 13:79–91
19. Blakemore WF, Gilson JM, Crang AJ (2000) Transplanted glial cells migrate over a greater distance and remyelinate demyelinated lesions more rapidly than endogenous remyelinating cells. J Neurosci Res 61:288–294
20. Blakemore WF, Gilson JM, Crang AJ (2003) The presence of astrocytes in areas of demyelination influences remyelination following transplantation of oligodendrocyte progenitors. Exp Neurol 184:955–963
21. Blakemore WF, Patterson RC (1978) Suppression of remyelination in the CNS by x-irradiation. Acta Neuropathol (Berl) 42:105–113

22. Brockschnieder D, Lappe-Siefke C, Goebbels S, Boesl MR, Nave KA, Riethmacher D (2004) Cell depletion due to diphtheria toxin fragment a after Cre-mediated recombination. Mol Cell Biol 24:7636–7642

23. Bunge MB, Bunge RP, Ris H (1961) Ultrastructural study of remyelination in an experimental lesion in adult cat spinal cord. J Biophys Biochem Cytol 10:67–94

24. Butzkueven H, Zhang JG, Soilu-Hanninen M, Hochrein H, Chionh F, Shipham KA, Emery B, Turnley AM, Petratos S, Ernst M, Bartlett PF, Kilpatrick TJ (2002) Lif receptor signaling limits immune-mediated demyelination by enhancing oligodendrocyte survival. Nat Med 8:613–619

25. Carroll WM, Jennings AR, Ironside LJ (1998) Identification of the adult resting progenitor cell by autoradiographic tracking of oligodendrocyte precursors in experimental CNS demyelination. Brain 121:293–302

26. Chandran S, Compston A, Jauniaux E, Gilson J, Blakemore W, Svendsen C (2004) Differential generation of oligodendrocytes from human and rodent embryonic spinal cord neural precursors. Glia 47:314–324

27. Chang A, Nishiyama A, Peterson J, Prineas J, Trapp BD (2000) Ng2-positive oligodendrocyte progenitor cells in adult human brain and multiple sclerosis lesions. J Neurosci 20:6404–6412

28. Chang A, Tourtellotte WW, Rudick R, Trapp BD (2002) Premyelinating oligodendrocytes in chronic lesions of multiple sclerosis. N Engl J Med 346:165–173

29. Chari DM, Blakemore WF (2002) New insights into remyelination failure in multiple sclerosis: Implications for glial cell transplantation. Mult Scler 8:271–277

30. Chari DM, Crang AJ, Blakemore WF (2003) Decline in rate of colonization of oligodendrocyte progenitor cell (OPC)-depleted tissue by adult OPCs with age. J Neuropathol Exp Neurol 62:908–916

31. Chari DM, Zhao C, Kotter MR, Blakemore WF, Franklin RJM (2006) Corticosteroids delay remyelination of experimental demyelination in the rodent central nervous system. J Neurosci Res 83:594–605

32. Crang AJ, Gilson J, Blakemore WF (1998) The demonstration by transplantation of the very restricted remyelinating potential of post-mitotic oligodendrocytes. J Neurocytol 27:541–553

33. Crang AJ, Gilson JM, Li WW, Blakemore WF (2004) The remyelinating potential and in vitro differentiation of MOG-expressing oligodendrocyte precursors isolated from the adult rat CNS. Eur J Neurosci 20:1445–1460

34. Dubois-Dalcq M, Ffrench-Constant C, Franklin RJ (2005) Enhancing central nervous system remyelination in multiple sclerosis. Neuron 48:9–12

35. Felts PA, Smith KJ (1992) Conduction properties of central nerve fibers remyelinated by Schwann cells. Brain Res 574:178–192

36. Foote AK, Blakemore WF (2005) Inflammation stimulates remyelination in areas of chronic demyelination. Brain 128:528–539

37. Franklin RJM, Blakemore WF (1993) Requirements for Schwann cell migration within CNS environments: A viewpoint. Int J Dev Neurosci 11:641–649

38. Franklin RJM, Goldman JE (2004) Remyelination by endogenous cells. In: Lazzarini RA (ed) Myelin biology and disorders. Elsevier, San Diego, 173–196

39. Ghasemlou N, Jeong SY, Lacroix S, David S (2007) T cells contribute to lysophosphatidylcholine-induced macrophage activation and demyelination in the CNS. Glia 55:294–302

40. Gilson JM, Blakemore WF (2002) Schwann cell remyelination is not replaced by oligodendrocyte remyelination following ethidium bromide induced demyelination. Neuroreport 13:1205–1208

41. Gledhill RF, McDonald WI (1977) Morphological characteristics of central demyelination and remyelination: A single-fiber study. Ann Neurol 1:552–560

42. Gout O, Gansmuller A, Baumann N, Gumpel M (1988) Remyelination by transplanted oligodendrocytes of a demyelinated lesion in the spinal cord of the adult shiverer mouse. Neurosci Lett 87:195–199

43. Graca DL, Blakemore WF (1986) Delayed remyelination in rat spinal cord following ethidium bromide injection. Neuropathol Appl Neurobiol 12:593–605
44. Grinspan JB, Edell E, Carpio DF, Beesley JS, Lavy L, Pleasure D, Golden JA (2000) Stage-specific effects of bone morphogenetic proteins on the oligodendrocyte lineage. J Neurobiol 43:1–17
45. Hall SM (1972) The effect of injections of lysophosphatidyl choline into white matter of the adult mouse spinal cord. J Cell Sci 10:535–546
46. Hinks GL, Chari DM, O'Leary MT, Zhao C, Keirstead HS, Blakemore WF, Franklin RJM (2001) Depletion of endogenous oligodendrocyte progenitors rather than increased availability of survival factors is a likely explanation for enhanced survival of transplanted oligodendrocyte progenitors in x-irradiated compared to normal CNS. Neuropathol Appl Neurobiol 27:59–67
47. Hinks GL, Franklin RJM (2000) Delayed changes in growth factor gene expression during slow remyelination in the CNS of aged rats. Mol Cell Neurosci 16:542–556
48. Ibanez C, Shields SA, El-Etr M, Baulieu EE, Schumacher M, Franklin RJ (2004) Systemic progesterone administration results in a partial reversal of the age-associated decline in CNS remyelination following toxin-induced demyelination in male rats. Neuropathol Appl Neurobiol 30:80–89
49. Irvine KA, Blakemore WF (2006) Age increases axon loss associated with primary demyelination in cuprizone-induced demyelination in c57bl/6 mice. J Neuroimmunol 175:69–76
50. Jasmin L, Janni G, Moallem TM, Lappi DA, Ohara PT (2000) Schwann cells are removed from the spinal cord after effecting recovery from paraplegia. J Neurosci 20:9215–9223
51. Jeffery ND, Blakemore WF (1997) Locomotor deficits induced by experimental spinal cord demyelination are abolished by spontaneous remyelination. Brain 120:27–37
52. Jeffery ND, Crang AJ, O'Leary MT, Hodge SJ, Blakemore WF (1999) Behavioural consequences of oligodendrocyte progenitor cell transplantation into experimental demyelinating lesions in the rat spinal cord. Eur J Neurosci 11:1508–1514
53. Jennings AR, Kirilak Y, Carroll WM (2002) In situ characterisation of oligodendrocyte progenitor cells in adult mammalian optic nerve. J Neurocytol 31:27–39
54. Johnson ES, Ludwin SK (1981) The demonstration of recurrent demyelination and remyelination of axons in the central nervous system. Acta Neuropathol (Berl) 53:93–98
55. Keirstead HS, Ben-Hur T, Rogister B, O'Leary MT, Dubois-Dalcq M, Blakemore WF (1999) Polysialylated neural cell adhesion molecule-positive CNS precursors generate both oligodendrocytes and Schwann cells to remyelinate the CNS after transplantation. J Neurosci 19:7529–7536
56. Keirstead HS, Blakemore WF (1997) Identification of post-mitotic oligodendrocytes incapable of remyelination within the demyelinated adult spinal cord. J Neuropathol Exp Neurol 56:1191–1201
57. Kerschensteiner M, Stadelmann C, Buddeberg BS, Merkler D, Bareyre FM, Anthony DC, Linington C, Bruck W, Schwab ME (2004) Targeting experimental autoimmune encephalomyelitis lesions to a predetermined axonal tract system allows for refined behavioral testing in an animal model of multiple sclerosis. Am J Pathol 164:1455–1469
58. Kotter MR, Li WW, Zhao C, Franklin RJ (2006) Myelin impairs CNS remyelination by inhibiting oligodendrocyte precursor cell differentiation. J Neurosci 26:328–332
59. Kotter MR, Setzu A, Sim FJ, Van Rooijen N, Franklin RJM (2001) Macrophage depletion impairs oligodendrocyte remyelination following lysolecithin-induced demyelination. Glia 35:204–212
60. Kotter MR, Zhao C, van Rooijen N, Franklin RJM (2005) Macrophage-depletion induced impairment of experimental cns remyelination is associated with a reduced oligodendrocyte progenitor cell response and altered growth factor expression. Neurobiol Dis 18:166–175
61. Lachapelle F, Bachelin C, Moissonnier P, Nait-Oumesmar B, Hidalgo A, Fontaine D, Baron-Van Evercooren A (2005) Failure of remyelination in the nonhuman primate optic nerve. Brain Pathol 15:198–207
62. Le Blanc K, Ringden O (2006) Mesenchymal stem cells: Properties and role in clinical bone marrow transplantation. Curr Opin Immunol 18:586–591

63. Li WW, Penderis J, Zhao C, Schumacher M, Franklin RJM (2006) Females remyelinate more efficiently than males following demyelination in the aged but not young adult CNS. Exp Neurol 202:250–254

64. Li WW, Setzu A, Zhao C, Franklin RJM (2005) Minocycline-mediated inhibition of microglia activation impairs oligodendrocyte progenitor cell responses and remyelination in a non-immune model of demyelination. J Neuroimmunol 158:58–66

65. Ludwin SK (1978) Central nervous system demyelination and remyelination in the mouse: An ultrastructural study of cuprizone toxicity. Lab Invest 39:597–612

66. Ludwin SK (1979) An autoradiographic study of cellular proliferation in remyelination of the central nervous system. Am J Pathol 95:683–696

67. Ludwin SK (1980) Chronic demyelination inhibits remyelination in the central nervous system. An analysis of contributing factors. Lab Invest 43:382–387

68. Ludwin SK, Johnson ES (1981) Evidence for a "dying-back" gliopathy in demyelinating disease. Ann Neurol 9:301–305

69. Ludwin SK, Sternberger NH (1984) An immunohistochemical study of myelin proteins during remyelination in the central nervous system. Acta Neuropathol (Berl) 63:240–248

70. Mason JL, Suzuki K, Chaplin DD, Matsushima GK (2001) Interleukin-1beta promotes repair of the CNS. J Neurosci 21:7046–7052

71. Mason JL, Toews A, Hostettler JD, Morell P, Suzuki K, Goldman JE, Matsushima GK (2004) Oligodendrocytes and progenitors become progressively depleted within chronically demyelinated lesions. Am J Pathol 164:1673–1682

72. Matsushima GK, Morell P (2001) The neurotoxicant, cuprizone, as a model to study demyelination and remyelination in the central nervous system. Brain Pathol 11:107–116

73. McKay JS, Blakemore WF, Franklin RJM (1998) Trapidil-mediated inhibition of CNS remyelination results from reduced numbers and impaired differentiation of oligodendrocytes. Neuropathol Appl Neurobiol 24:498–506

74. Morell P, Barrett CV, Mason JL, Toews AD, Hostettler JD, Knapp GW, Matsushima GK (1998) Gene expression in brain during cuprizone-induced demyelination and remyelination. Mol Cell Neurosci 12:220–227

75. Mujtaba T, Mayer-Proschel M, Rao MS (1998) A common neural progenitor for the CNS and PNS. Dev Biol 200:1–15

76. Murray JA, Blakemore WF (1980) The relationship between internodal length and fibre diameter in the spinal cord of the cat. J Neurol Sci 45:29–41

77. O'Leary MT, Blakemore WF (1997) Use of a rat y chromosome probe to determine the long-term survival of glial cells transplanted into areas of CNS demyelination. J Neurocytol 26:191–206

78. O'Leary MT, Hinks GL, Charlton HM, Franklin RJM (2002) Increasing local levels of IGF-I MRNA expression using adenoviral vectors does not alter oligodendrocyte remyelination in the CNS of aged rats. Mol Cell Neurosci 19:32–42

79. Penderis J, Shields SA, Franklin RJ (2003) Impaired remyelination and depletion of oligodendrocyte progenitors does not occur following repeated episodes of focal demyelination in the rat central nervous system. Brain 126:1382–1391

80. Penderis J, Woodruff RH, Lakatos A, Li WW, Dunning MD, Zhao C, Marchionni M, Franklin RJM (2003) Increasing local levels of neuregulin (glial growth factor-2) by direct infusion into areas of demyelination does not alter remyelination in the rat CNS. Eur J Neurosci 18:2253–2264

81. Raine CS, Diaz M, Pakingan M, Bornstein MB (1978) Antiserum-induced dissociation of myelinogenesis in vitro. An ultrastructural study. Lab Invest 38:397–403

82. Reynolds R, Wilkin GP (1993) Cellular reaction to an acute demyelinating/remyelinating lesion of the rat brain stem: Localisation of GD3 ganglioside immunoreactivity. J Neurosci Res 36:405–422

83. Sasaki M, Honmou O, Akiyama Y, Uede T, Hashi K, Kocsis JD (2001) Transplantation of an acutely isolated bone marrow fraction repairs demyelinated adult rat spinal cord axons. Glia 35:26–34

84. Shields SA, Gilson JM, Blakemore WF, Franklin RJM (1999) Remyelination occurs as extensively but more slowly in old rats compared to young rats following gliotoxin-induced CNS demyelination. Glia 28:77–83

85. Sim FJ, Hinks GL, Franklin RJM (2000) The re-expression of the homeodomain transcription factor Gtx during remyelination of experimentally-induced demyelinating lesions in young and old rat brain. Neuroscience 100:131–139

86. Sim FJ, Zhao C, Penderis J, Franklin RJM (2002) The age-related decrease in CNS remyelination efficiency is attributable to an impairment of both oligodendrocyte progenitor recruitment and differentiation. J Neurosci 22:2451–2459

87. Smith KJ, Blakemore WF, McDonald WI (1979) Central remyelination restores secure conduction. Nature 280:395–396

88. Smith KJ, Blakemore WF, McDonald WI (1981) The restoration of conduction by central remyelination. Brain 104:383–404

89. Smith KJ, Hall SM (1994) Central demyelination induced in vivo by the calcium ionophore ionomycin. Brain 117:1351–1356

90. Smith PM, Blakemore WF (2000) Porcine neural progenitors require commitment to the oligodendrocyte lineage prior to transplantation in order to achieve significant remyelination of demyelinated lesions in the adult CNS. Eur J Neurosci 12:2414–2424

91. Stidworthy MF, Genoud S, Suter U, Mantei N, Franklin RJM (2003) Quantifying the early stages of remyelination following cuprizone-induced demyelination. Brain Pathol 13:329–339

92. Talbott JF, Cao Q, Enzmann GU, Benton RL, Achim V, Cheng XX, Mills MD, Rao MS, Whittemore SR (2006) Schwann cell-like differentiation by adult oligodendrocyte precursor cells following engraftment into the demyelinated spinal cord is BMP-dependent. Glia 54:147–159

93. Talbott JF, Loy DN, Liu Y, Qiu MS, Bunge MB, Rao MS, Whittemore SR (2005) Endogenous nkx2.2+/olig2+ oligodendrocyte precursor cells fail to remyelinate the demyelinated adult rat spinal cord in the absence of astrocytes. Exp Neurol 192:11–24

94. Targett MP, Sussman J, Scolding N, O'Leary MT, Compston DA, Blakemore WF (1996) Failure to achieve remyelination of demyelinated rat axons following transplantation of glial cells obtained from the adult human brain. Neuropathol Appl Neurobiol 22:199–206

95. Tepavcevic V, Blakemore WF (2006) Haplotype matching is not an essential requirement to achieve remyelination of demyelinating CNS lesions. Glia 54:880–890

96. Wolswijk G (1998) Chronic stage multiple sclerosis lesions contain a relatively quiescent population of oligodendrocyte precursor cells. J Neurosci 18:601–699

97. Wolswijk G (2000) Oligodendrocyte survival, loss and birth in lesions of chronic-stage multiple sclerosis. Brain 123:105–115

98. Woodruff RH, Franklin RJM (1999) Demyelination and remyelination of the caudal cerebellar peduncle of adult rats following stereotaxic injections of lysolecithin, ethidium bromide, and complement/anti-galactocerebroside: A comparative study. Glia 25:216–228

99. Woodruff RH, Fruttiger M, Richardson WD, Franklin RJM (2004) Platelet-derived growth factor regulates oligodendrocyte progenitor numbers in adult CNS and their response following CNS demyelination. Mol Cell Neurosci 25:252–62

100. Yajima K, Suzuki K (1979) Demyelination and remyelination in the rat central nervous system following ethidium bromide injection. Lab Invest 41:385–392

101. Yao DL, Komoly S, Zhang QL, Webster HD (1994) Myelinated axons demonstrated in the CNS and PNS by anti-neurofilament immunoreactivity and Luxol fast blue counterstaining. Brain Pathol 4:97–100

102. Zhao C, Li WW, Franklin RJM (2006) Differences in the early inflammatory responses to toxin-induced demyelination are associated with the age-related decline in CNS remyelination. Neurobiol Aging 27:1298–1307

# Remyelination-Promoting Human IgMs: Developing a Therapeutic Reagent for Demyelinating Disease

A.E. Warrington(✉) and M. Rodriguez

**Abstract** Promoting remyelination following injury to the central nervous system (CNS) promises to be an effective neuroprotective strategy to limit the loss of surviving axons and prevent disability. Studies confirm that multiple sclerosis (MS) and spinal cord injury lesions contain myelinating cells and their progenitors. Recruiting these endogenous cells to remyelinate may be of therapeutic value. This review addresses the use of antibodies reactive to CNS antigens to promote remyelination. Antibody-induced remyelination in a virus-mediated model of chronic spinal cord injury was initially observed in response to treatment with CNS reactive antisera. Monoclonal mouse and human IgMs, which bind to the surface of oligodendrocytes and myelin, were later identified that were functionally equivalent to antisera. A recombinant form of a human remyelination-promoting IgM (rHIgM22) targets areas of CNS injury and promotes maximal remyelination within 5 weeks after a single low dose (25 µg/kg). The IgM isoform of this reparative antibody is required for in vivo function. We hypothesize that the IgM clusters membrane domains and

A.E. Warrington
Department of Neurology, Mayo Clinic College of Medicine, Rochester, MN 55905, USA
e-mail: Warrington.arthur@mayo.edu

M. Rodriguez (ed.), *Advances in Multiple Sclerosis and Experimental Demyelinating Diseases. Current Topics in Microbiology and Immunology 318.*
© Springer-Verlag Berlin Heidelberg 2008

associated signaling molecules on the surface of target cells. Current therapies for MS are designed to modulate inflammation. In contrast, remyelination promoting IgMs are the first potential therapeutic molecules designed to induce tissue repair by acting within the CNS at sites of damage on the cells responsible for myelin synthesis.

# 1   Multiple Sclerosis is a Disease of Myelin

Despite the recent re-examination of axon loss within the multiple sclerosis (MS) lesion, MS remains a disease primarily of myelin. Demyelination has long been the pathologic hallmark of the MS lesion. Loss of myelin is likely an early step [135] in a sequence of events leading to the loss of axons which can result in permanent neurologic deficits. Demyelination in MS is accompanied by varying degrees of inflammation, oligodendrocyte death, complement activation, antibody deposition, and gliosis [20, 79, 81, 152]. A hypothesis central to our therapeutic remyelinating strategies for MS is that demyelination is necessary but not sufficient for the development of disability. Demyelination likely predisposes axons to permanent injury via a second, immune-mediated assault [128, 129].

Models of human disease in animals confirm that demyelination is not sufficient for the development of neurologic deficits. In mice deficient in the major histocompatibility (MHC) Class I antigen-presenting arm of the immune system, virus-induced spinal cord disease results in chronic widespread demyelination without measurable neurologic deficits [125]. Axon function is largely preserved, likely due to the lack of a direct immune-mediated attack of the axon and an increase and redistribution of axonal ion channels. The implication of MHC Class I in neurologic deficit induction suggests that CD8[+] T cells are a pathologic immune effector that directly assaults demyelinated axons. CD8[+] T cells commonly mediate membrane lysis through the synthesis of perforin and Fas ligand, and perforin-deficient mice with persistent and chronic demyelination present with minimal neurologic deficits [101]. Similarly, humans with extensive CNS demyelination, identified by magnetic resonance imaging (MRI) and verified by pathologic examination of the tissue at biopsy or autopsy, can present with minimal or no neurologic deficits [93]. These data suggest that axons remain functional despite demyelination if subsequent damage is controlled. The primary function of mature myelinating oligodendrocytes may be to protect axons from external injury and to provide neurotrophic support. If true, then strategies that promote axon remyelination within a critical time period will ultimately be neuroprotective and limit permanent deficits.

# 2   Remyelination as a Normal Reparative Response

Spontaneous remyelination, visible pathologically as abnormally thin sheaths usually at the periphery of the lesion, occurs widely in patients with MS [42, 113, 149], and periods of remission may be associated with significant CNS remyelination.

Remyelination in acute MS lesions can be substantial [117]: up to 70% of MS lesions contain some degree of remyelination [80]. However, for the 50% of MS patients who suffer with progressive disease, remyelination is insufficient or may occur after the development of axonal deficits.

Remyelination in chronic MS lesions was thought to be limited, but a recent study [109] examining demyelinated lesions from 51 MS patients at autopsy reported that substantial remyelination, defined as the presence of shadow plaques, occurs in all clinical subtypes and at any time in disease progression. Therapeutic interventions to promote remyelination would ideally begin early in the disease course to limit disability, but therapy initiated late in disease may facilitate disability stabilization.

Why remyelination so often fails in MS is unclear; a number of reasons have been proposed, and the reason likely varies between individuals. Cells capable of remyelination, or factors that sustain their growth and differentiation, may be depleted from the lesion and adjacent CNS [44, 85]. In animal models of CNS damage, remyelination is accomplished by activating endogenous myelinating cells and recruiting progenitors from adjacent intact tissue [45, 102]. However, despite ineffective remyelination in MS, an abundant population of potential replacement cells, oligodendrocytes and their progenitors, are present even in chronic MS lesions [29, 30, 103, 170]. Why surviving cells fail to respond to the presence of tissue injury and demyelination is unknown, but their presence emphasizes that the lesion microenvironment is unsupportive of remyelination. Infiltrating immune cells or persistent virus infection may create a lesion environment containing a balance of inflammatory factors that inhibit remyelination. A progressive loss of axons also results in fewer substrates to remyelinate [129].

In contrast to what is observed in human disease, robust remyelination is the norm in most animal models of experimental demyelination. Demyelination can be induced by toxins such as cuprizone [21], ethidium bromide [172] or lysolecithin [51], autoimmune mechanisms (experimental autoimmune encephalomyelitis, EAE) [120], or by infection with corona virus, murine hepatitis virus (MHV) [53], or picornavirus (Theiler's murine encephalomyelitis virus or TMEV) [35, 134]. Complete spontaneous remyelination can occur in each of these models, suggesting that remyelination is a normal reparative response to injury. Lysolecithin-induced demyelination remyelinates rapidly and completely [18, 60], restoring axon conduction and recovery of motor function [61, 73, 144]. Repair is normally so quick in toxin-mediated models that it is far easier to identify agents that interfere with remyelination [16] than agents that accelerate it [18]. In most models, remyelination begins within 3 weeks of injury and is complete by 5 weeks.

An obvious difference between human MS and models of acute demyelination is a persistent activation of the immune system. MHV-induced demyelination is accompanied by ataxia and paralysis, deficits that reverse following virus clearance and remyelination [86, 148]. TMEV infection of the SJL mouse strain results in a persistent immune response directed against chronic virus antigens in the CNS. The extent of demyelination plateaus by three 3 months after virus infection [89] with limited spontaneous remyelination throughout the rest of the animal's lifespan, making this a useful model to design and test remyelination-enhancing therapies. TMEV-infected mice live with chronic demyelination for months to years. Spinal cord remyelination in the TMEV model plateaus at levels that are far from complete even after treatment with the most effective remyelination-promoting regents. The continued presence of Theiler's virus and progressive axonal injury and loss [155] likely account for the limits of histological repair and functional improvement. TMEV-infected mice develop progressive disability over the course of 3–9 months that can be measured with a number of objective performance tests [89, 125].

# 3 Strategies to Augment Remyelination

Current MS therapies have little effect on permanent and accumulating deficits. Most were designed to control the inflammation-based, MRI-visible aspects of the disease and were approved for clinical use based on a decrease in the relapse rate in short-term trials and a reduction of gadolinium-enhancing MRI lesions, a surrogate for reduced inflammation [68, 106]. Immunosuppressive therapies may not be efficacious in MS simply because inflammation is likely also required for CNS repair [19, 52]. Remyelination in active MS lesions [26] and in mouse models [17] proceeds in the presence of inflammation. The lesion environment consists of inflammatory elements that drive tissue repair as well as those that injure. Appropriate therapy depends on the clinical subtype of MS involved [80]. Patients with type II MS pathology (pronounced immunoglobulin, complement deposition, and a moderate loss of oligodendrocytes) will likely benefit from the removal of autoreactive antibodies. Type II MS patients respond to therapeutic plasma exchange more often than other subtypes with significant clinical improvement [69, 130, 167]. Improved treatments for MS must encourage rapid remyelination and selectively alter the inflammatory balance of the lesion.

## 3.1 Soluble Factors for Lesion Repair

Using soluble growth factors or cytokines to promote remyelination assumes that the injured CNS has cells capable of synthesizing myelin but that the environment does not support myelinogenesis. A number of factors important for oligodendrocyte survival, proliferation, and differentiation have been defined, including platelet-derived growth factor (PDGF-α) [105, 123], fibroblast growth factor 2 (FGF2) [10, 23, 119], neuregulin-1 [157], chemokine CXCL1 [126], insulin-like growth factor I (IGF-I) [90, 91] thyroid hormone [4, 43], neurotrophin-3 [13, 92], ciliary neurotrophic factor [14], and leukemia inhibitor factor [87]. In theory, administering the appropriate factor(s) to the demyelinated lesion could promote repair.

Soluble factor therapy to promote remyelination appears attractive but is presently unrealistic. While the existing industrial infrastructure can produce these small molecules at a reasonable price, several unresolved issues surround this type of therapy. Myelinogenesis requires combinations of multiple factors available to cells in a specific temporal sequence [46, 171]. The pathology of the lesions involved and the type of surviving myelinating cells need to be determined before deciding which factor to provide. Administering the incorrect factor may interfere with remyelination [48, 100]. If demyelinated lesions lack oligodendrocyte progenitors, then factors that recruit new progenitors to the lesion may be beneficial. However, administering soluble factors that induce oligodendrocyte progenitor proliferation to a lesion already replete with progenitors may suppress remyelination. There are clear differences to be resolved between human oligodendrocyte lineage cells and their better characterized mouse and rat counterparts; human oligodendrocyte progenitors do not respond to mitogens known to drive proliferation in rodent cells [6, 116]. Most studies defining soluble remyelination factors have been carried out in models of acute focal demyelination with transient inflammation. It is unclear whether growth factors and cytokines alter remyelination in the presence of chronic inflammation, as is the case in MS. The generally recognized pleiotropic effects of most cytokines and growth factors exacerbate all the above concerns. Sustained soluble factor delivery to the CNS would need to be controlled and targeted.

## 3.2 Cell Transplantation for Lesion Repair

The transplantation of remyelination-competent cells is a clinically relevant approach to repair lesions lacking endogenous oligodendrocytes. Numerous experimental studies have demonstrated that oligodendrocytes or their progenitors survive, proliferate, migrate, and myelinate when transplanted directly into dysmyelinated mutant animals or experimentally demyelinated lesions [22, 37, 162]. Remyelination by transplanted glial cells can restore spinal cord conduction [156] and neurologic function [62]. However, transplantation into an inflammatory milieu with myelin loss has been less effective.

There is a risk that transplanted cells, upon arrival at the lesion site, will be rendered incapable of remyelination similar to the endogenous cells. Therapies to alter the lesion environment to promote the survival of the transplanted cells will be required as well. In a multifocal disease such as MS, it is impractical to stereotactically implant cells directly into every demyelinated lesion. The most viable approach is a peripheral vascular delivery of cells that can enter into the CNS and target areas of damage. Soluble inflammatory factors released from the area of injury likely guide exogenous as well as endogenous reparative cells [102].

The choice of cell type to use for transplantation therapy will need to withstand the political and ethical scrutiny of society and the patient. The most promising candidates are embryonic stem (ES) cells, multipotential neural stem cells, and glial restricted precursors. Each have each been isolated from diverse regions of the rodent and human CNS [107], can be expanded almost without limit, differentiated in vitro [15] and when delivered intraspinally or intraventricularly can differentiate into myelinating cells in vivo [27, 47, 70, 78, 88, 115, 151, 173]. Appropriate Stem cells may be isolated from a patient's own bone marrow. Rodent bone marrow cells can differentiate into myelin-forming cells when transplanted into a focal demyelinated lesion [2, 3, 74, 137], and human bone marrow cells have a demonstrated neurogenic potential [94].

Of interest, studies administering neural stem cells intravenously into animals with CNS disease suggest that the transplanted cells induce repair by increasing the effectiveness of endogenous myelinating cells rather than by directly myelinating axons [115, 151]. Activated microglial cells concentrated at sites of CNS injury release soluble factors that direct neural stem cell migration and differentiation [1]. Similarly, dendritic cells transplanted into the injured spinal cord activate endogenous stem cells [95]. These studies suggest that a small number of transplanted cells, correctly targeted, may dramatically affect surviving oligodendrocyte progenitors and lesion repair by synthesizing cytokine and growth factors locally themselves or by stimulating other cells within the lesion to do so [59]. As with soluble factor-based repair strategies for MS, most cell transplantation-based strategies for remyelination have been tested only in dysmyelinating or acutely demyelinated lesions [40, 112, 169]. Limited data exist on the efficacy of cell transplantation to repair chronic immune-mediated demyelinating disease. For example, a clinical trial at Yale University stereotactically transplanting Schwann cells into MS patients was terminated prematurely after it was determined that none of the cells survived.

## 3.3   Immune-Mediated Lesion Repair

Clearly, manipulating cellular or humoral components of the immune system can promote endogenous CNS repair [34, 57, 99, 121, 132, 161] and increase repair by transplanted cells [141]. There are examples where interfering with immune cells and their effector molecules reduces myelin repair, suggesting that aspects of inflammation are important for remyelination [7, 75, 104]. Demyelination induced by lysolecithin in the spinal cord of B6 wild type mice remyelinates rapidly and completely, whereas remyelination in B6 Rag-1 mice, which lack mature T or B cells, is substantially impaired. Remyelination of spinal cord lesions is also greatly reduced in mice lacking CD4+ T cells, CD8+ T cells or macrophages [16, 75].

The transfer of activated immune cells can also potentiate repair of the injured CNS [54, 140]. When myelin basic protein-reactive T cells were injected peripherally into animals with spinal cord injury, T cells, B cells, and macrophages accumulated at the lesion site, and the local expression of macrophage- and astrocyte-associated neurotrophic factors increased [12]. T cells within demyelinated lesions may also drive remyelination by the local synthesis of oligodendrocyte modulatory factors [46, 71].

The phenomenon of preconditioning, an initial traumatic injury to the CNS (spinal cord) whereupon a subsequent injury at a distant site (optic nerve) facilitates an improvement in CNS repair [175], provides direct evidence of an innate organism-wide reparative system. The transfer of CNS antigen-activated splenocytes from CNS-lesioned animals substituted for a prior spinal cord lesion, leaving open the possibility that a protective immune response is either cellular or humoral (antibody) based. The immune response induced following CNS injury is likely a normal aspect of tissue repair. Damaged tissue and debris require removal, and an environment supportive of tissue repair needs to be established. However, the immune response repertoire varies across the human population [65], and therefore the response to injury varies as well.

Transient increases of the beneficial aspects of the immune response are likely safer than strategies designed to reduce detrimental aspects even if such therapy is required multiple times over the course of the disease. Therapies designed to restrict immune cells from the CNS for an extended period carry risks and may compromise immune control of latent virus infections [72, 96].

# 4 Antibodies Directed Against CNS Antigens Can be Pathogenic or Reparative

The existence of pathogenic autoantibodies has long been established in several peripheral neurologic syndromes including myasthenia gravis, Lambert Eaton syndrome, Guillain-Barré syndrome, acquired neuromyotonia [159] and, more recently, in the etiology of neuromyelitis optica or Devic's disease [76, 168]. In diseases mediated by pathogenic antibodies, reducing serum antibody levels by plasma exchange or immunosuppression should lead to clinical improvement. Resynthesis of pathogenic autoantibodies should lead to a return of clinical symptoms.

CNS-reactive antibodies also contribute to demyelination in MS. Active MS plaques contain a deposition of immunoglobulin and complement in 30%–50% of cases [82]. Plasma exchange, which reduces serum antibodies and complement, decreased the severity of fulminant MS exacerbations in all treated individuals demonstrating an antibody deposition pathologic phenotype (pattern II) [69]. This conclusively demonstrates the role of lesion antibody deposition in disease progression. The role of pathogenic demyelinating antibodies has been modeled in animals using anti-myelin oligodendrocyte glycoprotein (MOG). MOG antibodies administered to animals with established EAE increase disease severity and shift this predominately inflammatory model to a demyelinating disease [138].

Immunoglobulins are common within demyelinated lesions. Their presence may be due to an active immunoglobulin-based response to the CNS injury. Plasma cells, which secrete antibodies, are found within the demyelinated lesion itself [118], while oligoclonal bands have access to the entire CNS via the cerebrospinal fluid. Oligoclonal bands, one of the classic diagnostic criteria for MS, represent individually distinct, dominant antibody clones of IgG and IgM isotype that remain stable throughout the disease [176]. The reason for or function of oligoclonal bands remains elusive, but one hypothesis is that the bands display the heterogeneity of an antibody-based reparative response across the population. Although there is much evidence that high affinity IgGs are pathogenic, there is increasing evidence that IgMs activate repair mechanisms in the face of tissue injury. The presence of IgMs within the MS lesion may explain why some patients enter remission [5] or progress with mild disease. IgMs have traditionally been considered to be confined to the vasculature. At a molecular weight of close to 1 million, there is no known membrane transporter that can pass a molecule of this size. Approximately 90% of the B lymphocytes in the circulation synthesize IgM class antibodies. The polyreactive IgM is the first line of defense in the event of a bacterial infection. The low affinity and high valency of the IgM allow it to aggregate bacteria for lysis and bind to carbohydrate residues. IgMs typically have lower affinity but high avidity due to a pentameric structure that presents ten potential binding sites.

The initial observation that autoreactive antibodies can enhance endogenous remyelination was demonstrated using the TMEV-induced model of demyelination [134]. In an attempt to exacerbate TMEV-initiated demyelinating disease, chronically infected SJL mice were immunized with spinal cord homogenate (SCH) in incomplete Freund's adjuvant. Immunization with SCH induces a polyclonal antibody response directed against multiple CNS antigens. Rather than worsening the course of disease in virus-infected mice, as would be expected when increasing the titer of anti-CNS antibodies, the spinal cords of SCH-immunized mice contained four to five times more remyelination by area than nonimmunized mice. Remyelination could be equally enhanced by the passive transfer of antiserum [132] or purified immunoglobulin [131] from uninfected animals immunized with SCH, demonstrating a direct beneficial role of antibodies in promoting myelin repair for the first time.

TMEV infection in SJL mice leads to chronic immune-mediated demyelination and progressive disability very similar to that observed in chronic progressive MS. The strength of this animal model in testing remyelination strategies lies in the limited level of spontaneous remyelination. In the SJL mouse strain, spontaneous remyelination of spinal cord lesions occurs in less than 10% of the total demyelinated lesion area. This character is in stark contrast to toxin-induced models, where complete remyelination is generally swift and complete. Using a model of damage where remyelination is not the norm allowed the identification of a serum-based, remyelination-promoting response. Even though remyelination-promoting IgMs accelerate remyelination speed in a lysolecithin toxin model [18], a laborious measurement of the density of remyelinated axons was required to demonstrate this phenomenon. Using the TMEV model, the demyelinating and remyelinating effects of a given therapy can be quickly assessed using a blinded binary spinal cord quadrant grading system to provide a sampling of repair throughout the spinal cord [163].

Monoclonal antibodies (mAbs) can reproduce the reparative effect of polyclonal antisera. Hybridomas generated from the B cells of SCH-immunized mice were screened in an antigen-independent manner for their ability to reverse chronic demyelination; two mouse mAbs (SCH79.08 and SCH94.03), out of hundreds of screened clones, were efficacious in promoting remyelination [97]. Both mouse mAbs were IgMs (no IgGs were identified) and both bound to oligodendrocytes in culture. Subsequently, using binding to oligodendrocytes as the initial selection criteria, four additional mouse mAbs, all IgMs (A2B5, HNK-1, O1, and O4) [145] that promoted CNS remyelination in vivo, were identified [9, 161]. These IgMs are routinely used to identify and determine the maturation stage of oligodendrocytes. Given that binding to the surface of oligodendrocytes in culture could be used to select a group of mAbs for testing and that several of that group promoted remyelination, mAbs activity may involve direct stimulation of myelin-producing cells [8]. Because the antigens recognized by the mouse IgMs were all different and because the antigens appeared on the surface of oligodendrocytes at various times in maturation (from bipolar progenitor to postmitotic differentiated cells), it suggested that the in vivo effect was not antigen- or cell stage-specific.

# 5 Human Antibodies that Promote Remyelination

Using binding to oligodendrocytes as the initial screening criteria, human mAbs isolated from the sera of humans with lymphoproliferative disorders were tested for remyelination-promoting ability. The Mayo Clinic sera bank, a unique collection of over 125,000 samples collected over 40 years, was searched for samples with a monoclonal spike over 20 mg/ml from patients without evidence of antibody-based pathology. Antibodies isolated from serum provided serum-derived human monoclonal IgMs (sHIgM) and serum-derived human monoclonal IgGs (sHIgG). Of 102 mAbs preparations screened, six IgMs, but no IgGs, bound to the surface of oligodendrocytes in culture. All IgMs were tested in vivo for efficacy in promoting remyelination (Fig. 1A, B). sHIgM22 and sHIgM46 promoted significantly more remyelination than the other tested human IgMs [161]. Both IgMs bound to the surface of differentiated oligodendrocytes. sHIgM46 bound to multipolar cells clearly beyond the bipolar progenitor stage coincident with the expression of sulfatide. sHIgM22 bound to late-stage oligodendrocytes whose development coincided with the expression of MOG(Fig. 1E). This property mirrored the diversity of oligodendrocyte antigens and stages of differentiation recognized by reparative mouse IgMs.

Both positive human IgMs were isolated from patients with monoclonal gammopathy, a relatively common condition characterized by high concentrations of monoclonal serum antibody [33]. The remyelination-promoting human IgMs were not pathogenic to the patients that synthesize the molecules; neither presented with neurologic dysfunction despite carrying high levels of these IgMs for many years. The human IgMs identified in the initial screen all bind only to the surface of unfixed oligodendrocytes in a mixed glial culture; however, when incubated with unfixed slices of CNS tissue, five of the human IgMs bind to nonmyelin structures [19, 164]. This is also true of the well-characterized, remyelination-promoting mouse IgMs [165]. Only sHIgM22 retains a strong specific affinity for myelinated CNS tracts when used for immunocytochemistry on unfixed tissue slices (Fig. 1C, D).

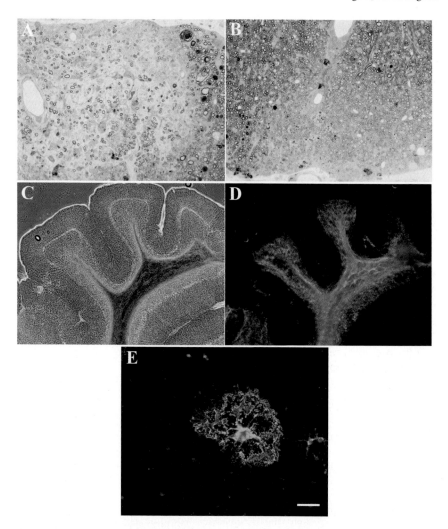

**Fig. 1** HIgM22-mediated promotion of remyelination in the Theiler's murine encephalomy-elitis virus-induced model of demyelination. SJL mice with chronic virus infection present pathologically with widespread demyelination, little remyelination, and clear neurologic defi-cits. The spinal cords of mice administered a single dose of rHIgM22 reproducibly contain significant remyelination when analyzed histologically 5 weeks after treatment. **A** An example of a demyelinated lesion from the spinal cord of an animal treated with saline. **B** An example of remyelination within a demyelinated lesion from the spinal cord of an animal treated with rHIgM22. Spinal cord cross-sections were stained for the presence of myelin using p-para-phenylenediamine. Remyelinated axons are thinner than normal and therefore stain lighter. The remyelination promoting human IgM, rHIgM22, binds to myelinated CNS tracts and the surface of oligodendrocytes. **C** Phase contrast image of a slice of mouse cerebellum immun-ofluorescently labeled in **D**. **D** rHIgM22 binds specifically to myelin in unfixed slices of CNS tissue. **E** rHIgM22 binds to the surface of an oligodendrocyte isolated from the cortex of an adult rat

## 6  Role of Anti-CNS Antibodies in Endogenous Repair

One of the established MS treatments may act, in part, through an antibody-mediated repair mechanism. Glatiramer acetate (GA, Copolymer-1 or Copaxone) is an immunogenic mixture of synthetic peptides effective in reducing MS exacerbations, lesion load, and disability [63, 64]. All patients treated with GA develop antibodies to GA, and a correlation exists between anti-GA serum titers and the therapeutic efficacy of GA within an individual [25].

The passive transfer of affinity-purified polyclonal antibodies against GA into chronically demyelinated mice increased spinal cord remyelination twofold [154]. Anti-GA antibodies are similar in character to remyelination-promoting antibodies, binding to oligodendrocytes, astrocytes, and neurons in the spinal cord and to early stages of oligodendrocytes and microglia in culture. Antibodies to GA cross-react with MBP [77, 150], and treatment with MBP antisera promotes remyelination [133].

CNS-reactive antibodies may also enhance axon outgrowth following CNS trauma. Rodents immunized with SCH prior to spinal cord hemisection or optic nerve crush demonstrated enhanced axonal regrowth in both lesion models [41, 57] with functional improvement after spinal cord injury. This SCH immunization strategy was identical to that used to identify remyelination-promoting antisera and similarly resulted in increased sera titers of myelin-reactive antibodies. Animals with the best axon regrowth contained the highest titers of myelin-reactive serum antibodies, which, when assayed in vitro, allowed axon outgrowth on immobilized CNS myelin, a substrate normally inhibitory to neurite extension. Unfortunately, CNS-reactive antibodies from animals with enhanced axon regeneration were not isolated and passively transferred to nonimmunized animals, so it is unknown whether antibodies alone mediate the reparative response.

There are similarities between remyelination-promoting monoclonal IgMs and the IN-1 mouse monoclonal IgM that promotes axon regrowth and functional recovery following CNS injury [24, 28, 31, 49]. IN-1 binds to oligodendrocytes and myelin [136] and may block myelin antigens inhibition to axon outgrowth [139, 166]. The remyelination-enhancing ability of IN-1 in models of chronic demyelination remains untested. However, there is a growing appreciation that encouraging remyelination plays an important role in repairing spinal cord impact injury [108, 153].

## 7  A Recombinant Human IgM Promotes Remyelination in vivo at Doses Comparable to Growth Factors

Recombinant forms of the two human IgMs, designated rHIgM22 and rHIgM46, have been synthesized [98]. The mRNA encoding each IgM was isolated from the cellular fraction of that patient's blood, reverse-transcribed, and the cDNA used to synthesize recombinant IgMs containing a mouse J chain. The presence of the mouse J chain may be of great utility in following the molecule in non-mouse recipients.

Both IgMs retain the immunohistochemical characteristics and in vivo reparative properties of the serum-derived versions. rHIgM22 binds myelinated tracts in slices of CNS tissue with even higher specificity than sHIgM22, which likely contains additional serum IgMs. rHIgM22 binds only to myelin in CNS slices obtained from the mouse, rat, rabbit, primate, and human (unpublished observations). Choosing an IgM to pursue for clinical trial in humans was decided by the availability of a production cell line that consistently synthesized high levels of IgM that could be easily assayed by immunocytochemistry or ELISA assays and was stable in long-term storage. rHIgM22 met these criteria better than rHIgM46.

Prior studies of induced remyelination have used bolus doses of 500 μg of IgM per mouse (25 mg/kg) administered intraperitoneally (i.p.), a dose based on earlier studies of remyelination induced by polyclonal antisera [132]. A comparable dose of IgM for adult humans treated at 25 mg/kg would be 2 g, a large amount of monoclonal antibody. A recent study clarified several important characteristics of rHIgM22-induced repair of chronically demyelinated lesions including the minimal effective dose to promote remyelination in mice with clear neurologic deficits [163]. A remarkable characteristic of rHIgM22 is the small amount of mAb in a single dose required for maximal long-term repair in the spinal cord. rHIgM22 effectively promoted remyelination down to a dose of 500 ng per mouse, a dose 1,000-fold lower than that used in prior studies. A regression analysis fitting the mean percent remyelination and dosing to a standard dose response curve (Fig. 2) resulted in a median effective dose (EC50) of 460 ng ± 74 per mouse.

An estimate of the systemic in vivo concentration of rHIgM22 at the $EC_{50}$ may be calculated by considering the treatment of a 20-g mouse with 460 ng of rHIgM22. Partition kinetics of the remyelination-promoting mouse IgM, SCH94.03 [58], determined that 0.1% of a 50-μg dose of $^{35}$S-labeled SCH94.03 entered the CNS of demyelinated mice. 0.1% of a 460-ng dose of rHIgM22 distributed throughout the 1-ml volume of the mouse CNS is 0.46 ng/ml. Although the concentration of rHIgM22 appears quite low when diluted throughout the blood stream, the concentration of IgM within target tissue may be considerably higher. MRI has demonstrated rHIgM22 accumulation within demyelinated lesions in vivo [114]. Soluble growth factors similarly localize in vivo by binding to specific extracellular matrix molecules [50, 122]. rHIgM22 tagged with biotin was tracked in vivo by the binding of avidin to ultrasmall superparamagnetic iron oxide particles and visualized by MR imaging. rHIgM22 entered and accumulated within CNS lesions of chronically demyelinated mice. Control human IgMs also entered the CNS of demyelinated mice but did not accumulate, presumably due to the lack of target antigens. $^{35}$S-labeled SCH94.03 also accumulated at demyelinated lesions in vivo as demonstrated by tissue section autoradiography [58]. These data suggest that the effective local concentration of rHIgM22 within the microenvironment of the demyelinated lesion is much higher than 0.5 ng/ml. The half-life of rHIgM22 in mouse sera was calculated to be 15 h, whereas the half-life of a normal mouse IgM in vivo is approximately 2 days [158]. Therefore, rHIgM22 must accumulate and signal in a short span of time.

rHIgM22-induced remyelination in the TMEV model occurs primarily between 3 and 5 weeks following treatment. This repair timeframe mimics precisely the

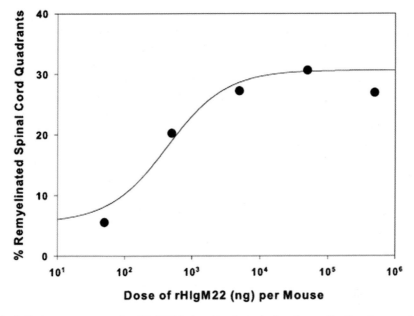

**Fig. 2** Dose response curve for rHIgM22-induced in vivo spinal cord remyelination. A regression analysis calculated a standard dose response curve for rHIgM22-induced remyelination (four parametric logistic function, SigmaPlot). The mean percent of spinal cord quadrants with more than 75% of the demyelinated area remyelinated is plotted vs the dose of rHIgM22 administered once intraperitoneally [163]. Each dosing group contained 15–18 mice. The analysis predicts a median effective dose (EC50) of 460 ng ± 74 per mouse. This is equivalent to a 23-μg/kg dose. A comparable dose for a 70-kg adult human would be 1.6 mg of IgM

time course of spontaneous remyelination observed after lysolecithin-induced demyelination, where the bulk of remyelination is also accomplished between 3 and 5 weeks following injury [18, 171]. Treatment with rHIgM22 appears to shift this virus-induced model of chronic demyelination, which normally presents with little spontaneous remyelination, to one that remyelinates at the same rate as a classic model of toxic injury. Mice in the dosing studies were treated with rHIgM22 6 months after infection, and therefore, demyelinated lesions existed without repair for at least 3 months prior [89]. Then, following a single dose of rHIgM22, substantial repair was observed throughout the spinal cord within 3 weeks. A second dose of rHIgM22 administered 5 weeks after the first was no more effective than a single dose. However, we now know that neutralizing antibodies to rHIgM22 are synthesized in animals within a week of treatment, and the second dose was likely quickly inactivated (unpublished observations).

A quantitative MRI analysis of lesion volume has followed rHIgM22-mediated lesion repair in the TMEV model [114]. Individual chronically demyelinated mice were MR imaged prior to treatment and again 5 weeks later. Mice receiving 500 ug of rHIgM22 contained a significantly smaller mean lesion load, decreasing by

40.6% compared to a lesion load increased by 13.6% in control-treated mice. Lesion volume decreased in each of 13 mice treated with rHIgM22, whereas lesion volume increased in seven of eight mice treated with saline.

Although controversial, rHIgM22 may be considered a novel class of growth factor. The classical definition of a growth factor is a molecule that binds to a target cell, induces a biologic effect, and functions at extremely dilute concentrations. This definition implies interaction of the factor with a specific receptor linked to an amplification system. rHIgM22 fulfills this definition. rHIgM22 binds to the surface of oligodendrocytes and the myelin sheath, localizes to lesion sites in vivo, acts directly on oligodendrocytes in vitro, inducing $Ca2^+$ influx [111] and protection from apoptosis [55], and effectively promotes remyelination at concentrations in the nanogram to milliliter range.

# 8 The IgM Character of Remyelination Promoting Antibodies is Vital for Function

A large body of evidence supports our hypothesis that the in vitro and in vivo biologic effects of remyelination-promoting antibodies require the pentameric IgM structure. First, we have been unable to identify an IgG, either mouse or human, which promotes remyelination. A large number of mouse IgGs, the result of hybridoma fusions, were screened in vivo for efficacy in remyelination, and none induced significant repair. A total of 100 human sera samples containing IgG monoclonal peaks were screened for binding to the surface of mixed cortical glial cells and to unfixed slices of cerebellum and cortex, and none were identified. Second, recombinant $IgG_4$ versions of rHIgM22 and rHIgM46 did bind to myelin in tissue slices or to the surface of oligodendrocytes in culture and did not promote remyelination in chronic demyelinated mice even at 1,000 times the least effective dose of rHIgM22.

Our research group evaluated the ability of IgM fragments of SCH94.03 and sHIgM22 to induce remyelination [32]. The two IgMs displayed different requirements for in vivo function; subfragments of sHIgM22 (monomeric IgM and $F(ab')_2$) promoted remyelination, whereas sub-fragments of SCH94.03 did not. These studies were conducted prior to rHIgM22-dosing studies that demonstrated the small amounts of IgM required for in vivo function. Consequently, animals received far more than the minimum effective dose. Mice received the same mass of IgM or fragments of human IgM, a single 500-μg dose of sHIgM22 or IgM fragments or five weekly 100g doses of mouse IgM or IgM fragments. The molecular weight of an Fv fragment is 25,000 kD and an intact IgM, 900,000. Considering that the $EC_{50}$ of rHIgM22 is 460 ng, a 1,000- to 36,000-fold dilution of intact IgM contaminating the test material could account for the observed in vivo remyelination. Therefore, it is erroneous to conclude that IgM fragments of sHIgM22 can induce remyelination.

Supporting the requirement of the IgM for biologic effect, intact pentameric sHIgM22 and SCH94.03 bound via immunocytochemistry to cultured oligodendrocytes and to cerebellar myelin tracts, whereas fragments of neither bound detectably. In addition, an isolated IgG1 spontaneous switch variant of antibody SCH94.03, in which the VDJ and VJ regions of the heavy and light chains of the IgM and IgG1 antibodies were identical, did not bind oligodendrocytes or cerebellar slices or promote remyelination.

Cross-linking IgGs into higher-order complexes may begin to approximate the pentameric structure of the IgM. When complexed with an anti-human γ chain secondary prior to immunocytochemistry, $rHIgG_422$ was weakly detected decorating the surface of oligodendrocytes in culture (unpublished observations). A similar observation is reported using the anti-MOG IgG, 8-18C5. The IgG is innocuous when added to oligodendrocytes in culture but when subsequently cross-linked using a secondary antibody MOG partitions of into subdomains of oligodendrocyte membrane, and severe process retraction is induced [83]. An additional example of this phenomenon is observed using mAbs to gangliosides on neurons [160]. The addition of an anti-GT1b IgM to neurons in culture can directly block neurite extension. High-affinity IgGs against GT1b and anti-GD1 bound to the neurons and attenuated CNS myelin inhibition of neurite extension, presumably by interfering with gangliosides on the surface of the neuron from binding to myelin antigens. However, the IgGs could not block neurite extension themselves. Only when the anti- ganglioside IgGs were precomplexed into multivalent aggregates and then added to the culture could the IgGs directly block neurite extension. Anti-ganglioside antibodies are associated with a number of human neuropathies. Endogenous cross-linking of these antibodies may contribute to disease progression.

# 9    Mechanisms of Antibody-Mediated CNS Repair

The therapeutic efficacy of remyelination promoting IgMs has been demonstrated in both immune- and nonimmune-mediated demyelination models [19, 110], indicating that the underlying mechanism is not a modulation of a model-specific pathogenesis but likely a fundamental physiologic stimulation of a reparative mechanism. The exact mechanism of how a single small dose of rHIgM22 promotes widespread remyelination in vivo remains unclear, but two general hypotheses, not mutually exclusive, are favored (Fig. 3).

Since all remyelination-promoting IgMs bind to oligodendrocytes and myelin [9, 161, 164], the recognition of those antigens in vivo is likely important for the mechanism of action. In the first alternative, remyelination-promoting IgMs directly target and signal oligodendrocytes and their progenitors within demyelinated lesions to facilitate their expansion and differentiation. Antisera reactive with CNS white matter antigens induce thymidine uptake when added to cultures of mixed CNS glia [132]. The direct binding of OL-specific antibodies initiate a variety of biochemical and morphological changes in these myelinating cells [11, 38, 84]. Electron microscopy of animals treated with anti-SCH immunoglobulin and pulsed with tritiated thymidine demonstrated proliferating cells with the

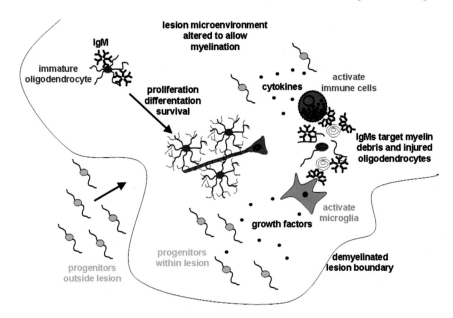

**Fig. 3** Potential in vivo mechanisms of action of remyelination-promoting IgMs. We propose that in vivo, reparative IgMs target to and accumulate at demyelinated CNS lesions and act directly on cells responsible for the synthesis of myelin by binding to surface antigens on oligodendrocyte progenitors, enhancing their proliferation, differentiation or survival. Alternatively, remyelination-promoting IgMs, concentrated at the lesion by affinity to myelin debris and injured or dying oligodendrocytes, act on other cells within the lesion. Resident microglia or immune cells may be induced to release cytokines and growth factors that (1) recruit oligodendrocyte progenitors to the site of damage, (2) increase oligodendrocyte progenitor proliferation, or (3) alter the lesion micro-environment to support remyelination

morphological features of oligodendrocyte progenitors[127]. Antibodies that bind to the oligodendrocyte-specific antigens galactocerebroside, sulfatide and myelin/oligodendrocyte-specific protein elicit biochemical and morphological changes in glial cells [39], which are preceded by a calcium influx [38]. Transient calcium fluxes are also observed in a subpopulation of astrocytes and immature oligodendrocytes following the addition of remyelination-promoting IgMs to the culture media [111]. The ability of an IgM to promote remyelination strongly correlates with its ability to stimulate calcium influx. rHIgM22 also protects immature oligodendrocytes in vitro from stressor molecules. In mice treated with rHIgM22, a decreased expression of caspase family members and increased expression of proteins associated with myelination is observed [55]. Remyelination-promoting IgMs may elicit similar signals at oligodendrocyte progenitors in damaged tissue. We and others have proposed that mAbs initiate signals by binding to plasma membrane microdomains [55]. The pentameric structure of the IgM, which binds and clusters disparate portions of the plasma membrane, is critical for in vivo remyelination.

Antibodies that bind to neurons also directly induce signals and alter cell morphology. mAbs against ganglioside GM1 suppress neurite outgrowth in vitro and in vivo [146, 147], whereas anti-idiotypic antibodies to GM1 induce neurite extension [124]. mAbs to the ganglioside GD3 (R24) or to the cerebellar granule cell surface protein (TAG-1) induce activation of the Src family kinase Lyn and result in similar alteration in protein tyrosine phosphorylation. Reducing the concentration of membrane GD3 by removing surface carbohydrates eliminates mAb-mediated signaling through both GD3 and TAG-1 [66, 67] suggesting that membrane glycosphingolipids are required for GPI-linked protein-mediated signaling.

In the second alternative, remyelination-promoting IgMs enhance myelin repair by initiating a cascade of events in cells other than oligodendrocytes upon accumulation within the demyelinated lesion. Reparative IgMs accumulating at the lesion may shift the microenvironment toward one that favors remyelination. This may be accomplished by inducing astrocytes [111] or immune cells to synthesize cytokines and growth factors supportive of myelination [23, 29, 92, 174]. Recall, for example, that rHIgM22 induces Ca flux in astrocytes and oligodendrocytes. IgM molecules are common within the oligoclonal immunoglobulin bands in MS patients [142, 143]. Since so little of the correct IgM is required for repair in our models, plasma cells situated within the demyelinated lesion may provide a sufficient concentration of antibody to activate a reparative response.

The myelin-binding character of the IgM-variable region targets the antibody to the lesion, where other IgM domains signal adjacent cells. In support of this concept, pentameric Fcμ fragments of human IgM suppress oligodendrocyte proliferation and alter transcription in mixed glial cultures, possibly through the synthesis of IL-1β from activated microglia [56]. Whether myelin-binding IgM initiates a similar upregulation in microglia and astrocytes within the lesion remains to be determined.

# 10 Therapeutic Goal: Alter the Balance of Inflammation to Favor Regeneration

We hope that remyelination promoting IgMs will soon be a clinical treatment option. The first patients to be treated with rHIgM22 will likely occur in late 2007– the initial study focusing on safety of the IgM. To date, remyelination-promoting human IgMs have exhibited no toxicity *in vitro* or *in vivo*. This will be the first clinical trial to attempt to induce repair of the central nervous system by directly targeting the cells of the brain and spinal cord rather than modulating the immune system. Demyelination is an aspect of many other human diseases involving axon damage. Stroke, peri-natal anoxia, leukodystrophies and spinal cord injuries will all likely benefit from increased remyelination. Future studies will determine whether remyelination promoting IgMs are efficacious in models of other human neurologic diseases.

Reparative CNS-binding IgMs represent a new class of therapeutics for human diseases. IgM based reagents offer a specificity of binding, and potentially of action, not possible with other molecules. The property of rHIgM22 to target to sites of CNS damage after peripheral administration presents additional applications of this IgM in the treatment of disease. The antibody may be reengineered as a vector to deliver additional reparative molecules to demyelinated lesions. in patients lacking a sufficient number of myelinating cells remyelination promoting IgMs may be combined with glial cell transplantation to improve the reparative potential of the additional cells. Human monoclonal IgMs that recognize neuronal surface antigens [164] may be used to target molecules to areas of axon pathology in neurodegenerative diseases such as Alzheimer's [36] and spinal cord injury.

Reparative CNS binding IgMs represent a new class of therapeutics for human diseases. IgM based reagents offer a specificity of binding, and potentially of action, not possible with other molecules. The property of rHIgM22 to target to sites of CNS damage after peripheral administration presents additional applications of this IgM in the treatment of disease. The antibody may be reengineered as a vector to deliver additional reparative molecules to demyelinated lesions. In patients lacking a sufficient number of myelinating cells remyelination promoting IgMs may be combined with glial cell transplantation to improve the reparative potential of the additional cells. Human monoclonal IgMs that recognize neuronal surface antigens [164] may be used to target molecules to areas of axon pathology in neurodegenerative diseases such as Alzheimer's [36] and spinal cord injury.

**Acknowledgements** The authors gratefully acknowledge the long-term support and confidence of the National Multiple Sclerosis Society (CA1011A8), the Multiple Sclerosis Society of Canada, and the National Institutes of Health (NS24180, NS32129). The authors also thank the generous support of the Hilton Foundation and Mr. and Mrs. Eugene Applebaum.

# References

1. Aarum J, Sandberg K, Haeberlein SL, Persson MA (2003) Migration and differentiation of neural precursor cells can be directed by microglia. Proc Natl Acad Sci USA 100:15983–15988
2. Akiyama Y, Radtke C, Honmou O, Kocsis JD (2002) Remyelination of the spinal cord following intravenous delivery of bone marrow cells. Glia 39:229–236
3. Akiyama Y, Radtke C, Kocsis JD (2002) Remyelination of the rat spinal cord by transplantation of identified bone marrow stromal cells. J Neurosci 22:6623–6630
4. Almazan G, Honegger P, Matthieu JM (1985) Triiodothyronine stimulation of oligodendroglial differentiation and myelination. A developmental study. Dev Neurosci 7:45–54
5. Annunziata P, Pluchino S, Martino T, Guazzi G (1997) High levels of cerebrospinal fluid IgM binding to myelin basic protein are associated with early benign course in multiple sclerosis. J Neuroimmunol 77:128–133
6. Armstrong RC, Dorn HH, Kufta CV, Friedman E, Dubois-Dalcq ME (1992) Pre-oligodendrocytes from adult human CNS. J Neurosci 12:1538–1547
7. Arnett HA, Mason J, Marino M, Suzuki K, Matsushima GK, Ting JP (2001) TNF alpha promotes proliferation of oligodendrocyte progenitors and remyelination. Nat Neurosci 4:1116–1122

8. Asakura K, Miller DJ, Murray K, Bansal R, Pfeiffer SE, Rodriguez M (1996) Monoclonal autoantibody SCH94.03, which promotes central nervous system remyelination, recognizes an antigen on the surface of oligodendrocytes. J Neurosci Res 43:273–281

9. Asakura K, Miller DJ, Pease LR, Rodriguez M (1998) Targeting of IgM kappa antibodies to oligodendrocytes promotes CNS remyelination. J Neurosci 18:7700–7708

10. Bansal R (2002) Fibroblast growth factors and their receptors in oligodendrocyte development: implications for demyelination and remyelination. Dev Neurosci 24:35–46

11. Bansal R, Winkler S, Bheddah S (1999) Negative regulation of oligodendrocyte differentiation by galactosphingolipids. J Neurosci 19:7913–7924

12. Barouch R, Schwartz M (2002) Autoreactive T cells induce neurotrophin production by immune and neural cells in injured rat optic nerve: implications for protective autoimmunity. FASEB J 16:1304–1306

13. Barres BA, Lazar MA, Raff MC (1994) A novel role for thyroid hormone, glucocorticoids and retinoic acid in timing oligodendrocyte development. Development 120:1097–1108

14. Barres BA, Schmid R, Sendtner M, Raff MC (1993) Multiple extracellular signals are required for long-term oligodendrocyte survival. Development 118:283–295

15. Ben-Hur T, Einstein O, Mizrachi-Kol R, Ben-Menachem O, Reinhartz E, Karussis D, Abramsky O (2003) Transplanted multipotential neural precursor cells migrate into the inflamed white matter in response to experimental autoimmune encephalomyelitis. Glia 41:73–80

16. Bieber AJ, Kerr S, Rodriguez M (2003) Efficient central nervous system remyelination requires T cells. Ann Neurol 53:680–684

17. Bieber AJ, Ure DR, Rodriguez M (2005) Genetically dominant spinal cord repair in a murine model of chronic progressive multiple sclerosis. J Neuropathol Exp Neurol 64:46–57

18. Bieber AJ, Warrington A, Asakura K, Ciric B, Kaveri SV, Pease LR, Rodriguez M (2002) Human antibodies accelerate the rate of remyelination following lysolecithin-induced demyelination in mice. Glia 37:241–249

19. Bieber AJ, Warrington A, Pease LR, Rodriguez M (2001) Humoral autoimmunity as a mediator of CNS repair. Trends Neurosci 24:S39–S44

20. Bjartmar C, Trapp BD (2001) Axonal and neuronal degeneration in multiple sclerosis: mechanisms and functional consequences. Curr Opin Neurol 14:271–278

21. Blakemore WF (1973) Demyelination of the superior cerebellar peduncle in the mouse induced by cuprizone. J Neurol Sci 20:63–72

22. Blakemore WF, Crang AJ (1988) Extensive oligodendrocyte remyelination following injection of cultured central nervous system cells into demyelinating lesions in adult central nervous system. Dev Neurosci 10:1–11

23. Bogler O, Wren D, Barnett SC, Land H, Noble M (1990) Cooperation between two growth factors promotes extended self-renewal and inhibits differentiation of oligodendrocyte-type-2 astrocyte (O-2A) progenitor cells. Proc Natl Acad Sci U S A 87:6368–6372

24. Bregman BS, Kunkel-Bagden E, Schnell L, Dai HN, Gao D, Schwab ME (1995) Recovery from spinal cord injury mediated by antibodies to neurite growth inhibitors. Nature 378:498–501

25. Brenner T, Arnon R, Sela M, Abramsky O, Meiner Z, Riven-Kreitman R, Tarcik N, Teitelbaum D (2001) Humoral and cellular immune responses to Copolymer 1 in multiple sclerosis patients treated with Copaxone. J Neuroimmunol 115:152–160

26. Bruck W, Kuhlmann T, Stadelmann C (2003) Remyelination in multiple sclerosis. J Neurol Sci 206:181–185

27. Brustle O, Jones KN, Learish RD, Karram K, Choudhary K, Wiestler OD, Duncan ID, McKay RD (1999) Embryonic stem cell-derived glial precursors: a source of myelinating transplants. Science 285:754–756

28. Caroni P, Schwab ME (1988) Antibody against myelin-associated inhibitor of neurite growth neutralizes nonpermissive substrate properties of CNS white matter. Neuron 1:85–96

29. Chang A, Nishiyama A, Peterson J, Prineas J, Trapp BD (2000) NG2-positive oligodendrocyte progenitor cells in adult human brain and multiple sclerosis lesions. J Neurosci 20:6404–6412

30. Chang A, Tourtellotte WW, Rudick R, Trapp BD (2002) Premyelinating oligodendrocytes in chronic lesions of multiple sclerosis. N Engl J Med 346:165–173
31. Chen MS, Huber AB, van der Haar ME, Frank M, Schnell L, Spillmann AA, Christ F, Schwab ME (2000) Nogo-A is a myelin-associated neurite outgrowth inhibitor and an antigen for monoclonal antibody IN-1. Nature 403:434–439
32. Ciric B, Howe CL, Paz Soldan M, Warrington AE, Bieber AJ, Van Keulen V, Rodriguez M, Pease LR (2003) Human monoclonal IgM antibody promotes CNS myelin repair independent of Fc function. Brain Pathol 13:608–616
33. Ciric B, VanKeulen V, Rodriguez M, Kyle RA, Gertz MA, Pease LR (2001) Clonal evolution in Waldenstrom macroglobulinemia highlights functional role of B-cell receptor. Blood 97:321–323
34. Cohen IR, Schwartz M (1999) Autoimmune maintenance and neuroprotection of the central nervous system. J Neuroimmunol 100:111–114
35. Dal Canto MC, Lipton HL (1977) Multiple sclerosis. Animal model: Theiler's virus infection in mice. Am J Pathol 88:497–500
36. Dodel R, Hampel H, Depboylu C, Lin S, Gao F, Schock S, Jackel S, Wei X, Buerger K, Hoft C, Hemmer B, Moller HJ, Farlow M, Oertel WH, Sommer N, Du Y (2002) Human antibodies against amyloid beta peptide: a potential treatment for Alzheimer's disease. Ann Neurol 52:253–256
37. Duncan ID (1996) Glial cell transplantation and remyelination of the central nervous system. Neuropathol Appl Neurobiol 22:87–100
38. Dyer CA (1993) Novel oligodendrocyte transmembrane signaling systems. Investigations utilizing antibodies as ligands. Mol Neurobiol 7:1–22
39. Dyer CA, Benjamins JA (1988) Redistribution and internalization of antibodies to galactocerebroside by oligodendroglia. J Neurosci 8:883–891
40. Einstein O, Karussis D, Grigoriadis N, Mizrachi-Kol R, Reinhartz E, Abramsky O, Ben-Hur T (2003) Intraventricular transplantation of neural precursor cell spheres attenuates acute experimental allergic encephalomyelitis. Mol Cell Neurosci 24:1074–1082
41. Ellezam B, Bertrand J, Dergham P, McKerracher L (2003) Vaccination stimulates retinal ganglion cell regeneration in the adult optic nerve. Neurobiol Dis 12:1–10
42. Feigin I, Popoff N (1966) Regeneration of myelin in multiple sclerosis. The role of mesenchymal cells in such regeneration and in myelin formation in the peripheral nervous system. Neurology 16:364–372
43. Fernandez M, Giuliani A, Pirondi S, D'Intino G, Giardino L, Aloe L, Levi-Montalcini R, Calza L (2004) Thyroid hormone administration enhances remyelination in chronic demyelinating inflammatory disease. Proc Natl Acad Sci U S A 101:16363–16368
44. Franklin RJ (2002) Why does remyelination fail in multiple sclerosis? Nat Rev Neurosci 3:705–714
45. Franklin RJ, Gilson JM, Blakemore WF (1997) Local recruitment of remyelinating cells in the repair of demyelination in the central nervous system. J Neurosci Res 50:337–344
46. Franklin RJ, Hinks GL, Woodruff RH, O'Leary MT (2001) What roles do growth factors play in CNS remyelination? Prog Brain Res 132:185–193
47. Gaiano N, Fishell G (1998) Transplantation as a tool to study progenitors within the vertebrate nervous system. J Neurobiol 36:152–161
48. Goddard DR, Berry M, Butt AM (1999) In vivo actions of fibroblast growth factor-2 and insulin-like growth factor-I on oligodendrocyte development and myelination in the central nervous system. J Neurosci Res 57:74–85
49. GrandPre T, Nakamura F, Vartanian T, Strittmatter SM (2000) Identification of the Nogo inhibitor of axon regeneration as a Reticulon protein. Nature 403:439–444
50. Guimond SE, Turnbull JE (1999) Fibroblast growth factor receptor signalling is dictated by specific heparan sulphate saccharides. Curr Biol 9:1343–1346
51. Hall SM (1972) The effect of injections of lysophosphatidyl choline into white matter of the adult mouse spinal cord. J Cell Sci 10:535–546

52. Hammarberg H, Lidman O, Lundberg C, Eltayeb SY, Gielen AW, Muhallab S, Svenningsson A, Linda H, van Der Meide PH, Cullheim S, Olsson T, Piehl F (2000) Neuroprotection by encephalomyelitis: rescue of mechanically injured neurons and neurotrophin production by CNS-infiltrating T and natural killer cells. J Neurosci 20:5283–5291

53. Herndon RM, Price DL, Weiner LP (1977) Regeneration of oligodendroglia during recovery from demyelinating disease. Science 195:693–694

54. Hohlfeld R, Kerschensteiner M, Stadelmann C, Lassmann H, Wekerle H (2000) The neuroprotective effect of inflammation: implications for the therapy of multiple sclerosis. J Neuroimmunol 107:161–166

55. Howe CL, Bieber AJ, Warrington AE, Pease LR, Rodriguez M (2004) Antiapoptotic signaling by a remyelination-promoting human antimyelin antibody. Neurobiol Dis 15:120–131

56. Howe CL, Mayoral S, Rodriguez M (2006) Activated microglia stimulate transcriptional changes in primary oligodendrocytes via IL-1beta. Neurobiol Dis 23:731–739

57. Huang DW, McKerracher L, Braun PE, David S (1999) A therapeutic vaccine approach to stimulate axon regeneration in the adult mammalian spinal cord. Neuron 24:639–647

58. Hunter SF, Miller DJ, Rodriguez M (1997) Monoclonal remyelination-promoting natural autoantibody SCH 94.03: pharmacokinetics and in vivo targets within demyelinated spinal cord in a mouse model of multiple sclerosis. J Neurol Sci 150:103–113

59. Imitola J, Comabella M, Chandraker AK, Dangond F, Sayegh MH, Snyder EY, Khoury SJ (2004) Neural stem/progenitor cells express costimulatory molecules that are differentially regulated by inflammatory and apoptotic stimuli. Am J Pathol 164:1615–1625

60. Jeffery ND, Blakemore WF (1995) Remyelination of mouse spinal cord axons demyelinated by local injection of lysolecithin. J Neurocytol 24:775–781

61. Jeffery ND, Blakemore WF (1997) Locomotor deficits induced by experimental spinal cord demyelination are abolished by spontaneous remyelination. Brain 120:27–37

62. Jeffery ND, Crang AJ, O'Leary M T, Hodge SJ, Blakemore WF (1999) Behavioural consequences of oligodendrocyte progenitor cell transplantation into experimental demyelinating lesions in the rat spinal cord. Eur J Neurosci 11:1508–1514

63. Johnson KP, Brooks BR, Cohen JA, Ford CC, Goldstein J, Lisak RP, Myers LW, Panitch HS, Rose JW, Schiffer RB (1995) Copolymer 1 reduces relapse rate and improves disability in relapsing-remitting multiple sclerosis: results of a phase III multicenter, double-blind placebo-controlled trial. The Copolymer 1 Multiple Sclerosis Study Group. Neurology 45:1268–1276

64. Johnson KP, Brooks BR, Ford CC, Goodman A, Guarnaccia J, Lisak RP, Myers LW, Panitch HS, Pruitt A, Rose JW, Kachuck N, Wolinsky JS (2000) Sustained clinical benefits of glatiramer acetate in relapsing multiple sclerosis patients observed for 6 years. Copolymer 1 Multiple Sclerosis Study Group. Mult Scler 6:255–266

65. Jones TB, Basso DM, Sodhi A, Pan JZ, Hart RP, MacCallum RC, Lee S, Whitacre CC, Popovich PG (2002) Pathological CNS autoimmune disease triggered by traumatic spinal cord injury: implications for autoimmune vaccine therapy. J Neurosci 22:2690–2700

66. Kasahara K, Watanabe K, Takeuchi K, Kaneko H, Oohira A, Yamamoto T, Sanai Y (2000) Involvement of gangliosides in glycosylphosphatidylinositol-anchored neuronal cell adhesion molecule TAG-1 signaling in lipid rafts. J Biol Chem 275:34701–34709

67. Kasahara K, Watanabe Y, Yamamoto T, Sanai Y (1997) Association of Src family tyrosine kinase Lyn with ganglioside GD3 in rat brain. Possible regulation of Lyn by glycosphingolipid in caveolae-like domains. J Biol Chem 272:29947–29953

68. Keegan BM, Noseworthy JH (2002) Multiple sclerosis. Annu Rev Med 53:285–302

69. Keegan M, Konig F, McClelland R, Bruck W, Morales Y, Bitsch A, Panitch H, Lassmann H, Weinshenker B, Rodriguez M, Parisi J, Lucchinetti CF (2005) Relation between humoral pathological changes in multiple sclerosis and response to therapeutic plasma exchange. Lancet 366:579–582

70. Keirstead HS, Blakemore WF (1999) The role of oligodendrocytes and oligodendrocyte progenitors in CNS remyelination. Adv Exp Med Biol 468:183–197

71. Kerschensteiner M, Gallmeier E, Behrens L, Leal VV, Misgeld T, Klinkert WE, Kolbeck R, Hoppe E, Oropeza-Wekerle RL, Bartke I, Stadelmann C, Lassmann H, Wekerle H, Hohlfeld R (1999) Activated human T cells, B cells, and monocytes produce brain-derived neurotrophic factor in vitro and in inflammatory brain lesions: a neuroprotective role of inflammation? J Exp Med 189:865–870

72. Khalili K, White MK, Lublin F, Ferrante P, Berger JR (2007) Reactivation of JC virus and development of PML in patients with multiple sclerosis. Neurology 68:985–990

73. Kohama I, Lankford KL, Preiningerova J, White FA, Vollmer TL, Kocsis JD (2001) Transplantation of cryopreserved adult human Schwann cells enhances axonal conduction in demyelinated spinal cord. J Neurosci 21:944–950

74. Koshizuka S, Okada S, Okawa A, Koda M, Murasawa M, Hashimoto M, Kamada T, Yoshinaga K, Murakami M, Moriya H, Yamazaki M (2004) Transplanted hematopoietic stem cells from bone marrow differentiate into neural lineage cells and promote functional recovery after spinal cord injury in mice. J Neuropathol Exp Neurol 63:64–72

75. Kotter MR, Setzu A, Sim FJ, Van Rooijen N,Franklin RJ (2001) Macrophage depletion impairs oligodendrocyte remyelination following lysolecithin-induced demyelination. Glia 35:204–212

76. Lennon VA, Wingerchuk DM, Kryzer TJ, Pittock SJ, Lucchinetti CF, Fujihara K, Nakashima I, Weinshenker BG (2004) A serum autoantibody marker of neuromyelitis optica: distinction from multiple sclerosis. Lancet 364:2106–2112

77. Lisak RP, Zweiman B, Blanchard N, Rorke LB (1983) Effect of treatment with Copolymer 1 (Cop-1) on the in vivo and in vitro manifestations of experimental allergic encephalomyelitis (EAE). J Neurol Sci 62:281–293

78. Liu S, Qu Y, Stewart TJ, Howard MJ, Chakrabortty S, Holekamp TF, McDonald JW (2000) Embryonic stem cells differentiate into oligodendrocytes and myelinate in culture and after spinal cord transplantation. Proc Natl Acad Sci U S A 97:6126–6131

79. Lucchinetti C, Bruck W (2004) The pathology of primary progressive multiple sclerosis. Mult Scler 10 [Suppl 1]:S23–S30

80. Lucchinetti C, Bruck W, Parisi J, Scheithauer B, Rodriguez M, Lassmann H (1999) A quantitative analysis of oligodendrocytes in multiple sclerosis lesions. A study of 113 cases. Brain 122:2279–2295

81. Lucchinetti C, Bruck W, Parisi J, Scheithauer B, Rodriguez M, Lassmann H (2000) Heterogeneity of multiple sclerosis lesions: implications for the pathogenesis of demyelination. Ann Neurol 47:707–717

82. Lucchinetti CF, Brueck W, Rodriguez M, Lassmann H (1998) Multiple sclerosis: lessons from neuropathology. Semin Neurol 18:337–349

83. Marta CB, Montano MB, Taylor CM, Taylor AL, Bansal R, Pfeiffer SE (2005) Signaling cascades activated upon antibody cross-linking of myelin oligodendrocyte glycoprotein: potential implications for multiple sclerosis. J Biol Chem 280:8985–8993

84. Marta CB, Taylor CM, Coetzee T, Kim T, Winkler S, Bansal R, Pfeiffer SE (2003) Antibody cross-linking of myelin oligodendrocyte glycoprotein leads to its rapid repartitioning into detergent-insoluble fractions, and altered protein phosphorylation and cell morphology. J Neurosci 23:5461–5471

85. Mason JL, Toews A, Hostettler JD, Morell P, Suzuki K, Goldman JE, Matsushima GK (2004) Oligodendrocytes and progenitors become progressively depleted within chronically demyelinated lesions. Am J Pathol 164:1673–1682

86. Matthews AE, Weiss SR, Paterson Y (2002) Murine hepatitis virus – a model for virus-induced CNS demyelination. J Neurovirol 8:76–85

87. Mayer M, Bhakoo K, Noble M (1994) Ciliary neurotrophic factor and leukemia inhibitory factor promote the generation, maturation and survival of oligodendrocytes in vitro. Development 120:143–153

88. McDonald JW, Liu XZ, Qu Y, Liu S, Mickey SK, Turetsky D, Gottlieb DI, Choi DW (1999) Transplanted embryonic stem cells survive, differentiate and promote recovery in injured rat spinal cord. Nat Med 5:1410–1412

89. McGavern DB, Murray PD, Rivera-Quinones C, Schmelzer JD, Low PA, Rodriguez M (2000) Axonal loss results in spinal cord atrophy, electrophysiological abnormalities and neurological deficits following demyelination in a chronic inflammatory model of multiple sclerosis. Brain 123:519–531

90. McMorris FA, Dubois-Dalcq M (1988) Insulin-like growth factor I promotes cell proliferation and oligodendroglial commitment in rat glial progenitor cells developing in vitro. J Neurosci Res 21:199–209

91. McMorris FA, Mozell RL, Carson MJ, Shinar Y, Meyer RD, Marchetti N (1993) Regulation of oligodendrocyte development and central nervous system myelination by insulin-like growth factors. Ann N Y Acad Sci 692:321–334

92. McTigue DM, Horner PJ, Stokes BT, Gage FH (1998) Neurotrophin-3 and brain-derived neurotrophic factor induce oligodendrocyte proliferation and myelination of regenerating axons in the contused adult rat spinal cord. J Neurosci 18:5354–5365

93. Mews I, Bergmann M, Bunkowski S, Gullotta F, Bruck W (1998) Oligodendrocyte and axon pathology in clinically silent multiple sclerosis lesions. Mult Scler 4:55–62

94. Mezey E, Chandross KJ, Harta G, Maki RA, McKercher SR (2000) Turning blood into brain: cells bearing neuronal antigens generated in vivo from bone marrow. Science 290:1779–1782

95. Mikami Y, Okano H, Sakaguchi M, Nakamura M, Shimazaki T, Okano HJ, Kawakami Y, Toyama Y, Toda M (2004) Implantation of dendritic cells in injured adult spinal cord results in activation of endogenous neural stem/progenitor cells leading to de novo neurogenesis and functional recovery. J Neurosci Res 76:453–465

96. Miller DH, Khan OA, Sheremata WA, Blumhardt LD, Rice GP, Libonati MA, Willmer-Hulme AJ, Dalton CM, Miszkiel KA, O'Connor PW (2003) A controlled trial of natalizumab for relapsing multiple sclerosis. N Engl J Med 348:15–23

97. Miller DJ, Sanborn KS, Katzmann JA, Rodriguez M (1994) Monoclonal autoantibodies promote central nervous system repair in an animal model of multiple sclerosis. J Neurosci 14:6230–6238

98. Mitsunaga Y, Ciric B, Van Keulen V, Warrington AE, Paz Soldan M, Bieber AJ, Rodriguez M, Pease LR (2002) Direct evidence that a human antibody derived from patient serum can promote myelin repair in a mouse model of chronic-progressive demyelinating disease. FASEB J 16:1325–1327

99. Moalem G, Monsonego A, Shani Y, Cohen IR, Schwartz M (1999) Differential T cell response in central and peripheral nerve injury: connection with immune privilege. FASEB J 13:1207–1217

100. Muir DA, Compston DA (1996) Growth factor stimulation triggers apoptotic cell death in mature oligodendrocytes. J Neurosci Res 44:1–11

101. Murray PD, Pavelko KD, Leibowitz J, Lin X, Rodriguez M (1998) CD4(+) and CD8(+) T cells make discrete contributions to demyelination and neurologic disease in a viral model of multiple sclerosis. J Virol 72:7320–7329

102. Nait-Oumesmar B, Decker L, Lachapelle F, Avellana-Adalid V, Bachelin C, Van Evercooren AB (1999) Progenitor cells of the adult mouse subventricular zone proliferate, migrate and differentiate into oligodendrocytes after demyelination. Eur J Neurosci 11:4357–4366

103. Nait-Oumesmar B, Picard-Riera N, Kerninon C, Decker L, Seilhean D, Hoglinger GU, Hirsch EC, Reynolds R, Baron-Van Evercooren A (2007) Activation of the subventricular zone in multiple sclerosis: evidence for early glial progenitors. Proc Natl Acad Sci USA 104:4694–4699

104. Njenga MK, Murray PD, McGavern D, Lin X, Drescher KM, Rodriguez M (1999) Absence of spontaneous central nervous system remyelination in class II-deficient mice infected with Theiler's virus. J Neuropathol Exp Neurol 58:78–91

105. Noble M, Murray K, Stroobant P, Waterfield MD, Riddle P (1988) Platelet-derived growth factor promotes division and motility and inhibits premature differentiation of the oligodendrocyte/type-2 astrocyte progenitor cell. Nature 333:560–562

106. Noseworthy JH, Gold R, Hartung HP (1999) Treatment of multiple sclerosis: recent trials and future perspectives. Curr Opin Neurol 12:279–293

107. Nunes MC, Roy NS, Keyoung HM, Goodman RR, McKhann G 2nd, Jiang L, Kang J, Nedergaard M, Goldman SA (2003) Identification and isolation of multipotential neural progenitor cells from the subcortical white matter of the adult human brain. Nat Med 9:439–447

108. Pannu R, Christie DK, Barbosa E, Singh I, Singh AK (2007) Post-trauma Lipitor treatment prevents endothelial dysfunction, facilitates neuroprotection, and promotes locomotor recovery following spinal cord injury. J Neurochem 101:182–200

109. Patrikios P, Stadelmann C, Kutzelnigg A, Rauschka H, Schmidbauer M, Laursen H, Sorensen PS, Bruck W, Lucchinetti C, Lassmann H (2006) Remyelination is extensive in a subset of multiple sclerosis patients. Brain 129:3165–3172

110. Pavelko KD, van Engelen BG, Rodriguez M (1998) Acceleration in the rate of CNS remyelination in lysolecithin-induced demyelination. J Neurosci 18:2498–2505

111. Paz Soldan MM, Warrington AE, Bieber AJ, Ciric B, Van Keulen V, Pease LR, Rodriguez M (2003) Remyelination-promoting antibodies activate distinct Ca2+ influx pathways in astrocytes and oligodendrocytes: relationship to the mechanism of myelin repair. Mol Cell Neurosci 22:14–24

112. Penderis J, Shields SA, Franklin RJ (2003) Impaired remyelination and depletion of oligodendrocyte progenitors does not occur following repeated episodes of focal demyelination in the rat central nervous system. Brain 126:1382–1391

113. Perier O, Gregoire A (1965) Electron microscopic features of multiple sclerosis lesions. Brain 88:937–952

114. Pirko I, Ciric B, Gamez J, Bieber AJ, Warrington AE, Johnson AJ, Hanson DP, Pease LR, Macura SI, Rodriguez M (2004) A human antibody that promotes remyelination enters the CNS and decreases lesion load as detected by T2-weighted spinal cord MRI in a virus-induced murine model of MS. FASEB J 18:1577–1579

115. Pluchino S, Quattrini A, Brambilla E, Gritti A, Salani G, Dina G, Galli R, Del Carro U, Amadio S, Bergami A, Furlan R, Comi G, Vescovi AL, Martino G (2003) Injection of adult neurospheres induces recovery in a chronic model of multiple sclerosis. Nature 422:688–694

116. Prabhakar S, D'Souza S, Antel JP, McLaurin J, Schipper HM, Wang E (1995) Phenotypic and cell cycle properties of human oligodendrocytes in vitro. Brain Res 672:159–169

117. Prineas JW, Barnard RO, Kwon EE, Sharer LR, Cho ES (1993) Multiple sclerosis: remyelination of nascent lesions. Ann Neurol 33:137–151

118. Prineas JW, Wright RG (1978) Macrophages, lymphocytes, and plasma cells in the perivascular compartment in chronic multiple sclerosis. Lab Invest 38:409–421

119. Qian X, Davis AA, Goderie SK, Temple S (1997) FGF2 concentration regulates the generation of neurons and glia from multipotent cortical stem cells. Neuron 18:81–93

120. Raine CS, Stone SH (1977) Animal model for multiple sclerosis. Chronic experimental allergic encephalomyelitis in inbred guinea pigs. N Y State J Med 77:1693–1696

121. Rapalino O, Lazarov-Spiegler O, Agranov E, Velan GJ, Yoles E, Fraidakis M, Solomon A, Gepstein R, Katz A, Belkin M, Hadani M, Schwartz M (1998) Implantation of stimulated homologous macrophages results in partial recovery of paraplegic rats. Nat Med 4:814–821

122. Rapraeger AC, Krufka A, Olwin BB (1991) Requirement of heparan sulfate for bFGF-mediated fibroblast growth and myoblast differentiation. Science 252:1705–1758

123. Richardson WD, Pringle N, Mosley MJ, Westermark B, Dubois-Dalcq M (1988) A role for platelet-derived growth factor in normal gliogenesis in the central nervous system. Cell 53:309–319

124. Riggott MJ, Matthew WD (1997) Neurite outgrowth is enhanced by anti-idiotypic monoclonal antibodies to the ganglioside GM1. Exp Neurol 145:278–287

125. Rivera-Quinones C, McGavern D, Schmelzer JD, Hunter SF, Low PA, Rodriguez M (1998) Absence of neurological deficits following extensive demyelination in a class I-deficient murine model of multiple sclerosis. Nat Med 4:187–193

126. Robinson S, Tani M, Strieter RM, Ransohoff RM, Miller RH (1998) The chemokine growth-regulated oncogene-alpha promotes spinal cord oligodendrocyte precursor proliferation. J Neurosci 18:10457–10563

127. Rodriguez M (1991) Immunoglobulins stimulate central nervous system remyelination: electron microscopic and morphometric analysis of proliferating cells. Lab Invest 64:358–370

128. Rodriguez M (2003) A function of myelin is to protect axons from subsequent injury: implications for deficits in multiple sclerosis. Brain 126:751–752

129. Rodriguez M (2007) Effectors of demyelination and remyelination in the CNS: Implications for multiple sclerosis. Brain Pathol 17:219–229

130. Rodriguez M, Karnes WE, Bartleson JD, Pineda AA (1993) Plasmapheresis in acute episodes of fulminant CNS inflammatory demyelination. Neurology 43:1100–1104

131. Rodriguez M, Lennon VA (1990) Immunoglobulins promote remyelination in the central nervous system. Ann Neurol 27:12–17

132. Rodriguez M, Lennon VA, Benveniste EN, Merrill JE (1987) Remyelination by oligodendrocytes stimulated by antiserum to spinal cord. J Neuropathol Exp Neurol 46:84–95

133. Rodriguez M, Miller DJ, Lennon VA (1996) Immunoglobulins reactive with myelin basic protein promote CNS remyelination. Neurology 46:538–545

134. Rodriguez M, Oleszak E, Leibowitz J (1987) Theiler's murine encephalomyelitis: a model of demyelination and persistence of virus. Crit Rev Immunol 7:325–365

135. Rodriguez M, Scheithauer BW, Forbes G, Kelly PJ (1993) Oligodendrocyte injury is an early event in lesions of multiple sclerosis. Mayo Clin Proc 68:627–636

136. Rubin BP, Dusart I, Schwab ME (1994) A monoclonal antibody (IN-1) which neutralizes neurite growth inhibitory proteins in the rat CNS recognizes antigens localized in CNS myelin. J Neurocytol 23:209–217

137. Sasaki M, Honmou O, Akiyama Y, Uede T, Hashi K, Kocsis JD (2001) Transplantation of an acutely isolated bone marrow fraction repairs demyelinated adult rat spinal cord axons. Glia 35:26–34

138. Schluesener HJ, Sobel RA, Linington C, Weiner HL (1987) A monoclonal antibody against a myelin oligodendrocyte glycoprotein induces relapses and demyelination in central nervous system autoimmune disease. J Immunol 139:4016–4021

139. Schwab ME (1996) Structural plasticity of the adult CNS. Negative control by neurite growth inhibitory signals. Int J Dev Neurosci 14:379–385

140. Schwartz M, Moalem G, Leibowitz-Amit R, Cohen IR (1999) Innate and adaptive immune responses can be beneficial for CNS repair. Trends Neurosci 22:295–299

141. Setzu A, Lathia JD, Zhao C, Wells K, Rao MS, Ffrench-Constant C, Franklin RJ (2006) Inflammation stimulates myelination by transplanted oligodendrocyte precursor cells. Glia 54:297–303

142. Sindic CJ, Cambiaso CL, Depre A, Laterre EC, Masson PL (1982) The concentration of IgM in the cerebrospinal fluid of neurological patients. J Neurol Sci 55:339–350

143. Sindic CJ, Monteyne P, Laterre EC (1994) Occurrence of oligoclonal IgM bands in the cerebrospinal fluid of neurological patients: an immunoaffinity-mediated capillary blot study. J Neurol Sci 124:215–219

144. Smith EJ, Blakemore WF, McDonald WI (1979) Central remyelination restores secure conduction. Nature 280:395–396

145. Sommer I, Schachner M (1981) Monoclonal antibodies (O1 to O4) to oligodendrocyte cell surfaces: an immunocytological study in the central nervous system. Dev Biol 83:311–327

146. Spirman N, Sela BA, Gitler C, Calef E, Schwartz M (1984) Regenerative capacity of the goldfish visual system is affected by antibodies specific to gangliosides injected intraocularly. J Neuroimmunol 6:197–207

147. Spirman N, Sela BA, Schwartz M (1982) Antiganglioside antibodies inhibit neuritic outgrowth from regenerating goldfish retinal explants. J Neurochem 39:874–877

148. Stohlman SA, Hinton DR (2001) Viral induced demyelination. Brain Pathol 11:92–106

149. Suzuki K, Andrews JM, Waltz JM, Terry RD (1969) Ultrastructural studies of multiple sclerosis. Lab Invest 20:444–454

150. Teitelbaum D, Aharoni R, Sela M, Arnon R (1991) Cross-reactions and specificities of monoclonal antibodies against myelin basic protein and against the synthetic copolymer 1. Proc Natl Acad Sci U S A 88:9528–9532
151. Totoiu MO, Nistor GI, Lane TE, Keirstead HS (2004) Remyelination, axonal sparing, and locomotor recovery following transplantation of glial-committed progenitor cells into the MHV model of multiple sclerosis. Exp Neurol 187:254–265
152. Trapp BD, Peterson J, Ransohoff RM, Rudick R, Mork S, Bo L (1998) Axonal transection in the lesions of multiple sclerosis. N Engl J Med 338:278–285
153. Tripathi R, McTigue DM (2007) Prominent oligodendrocyte genesis along the border of spinal contusion lesions. Glia 55:698–711
154. Ure DR, Rodriguez M (2002) Polyreactive antibodies to glatiramer acetate promote myelin repair in murine model of demyelinating disease. FASEB J 16:1260–1262
155. Ure DR, Rodriguez M (2002) Preservation of neurologic function during inflammatory demyelination correlates with axon sparing in a mouse model of multiple sclerosis. Neuroscience 111:399–411
156. Utzschneider DA, Archer DR, Kocsis JD, Waxman SG, Duncan ID (1994) Transplantation of glial cells enhances action potential conduction of amyelinated spinal cord axons in the myelin-deficient rat. Proc Natl Acad Sci U S A 91:53–57
157. Vartanian T, Fischbach G, Miller R (1999) Failure of spinal cord oligodendrocyte development in mice lacking neuregulin. Proc Natl Acad Sci U S A 96:731–735
158. Vieira P, Rajewsky K (1988) The half-lives of serum immunoglobulins in adult mice. Eur J Immunol 18:313–316
159. Vincent A, Lily O, Palace J (1999) Pathogenic autoantibodies to neuronal proteins in neurological disorders. J Neuroimmunol 100:169–180
160. Vyas AA, Patel HV, Fromholt SE, Heffer-Lauc M, Vyas KA, Dang J, Schachner M, Schnaar RL (2002) Gangliosides are functional nerve cell ligands for myelin-associated glycoprotein (MAG), an inhibitor of nerve regeneration. Proc Natl Acad Sci U S A 99:8412–8417
161. Warrington AE, Asakura K, Bieber AJ, Ciric B, Van Keulen V, Kaveri SV, Kyle RA, Pease LR, Rodriguez M (2000) Human monoclonal antibodies reactive to oligodendrocytes promote remyelination in a model of multiple sclerosis. Proc Natl Acad Sci USA 97:6820–6825
162. Warrington AE, Barbarese E, Pfeiffer SE (1993) Differential myelinogenic capacity of specific developmental stages of the oligodendrocyte lineage upon transplantation into hypomyelinating hosts. J Neurosci Res 34:1–13
163. Warrington AE, Bieber AJ, Ciric B, Pease LR, Van Keulen V, Rodriguez M (2007) A recombinant human IgM promotes myelin repair after a single, very low dose. J Neurosci Res 85:967–976
164. Warrington AE, Bieber AJ, Van Keulen V, Ciric B, Pease LR, Rodriguez M (2004) Neuronbinding human monoclonal antibodies support central nervous system neurite extension. J Neuropathol Exp Neurol 63:461–473
165. Warrington AE, Pfeiffer SE (1992) Proliferation and differentiation of O4+ oligodendrocytes in postnatal rat cerebellum: analysis in unfixed tissue slices using anti-glycolipid antibodies. J Neurosci Res 33:338–353
166. Weibel D, Cadelli D, Schwab ME (1994) Regeneration of lesioned rat optic nerve fibers is improved after neutralization of myelin-associated neurite growth inhibitors. Brain Res 642:259–266
167. Weinshenker BG, O'Brien PC, Petterson TM, Noseworthy JH, Lucchinetti CF, Dodick DW, Pineda AA, Stevens LN, Rodriguez M (1999) A randomized trial of plasma exchange in acute central nervous system inflammatory demyelinating disease. Ann Neurol 46:878–886
168. Weinshenker BG, Wingerchuk DM, Pittock SJ, Lucchinetti CF, Lennon VA (2006) NMO-IgG: a specific biomarker for neuromyelitis optica. Dis Markers 22:197–206
169. Windrem MS, Nunes MC, Rashbaum WK, Schwartz TH, Goodman RA, McKhann G 2nd, Roy NS, Goldman SA (2004) Fetal and adult human oligodendrocyte progenitor cell isolates myelinate the congenitally dysmyelinated brain. Nat Med 10:93–97

170. Wolswijk G (1997) Oligodendrocyte precursor cells in chronic multiple sclerosis lesions. Mult Scler 3:168–169
171. Woodruff RH, Franklin RJ (1997) Growth factors and remyelination in the CNS. Histol Histopathol 12:459–466
172. Yajima K, Suzuki K (1979) Demyelination and remyelination in the rat central nervous system following ethidium bromide injection. Lab Invest 41:385–392
173. Yandava BD, Billinghurst LL, Snyder EY (1999) "Global" cell replacement is feasible via neural stem cell transplantation: evidence from the dysmyelinated shiverer mouse brain. Proc Natl Acad Sci U S A 96:7029–7034
174. Yao DL, Liu X, Hudson LD, Webster HD (1995) Insulin-like growth factor I treatment reduces demyelination and up-regulates gene expression of myelin-related proteins in experimental autoimmune encephalomyelitis. Proc Natl Acad Sci U S A 92:6190–194
175. Yoles E, Hauben E, Palgi O, Agranov E, Gothilf A, Cohen A, Kuchroo V, Cohen IR, Weiner H, Schwartz M (2001) Protective autoimmunity is a physiological response to CNS trauma. J Neurosci 21:3740–3748
176. Ziemssen T, Ziemssen F (2005) The role of the humoral immune system in multiple sclerosis (MS) and its animal model experimental autoimmune encephalomyelitis (EAE). Autoimmun Rev 4:460–467

# Neuroimaging of Demyelination
# and Remyelination Models

I. Pirko(✉) and A.J. Johnson

**Abstract** Small-animal magnetic resonance imaging is becoming an increasingly utilized noninvasive tool in the study of animal models of MS including the most commonly used autoimmune, viral, and toxic models. Because most MS models are induced in rodents with brains and spinal cords of a smaller magnitude than humans, small-animal MRI must accomplish much higher resolution acquisition in order to generate useful data. In this review, we discuss key aspects and important differences between high field strength experimental and human MRI. We describe the role of conventional imaging sequences including T1, T2, and proton density-weighted imaging, and we discuss the studies aimed at analyzing blood–brain barrier (BBB) permeability and acute inflammation utilizing gadolinium-enhanced

I. Pirko
Department of Neurology, Waddell Center for Multiple Sclerosis, University of Cincinnati,
260 Stetson St, Suite 2300, Cincinnati, OH 45267-0525, USA
e-mail: Istvan.Pirko@uc.edu

M. Rodriguez (ed.), *Advances in Multiple Sclerosis and Experimental*
*Demyelinating Diseases. Current Topics in Microbiology and Immunology 318.*
© Springer-Verlag Berlin Heidelberg 2008

MRI. Advanced MRI methods, including diffusion-weighted and magnetization transfer imaging in monitoring demyelination, axonal damage, and remyelination, and studies utilizing in vivo T1 and T2 relaxometry, provide insight into the pathology of demyelinating diseases at previously unprecedented details. The technical challenges of small voxel in vivo MR spectroscopy and the biologically relevant information obtained by analysis of MR spectra in demyelinating models is also discussed. Novel cell-specific and molecular imaging techniques are becoming more readily available in the study of experimental MS models. As a growing number of tissue restorative and remyelinating strategies emerge in the coming years, noninvasive monitoring of remyelination will be an important challenge in small-animal imaging. High field strength small-animal experimental MRI will continue to evolve and interact with the development of new human MR imaging and experimental NMR techniques.

# 1 Introduction

## 1.1 Animal Models of Multiple Sclerosis

Multiple sclerosis is an inflammatory demyelinating disease of the central nervous system. It is the leading cause of disability among young adults in the Western world [45]. While the number of MS-related scientific publications has grown exponentially over the last few decades, the etiology of MS remains elusive. Ideally, the best way to study MS is by studying the human disease itself. However, access to MS tissue is limited because MS patients only rarely get biopsied. Autopsy samples are inherently biased toward a chronic, more burnt-out stage of lesion formation, which hampers our ability to characterize the various pathomechanisms involved in the generation of MS lesions. In addition, studying human diseases in general does not allow for comprehensive studies of effector mechanisms, as the experimental circumstances cannot be readily modified. Animal models of disease, especially small rodent models, represent the most common pathway to investigate the pathomechanism of selected features of human diseases. Frequently studied models of MS include (1) the autoimmune model experimental allergic encephalomyelitis (EAE), (2) the viral-induced models including Theiler's murine encephalitis virus (TMEV) infection, and (3) toxin-induced models, which include the administration of cuprizone or lysolecithin. The autoimmune disease EAE is clearly the most commonly studied MS model. However, it is important to realize that, in general, human MS does not behave like a classic autoimmune disease. In the broad sense of autoimmunity, in which the immune response is harmful to the host, MS can be considered an autoimmune disease. However, strong antigens that could also serve as serum test for MS have not yet been identified. In addition, the overlap syndromes frequently seen in classic autoimmune diseases are not typically observed in MS. However, they may be seen in neuromyelitis optica (NMO), which is distinct from MS from the standpoint of pathology, radiology, epidemiology, and response to therapy and is similar to classic autoimmune diseases in its strong serum marker, the NMO antibody [33]. Studies conducted in EAE have clearly contributed greatly to our understanding of neuroinflammation and to the development of some of the currently available, partially effective MS therapies [60]. Despite these important contributions from studies in EAE, several aspects of MS may require alternative animal models. Some features of EAE are inconsistent with basic observations in MS and emphasize the importance of the lesser studied viral models of the disease [31, 43, 58]. In the coming years, models that better characterize the neurodegenerative and chronic progressive features of MS may gain more importance and complement the studies currently conducted in EAE.

## 1.2    The Role of MR in Animal Models of MS

Magnetic resonance imaging (MRI) of the central nervous system has become a critically important diagnostic modality in establishing the diagnosis and monitoring the disease course of MS [65, 66]. The newest change introduced with the currently used McDonald's criteria for MS is the inclusion of MRI findings [35, 55]. MRI is also commonly used as an outcome measure in clinical trials of MS [34]. It is important to understand how the MRI signal is generated in order to use MRI-provided information in our studies of MS and its models. In standard clinical MRI applications, the MRI signal originates from $^1$H proton nuclei. It is possible to study other nuclei as well. However, protons are the most abundant in biological systems. There are several proton-containing molecules in living organisms, but presumably water protons dominate signal in MRI studies. In applying MRI to animal models of MS (most commonly in small rodents requiring high-resolution studies), there are four important factors to consider: (1) spatial resolution, (2) signal-to-noise ratio (SNR), (3) image contrast, and (4) acquisition time. The theoretical limit of resolution is about 10 μm in each direction. This is the estimated length of water molecule movements at normal body temperature during typical MR measurement times (10–100 ms). In real-life circumstances, this resolution is very difficult to achieve because water signal from such small voxels is associated with a very poor SNR. The only way to overcome this at a given field strength is by oversampling, which increases the SNR by the square root of the number of acquisitions, which can easily result in very long acquisition times. In addition to the molecular movements of water, in vivo imaging is associated with other, larger-scale movements. These occur even with a perfectly anesthetized and immobilized animal. Motion related to pulsation of blood vessels, CSF, respiration, and involuntary muscle activity all contribute to subtle movements. Therefore, the goal for minimal resolution is in the 100-μm range for in vivo acquisition, which also allows for reasonably short acquisition times and optimal SNR.

To understand image contrast in MRI (our ability to distinguish between different tissue segments or anatomical regions), we need to consider that two anatomical regions cannot be distinguished from each other by MRI, no matter how high the resolution or SNR unless they contain water molecules with different physical or chemical properties. In order to generate MR contrast based on the physical properties of water molecules, T1 and T2 relaxation times, proton density (PD), and the diffusion coefficient (D) are widely used. T1 and T2 are signal relaxation times after excitation, which are related to the molecular environment of the proton signal. Proton density represents water concentration in a given voxel of interest. The term "diffusion" represents Brownian (or thermal) motion of water molecules, which can vary greatly between tissue segments and under pathological circumstances.

A full review of the strength and limitations of small-animal imaging are beyond the scope of this manuscript; however, a few facts are important to consider. Small-animal MRI studies are most commonly conducted in dedicated narrow-bore, high field strength small-animal systems. It is not uncommon to conduct studies at field strengths as high as 4.7–11 Tesla. Higher field strength does not translate into higher resolution but results in higher SNR, which allows for the acquisition of higher-resolution signal in shorter amounts of time. The actual resolution of a study greatly depends on the gradient field strength, which is independent of the field strength of the static cryomagnet. The gradient field strength is the force of the variable electromagnetic fields that allow for spatial encoding during MRI acquisition. SNR also depends on the characteristics of the radiofrequency coils used for excitation and acquisition. Therefore, it is critically important to use appropriate gradient sets and RF coils in small-animal imaging. Higher field strength will also result in different contrast-to-noise ratios and higher likelihood for susceptibility artifacts. These must be considered when analyzing images acquired at high field strength [51].

## 2 Conventional MRI Studies

### 2.1 Structural Studies Utilizing T1-, T2-, and Proton Density-Weighted MRI Sequences

The presence of inflammatory infiltrates in the central nervous system is the hallmark of MS. These infiltrates presumably result in demyelination and, to a lesser extent, axonal damage. In most cases, the inflammatory infiltrates appear perivascularly. Early perivascular infiltration can be visualized in animal models of MS. In an ex vivo high field strength MRI study conducted at 9.4-Tesla field strength and utilizing a whole CNS homogenate-induced guinea pig EAE model, perivascular cuffing was visualized by high-resolution T1-weighted sequences. This study did not look at demyelination or other features of EAE [13] (Fig. 1).

Extrapolating from human MRI studies, we expect to find CNS lesions in animal models on T2-weighted sequences. While T2-weighted scans are sensitive to a broad array of pathology, they are nonspecific; several different tissue processes result in similar features on T2-weighted images. Edema, cellular infiltration, gliosis,

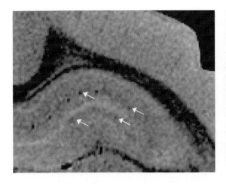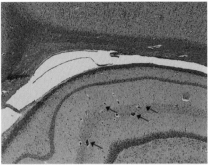

**Fig. 1** Perivascular cuffing in an EAE model as visualized by noncontrast MRI. MRI of the hippocampus (*left panel*) and histology of matching area from same animal (right panel, H&E stain to assess cellular infiltration and with SoloChrome-R-cyanin [SCR] to demonstrate myelin). Layers of the hippocampus (*left panel*) are apparent as bands above and below the hippocampal fissure. Small blood vessels (*arrows*) appear as solid black structures. Not all vessels apparent in the histology stain appear in the MR image. This may represent mismatch between the 20-μm-thick SCR stain and the 230-μm-thick T1 stain. Adopted from [13] with permission

demyelination, and severe necrosis all result in T2 hyperintensities. The nonspecific nature of T2-weighted change was also demonstrated in an EAE study conducted in guinea pigs, where perivascular cuffing was visualized in vivo as T2 hyperintensities and confirmed by ex vivo tissue studies. Histologically, the areas of cuffing were not associated with demyelination, only with cellular infiltration, However, the same T2 hyperintensity was observed as would be expected with demyelination [16]. An ex vivo study looked at the chronic relapsing EAE model induced by spinal cord homogenate injection in Lewis rats experiencing two to three relapses over the first 40 days of the disease and found MRI-detectable lesion formation in the spine. The lesions were most abundant in the cervical and thoracic regions. While the utilized proton density (PD)-weighted multislice high-resolution ($40\times40\times500$-μm) MRI sequences at 7-Tesla field strength were able to detect lesions, they could not distinguish between demyelination, remyelination, inflammation, or edema when matching histology slides were studied. In addition, no lesions were seen in the gray matter of these animals, although such lesions were present in histology [30]. Similar imaging features were described in a PLP-induced EAE model in Lewis rats [40] and in a marmoset EAE model induced by adoptive transfer of naturally occurring major basic protein (MBP)-reactive T cells [14]. In a very-high-resolution ($40\times40\times380\,\mu$m) ex vivo study conducted at 4.7 Tesla in a chronic guinea pig EAE model triggered by spinal cord homogenate, proton density- and T2-weighted images visualized areas of demyelination confirmed by matching histology [48] (Fig. 2).

The above studies suggest that conventional MRI sequences cannot differentiate between inflammation and demyelination, two key aspects of human MS. However, by intuitive combinations of pulse sequences coupled with sophisticated analytical

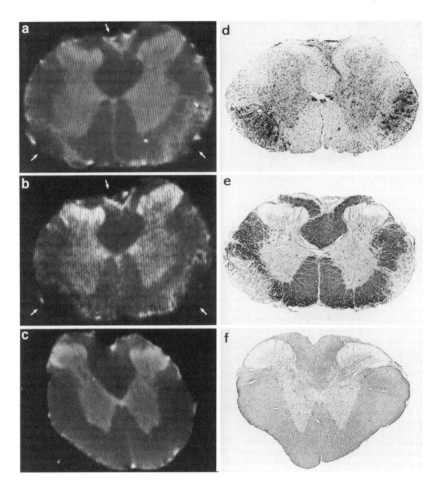

**Fig. 2** **a** Transverse nuclear magnetic resonance (NMR) ex vivo image of a spinal cord (PD-weighted spin echo sequence, TR: 3 s, TE: 20 ms, 40×40×380 μm). Note the three lesions identified by *arrows*. **b** Transverse NMR image of a diseased spinal cord, same localization as (**a**) with T2-weighted imaging (TR: 3 s, TE: 60 ms). The difference in image contrast is apparent (*arrows*). **c** Transverse NMR image of a normal region of the spinal cord (same PD-weighted sequence as for **a**). **d** Light microscopic view of perivascular infiltrations of lymphocytes and macrophages. There is a striking agreement with the NMR images (**a, b**); for example, both show a band of largely unaffected white matter between the lesion on the right and the ventral horn of the gray matter. **e** Light microscopic view showing large areas of demyelination. **f** Light microscopic view of a normal region of the diseased spinal cord. (**d** cresyl violet; **e, f** anti-MBP stain). Reproduced from [48] with permission

techniques, a distinction may be possible even without advanced MRI techniques. In a study conducted in a Hartley guinea pig EAE model induced by isologous CNS homogenate injection, several conventional pulse sequences visualized cord lesions at 1.5 Tesla. Fast spin echo (FSE), conventional spin echo (CSE)-based T2, PD sequences, FSE-based FLAIR (fluid attenuated inversion recovery) and STIR (short tau inversion recovery) sequences and CSE T1 studies, including pre- and post-gadolinium studies, were conducted. Following image acquisition, the cords were removed and analyzed histologically. Signal-to-noise ratio analysis based on histologically identified regions of interest was performed. Investigators concluded that STIR-FSE and PD-CSE could differentiate tissue containing cellular infiltrates with a high degree of accuracy. They also found reduced SNR of PD-CSE and T1-CSE with gadolinium in demyelinated lesions containing inflammation. They suggested that a combination of STIR-FSE, PD-CSE, and T1 CSE with gadolinium might be useful for differentiating lesions containing inflammation from lesions that also show demyelination [5] (Fig. 3). The limitations of this study are the relatively low field strength for animal studies. From the standpoint of correlating small-animal and human MRI, however, low field strength studies may be more appropriate. The currently approved highest field strength for human studies is 4 Tesla, with the majority of routine clinical scans conducted at 1.5 Tesla. This is in stark contrast to small-animal MRI, in which field strength is generally between 4.7 and 11 Tesla.

TMEV infection of IFN-$\gamma$R$^{-/-}$ mice allows the study of an acutely progressive demyelinating model that results in death 6–8 weeks after infection. In this model, four different types of T2 hyperintense lesions were identified based on characteristics on 3D volumetry studies. Each treated animal developed T2 hyperintense lesions characterized by (1) continuous enlargement, (2) enlargement followed by retraction, (3) fluctuating enlargement and retraction, and (4) stable lesions. In these animals, the overall lesion volume grew linearly until the last week of life, when it grew exponentially. It is not known if different immune mechanisms generate the four lesion types. Continuously expanding and fluctuating lesions contributed much more to the overall lesion volume in this model [52] (Fig. 4).

## 2.2 T1-Weighted Post-Contrast Studies

Gadolinium-enhanced T1-weighted studies are useful in gathering information about acute inflammation in MS. In a canine model of EAE, multiple new lesions were visualized with each clinical episode on T2-weighted imaging. T2-weighted images could not differentiate between the chronicity of lesions. However, as in human MS, gadolinium enhancement helped differentiate the lesion by age with contrast dye uptake most commonly observed in acute lesions [29]. This study also reminds us that while EAE models may seem to reflect several features of MS, the development of many new lesions is highly unusual in clinical episodes of human MS, in which a new clinical event is typically associated with the formation of one single new lesion.

Overall, gadolinium (Gd) enhancement is considered an early event in the formation of MS lesions. Several studies conducted in EAE or experimental optic neuritis (EON) models have investigated the relationship between gadolinium enhancement and tissue pathology. In an EAE model induced in guinea pigs, gadolinium enhancement of the optic nerves appeared 5–8 days following disease

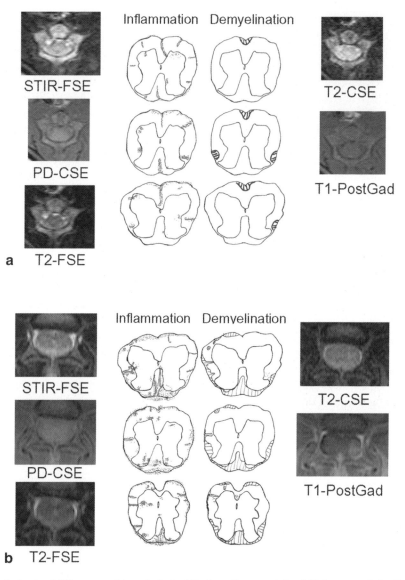

**Fig. 3** In vivo MRI compared to pathological findings. Representative MR images and distribution of pathological changes from (**a**) acute and (**b**) chronic EAE animals. The MR images are labeled for each sequence: STIR-FSE, PD-CSE, T2-FSE, T2-CSE, and T1 post-Gd. The schematic diagrams depict the distribution of inflammation and demyelination on the three anatomical slides that correlate with the imaging slice location. STIR-FSE, PD-CSE, and T1 CSE with gadolinium images are suggested as the most useful sequences in differentiating inflammation and demyelination on conventional MRI studies. Reprinted from [5] with permission

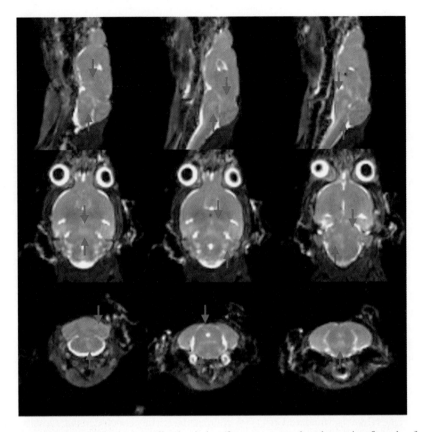

**Fig. 4** TMEV-induced brain demyelination in interferon-γ receptor knockout mice, 5 weeks after disease induction. Representative sagittal (*top row*), axial (*middle row*), and coronal images (*bottom row*) extracted from a 3D data set acquired in vivo, using a T2-weighted RARE pulse sequence (TR 2000, TE 65). The lesion load is very high at this time point. Larger hyperintense lesions are identified by *red arrows*

induction but before the onset of clinically detectable motor dysfunction. On matching histology, demyelination of the optic nerves was not seen, although scant inflammatory cell foci were visualized. The study concluded that the earliest event in EAE lesion formation is gadolinium leakage signifying cellular infiltration but not necessarily demyelination [18]. However, it remains controversial whether gadolinium leakage always accompanies the formation of T2 visible lesions. In a study comparing acute and chronic EAE models in guinea pigs, using 1.89-Tesla MRI systems, gadolinium-enhancing lesions were only observed in the acute EAE model, even though T2 lesions were detected in both cases. In the acute model, gadolinium-enhancing lesions always became visible between days 14 and 24. Based on this study, gadolinium permeability appears to be an inherent feature of lesion formation in the acute but not in the chronic model [25]. However, another study comparing acute and chronic relapsing EAE determined a linear relationship between enhancing lesions and severity of clinical disability in the chronic relapsing model. Lesions in animals in the progressive phase showed the most sustained BBB breakdown as detected by gadolinium enhancement. In the acute model, the duration of relapse overlapped with the duration of enhancement. However, unlike in the chronic model, where enhancement was seen in distinct lesions, diffuse leakage was detected in the acute model [21]. In an EON study investigating the duration of gadolinium enhancement, contrast dye uptake appeared between 3 days and 14 days with increasing intensity, starting at the apex and progressing toward the chiasm. The enhancement persisted at the last studied time point of 30 days and preceded the onset of T2-weighted abnormalities in the optic nerves. Histologically, the expansion of extracellular space and inflammatory infiltrates corresponded with the intensity of enhancement. The degree of demyelination correlated well with the presence of T2 hyperintensities [17]. The persistent enhancement seen in this model at 30 days would be unusual in human MS. The last two models show poor correlation with the pathology of human MS; diffuse enhancement is not seen in any stage of MS, while focal enhancement characterizes new lesion formation in relapsing-remitting MS. In chronic progressive forms of MS, persistent gadolinium enhancement is not seen. In fact, persistently enhancing lesions would trigger investigations for an alternative diagnosis.

Another study compared chronic relapsing and acute EAE models in a 0.5-Tesla scanner using custom-built small-animal coils. The investigators concluded that the duration of enhancement is very short (less than 5 days) in acute EAE but might last up to 5 weeks in chronic EAE. This study also utilized Gd-labeled albumin in an effort to distinguish between BBB permeability to large molecules and small molecules (like the standard Gd-DTPA contrast dye). They concluded that Gd-albumin was not always detectable in areas of leakage of the smaller molecular weight compound. They also noted that addition of immunoglobulins to the small molecular-weight gadolinium complex led to enhancement of lesions not seen with gadolinium-albumin or gadolinium-DTPA alone. Based on this study, there appear to be different degrees of BBB permeability in EAE models [23].

In a TMEV infection-induced acute progressive demyelinating model in IFN-$\gamma$R$^{-/-}$ mice, gadolinium enhancement was seen early in the disease process with the development of each new lesion. However, later in the disease, gadolinium leakage was not always observed, even though the animals continued to develop large, easily identifiable lesions on T2-weighted images [52]. In general, gadolinium enhancement means inflammation and not demyelination, and thus the appearance of enhancing lesions on standard T1-weighted gadolinium-DTPA studies do not provide any specificity about the inflammatory processes visualized [23].

Based on the above studies, gadolinium enhancement accompanies acute inflammation in the CNS; however, the mechanism and the duration of enhancement, plus the fact that enhancement is not always detectable despite ongoing new lesion formation, remains controversial. To clarify the action mechanism of MRI contrast dye enhancement, gadolinium and lanthanum enhancement was compared to the presence of gadolinium and lanthanum in the tissue following MRI studies in a chronic EAE model. The areas of gadolinium enhancement showed evidence of vesicular transportation of lanthanid metals into endothelial cells with subsequent deposition of tracers to the perivascular space. However, interendothelial junctions remained intact. Perfusion with 2,4-dinitrophenol, a metabolic inhibitor, suppressed the appearance of endothelial vesicles. The 2, 4-dinitrophenol effectively reduces the proton gradient across mitochondria and collapses the proton motive force that cells use for ATP production. Therefore, endothelial cells metabolically regulate gadolinium enhancement in this model. Further, gadolinium enhancement is not a sign of full disruption of endothelial junctions but may relate to an active process of gadolinium uptake by the endothelial cells under specific circumstances [22].

## 2.3   The Role of Conventional MRI in Monitoring Therapeutical Interventions

Similar to MRI in human clinical trials, small-animal MRI has been used to assess the effects of novel therapeutic agents in MS models. In most cases, studies monitor conventional MRI measures, such as decreased T2 hyperintense lesion load compared to controls, or decreased gadolinium enhancement on T1-weighted images. Examples of MRI monitoring in studies of novel therapeutic agents tested after disease induction in the EAE model include the small molecular inhibitor of alpha-4 integrin [49], anti-CD18 antibodies directed at the common beta chain of leukocyte integrin [57], antibodies against ICAM-1 [38], neurotrophic ACTH analog [10], PEG-catalase to reduce oxidative stress [19], and the iron chelator deferoxamine [20]. New agents to prevent disease onset in EAE have also been monitored by small-animal MRI, including a chimeric human myelin basic protein and proteolipid protein [36], acylated MBP [26], and the phosphodiesterase inhibitor rolipram [15].

Conventional MRI sequences allow insights into the pathogenesis of MS animal models. As small-animal MRI systems become more easily available to most research institutions, the use of standard sequences will increase greatly in the coming years.

## 3   Advanced MRI Methods for Visualizing Demyelinating Diseases

### 3.1   Diffusion-Weighted Imaging and Diffusion Tensor Imaging

Diffusion-weighted MRI (DWI) and diffusion tensor imaging (DTI) offer insight into the molecular movements of water in the studied tissue, allowing a very sensitive and unique insight into the pathology of several diseases. In general, DWI of the brain takes advantage of the fact that myelinated tracts of the brain are anisotropic with regard to water diffusion. Water diffuses much more easily along the fibers than across the fibers. Monitoring changes in free and restricted diffusion of water can identify various pathologic processes including stroke, ischemia, brain tumors, and white matter diseases. DTI studies can investigate the actual directions of fiber tracts and perform very detailed anatomical tractography. In a MBP-induced macaque EAE model, diffusion-weighted imaging was performed in a 2.0-Tesla clinical system with the goal of identifying pathological changes to internal capsule fibers. The internal capsule was chosen for its highly organized fiber directionality, which makes it a good medium for diffusion directionality and DTI studies. The authors saw changes on DWI the day of and the day before the onset of T2 hyper-intensities, which suggested higher sensitivity to the changes compared to T2-weighted imaging. The authors also demonstrated DWI visualization of areas of abnormal signal that otherwise look normal on standard T2-weighted imaging [24]. Another paper investigating the sensitivity of DWI drew similar conclusions; in excised spinal cords from a MBP-induced model of EAE in pigs, T1 and T2 studies conducted at 8.4 Tesla, they only found abnormalities in 50% of cords, whereas DWI found pathology in all of them, including in areas of normal-appearing white matter (NAWM) [3] (Fig. 5).

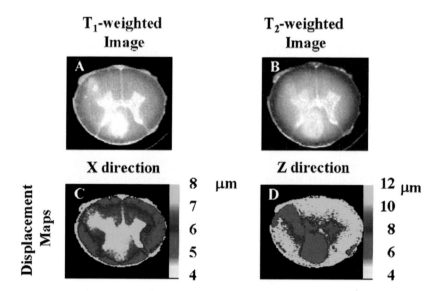

**Fig. 5** **A** T1- and **B** T2-weighted images and **C–D** q-space-analyzed DWI images of a representative swine spinal cord with EAE: (**C, D**) displacement maps obtained perpendicular (x) (**C**) and parallel (z) (**D**) to the long axis of the spinal cord. Image **C** offers more details about presumed demyelinating lesions compared to T1- or T2-weighted images (*areas in red*). Image **D** also shows areas of presumed axonal perturbation (*areas in red* in the white matter). Adopted from [3] with permission

In an EAE model of transgenic mice with T-cell receptors that recognize MBP, an ex vivo study was done at 11.7 Tesla including T2*-weighted imaging, DTI, and comparative microscopy. The authors report reduced diffusion anisotropy in the hyperintense regions, representing a loss in the normally seen directional diffusion of water [1]. Another study focusing on internal capsule fibers conducted at 7 Tesla, which utilized MBP-induced EAE in monkeys, identified acute EAE lesions by a decrease in the diffusion MR image signal with the diffusion-sensitizing gradient in all three orthogonal directions. Multiple inflammatory attacks preceded chronic demyelinating lesions in this model, as did a decrease in diffusion MRI signal with the diffusion-sensitizing gradient in the two orthogonal planes perpendicular to the direction of fiber in the internal capsule. With gradients parallel to fibers, no change was seen. This suggests that the integrity of the axons was preserved (parallel gradients), while demyelination was present (perpendicular gradients). In brain areas where the fiber directionality is well characterized, such as in the internal capsule, diffusion-based techniques may allow for the differentiation between myelin and axonal changes [56]. Contradicting these findings, another study utilizing the same presumptions investigated in vivo spinal cords in a MOG peptide-induced EAE model with diffusion tensor imaging at 4.7 Tesla. In this model, axial diffusivity (axonal component) decreased whereas radial (myelin component) was the same as in controls. The authors suggest that axonal damage in EAE is more widespread than previously thought, although it is difficult to imagine that demyelination is unseen in a model where most pathological changes relate to demyelination rather than axonal damage of the spinal cord [28].

DWI and DTI studies allow for very detailed noninvasive visualization of axonal and myelin damage in MS models. Therefore, their utilization in the studies of MS models is expected to grow.

## 3.2  Magnetization Transfer Imaging

Magnetization transfer imaging (MTI) is a newer imaging modality first introduced to the field of MS by Dousset et al. [9]. Most MRI pulse sequences used in biological research investigate protons in liquids or gels, and the usual minimum echo times range from 2 to 10 ms. If the T2 relaxation time of the studied protons in a material is less than 1–2 ms, those protons cannot be detected directly in clinical MRI systems. However, a technique called solid-state NMR/MRI can detect such substances. Biologically important macromolecules, including large proteins or myelin, have very short T2 relaxation times. The mobile protons of water are in constant motion and come into contact with these macromolecules. Using an RF pulse with a frequency designed to excite the macromolecular spins while leaving the liquid spins largely unaffected, one can saturate the macromolecular spins. If some of this saturated magnetization transfers to the liquid protons as a result of the constant interaction between mobile protons and the large molecules, then the mobile protons also become partially saturated. This results in reduced signal intensity from the mobile (small molecular) protons and serves as the basis of MT imaging.

MT imaging is a technique especially suited to study the influence of macromolecules, including myelin, on their environment. MT is becoming an important imaging modality in human MS and its animal models. In a study comparing a spinal cord homogenate-induced EAE model in Hartley guinea pigs with data acquired from healthy human volunteers conducted in a 1.5T standard clinical scanner, the magnetization transfer ratio (MTR) of normal white matter was 42%–44% with 2.5% variability. In an EAE model with almost no demyelination but significant edema, a 5%–8% MTR decrease was seen compared to before induction. In human MS, a 25% MTR decrease is typically seen, which is likely due to demyelination. Therefore, MTR may differentiate between inflammatory infiltrates and areas of demyelination. However, the MTR of the NAWM also may decrease, suggesting that MTR-based techniques are more sensitive than conventional spin echo or gradient echo-based MR imaging sequences [9] (Fig. 6).

In a CNS homogenate-induced chronic-progressive EAE model in Hartley guinea pigs, lumbar MRI was conducted at 4.0 Tesla using conventional sequences and MTI. On regions of interest analysis on matching histological samples and MRI, water phantom matched MTR, and proton density correlated well with axonal density. In NAWM and lesions, the MTR was decreased. The authors conclude that MTR is more sensitive than conventional techniques and can reveal axonal changes as well as changes in myelin [6].

The high sensitivity of MTR also allows for therapy monitoring. In a CNS homogenate-induced chronic progressive EAE model in Hartley guinea pigs, treatment with integrin antibodies was followed by MRI using a combination of magnetization transfer imaging and T2 relaxometry. Reductions in MTR were prevented or reversed by antibody in NAWM of the study animals. On multicomponent T2 relaxometry, no change was seen in myelin water percentage, as determined by the

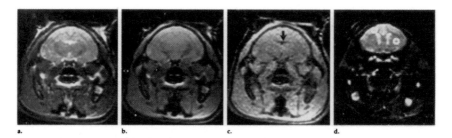

**Fig. 6** MR images of a normal guinea pig brain in the coronal plane. Images obtained with MTI (TR ms/TE ms=70/7) (**a**) and without (**b**) the radio-frequency saturating pulse. **c** Subtracted image of image **a** from image **b**; the magnitude of the signal intensity is proportional to the intensity of saturation transfer. Note that the CSF in the ventricle (*arrow*) has a low magnetization transfer, while gray and white matters have a high magnetization transfer. **d** MTI obtained at the level of the frontal lobes, with two cursors indicating the regions of interest. The two MTR values calculated in those areas are 41% for the left and 43.7% for the right. Reprinted from [9] with permission

short T2 component. The authors conclude that the short T2 component on relaxometry is more sensitive to the overall myelin content in tissue, whereas MTR is more sensitive to changes to myelin induced by inflammation [12].

MTI is easily applicable in the study of MS models. With the advent of therapeutic approaches to promote remyelination, the importance of this technique will likely continue to grow.

## 4   T1 and T2 Relaxometry

The actual measurement of T1 and T2 relaxation times in tissue may offer more insight into tissue pathology than conventional imaging methods. This technique can follow the developmental changes in myelination in experimental animals. It has been established that the age of animals at EAE induction significantly alters the disease course. Adult guinea pigs typically develop acute fulminant EAE, whereas a relapsing-remitting course is seen if induction is performed in the first 2 weeks of life. The T1 and T2 relaxation times were prolonged after birth, shortened in the first few weeks and reached adult levels by 6–11 weeks. Interestingly, by histology, myelination remained unchanged over this period, whereas gray–white differentiation was poor at birth and increased with time. The authors conclude that EAE susceptibility may be related to changes in gray matter myelination changes rather than myelination in the white matter [44]. Immune maturity may also play a role in this phenomenon.

A MBP-induced guinea pig EAE model studied BBB leakage to gadolinium-DTPA. Gadolinium-DTPA resulted in decreased T1 relaxation time in the thoracolumbar spine. Prior to the gadolinium injection, T1 and T2 relaxation times were prolonged, consistent with observations that demyelinating and inflammatory pathology results in prolonged relaxation time [47]. Ultrafast MRI methods measure T1 and T2 relaxation times in vivo. An MRI study conducted at 7 Tesla using adoptive transfer EAE reported an increase of relaxation times that paralleled the appearance of albumin in tissue on histology. This increase was detected before the onset of immune cell infiltration. After gadolinium injection, a decrease in T1 times was observed, which paralleled macrophage infiltration in this study. Therefore, serial T1 relaxation time measurements may allow differentiation between the early phase of edema formation and a later phase of cellular infiltration in EAE [39]. Similar findings were reported in MBP-induced EAE in Lewis rats, where the positive animals showed increased relaxation times and BBB permeability as time progressed. This was more pronounced on days 10 and 11, when clinical features such as paraplegia developed [41]. However, the measurement of relaxation times without concomitant imaging with other modalities may be misleading. In a relapsing-remitting guinea pig EAE model, T1 and T2 relaxation times were measured in the early stage (first attack) and in relapses and remission. Relaxation times could not distinguish between these stages because of a wide range of variety of the parameters independent of the stage studied [27].

An ex vivo relaxometry study reported the ability to differentiate between hyperacute EAE and less severe forms. Cervical cord and brain samples were studied with in vitro T1, T2 and multicomponent T2 relaxometry. The hyperacute form was easily differentiated on the bi-exponential T2 measurements [64]. The authors conclude that the severity of EAE may be demonstrated by studying the short T2 component; however, a sufficient number of echoes (acquisitions) are needed, which may result in prolonged acquisition times. These, in turn, can limit the use of this technique in vivo. In human MS, similar techniques have been successfully used in vivo to determine the short T2 (myelin) water component in white matter areas of interest [32].

Relaxometry has also been used as a therapy-monitoring tool. In an MBP-specific T cell-induced adoptive transfer EAE model, PPD-specific T cells were transferred along with MBP-specific T cells of different specificity to study their effect in disease induction. The changes seen were dependent on the number and specificity of transferred cells. As the specificity of the transferred MBP-specific T cells became higher, fewer were needed to induce clinically significant changes. If a low number of MBP-specific T cells were used, the addition of PPD-specific T cells resulted in a more disabling disease course. On MRI relaxometry studies, MBP-specific T cells with a lower specificity were able to produce significant BBB leakage in the brain compared to cells with higher specificity. The authors concluded that MBP T cells with higher specificity were more likely to cause new lesion formation in the spinal cord, which resulted in more clinical disability. The cord was not studied by MRI due to technical limitations. The authors propose a synergy between PPD- and MBP-specific T cells and suggest it is part of the mechanism of action of mycobacteria in complete Freund's adjuvant [42].

The advent of ultrafast techniques allows relaxometry on several slices or the entire brain within a reasonable amount of time. The utilization of this MRI technique in MS models will likely grow in the coming years.

# 5   Magnetic Resonance Spectroscopy

Magnetic resonance spectroscopy (MRS) allows insight into the chemical ingredients of a studied voxel or voxels of interest. The most commonly studied nuclei are proton and phosphorus. MRS is derived directly from NMR spectroscopy. The only technical difference between NMR spectroscopy and MRS is that the former is usually conducted on homogenous substances such as liquid extracts, whereas the latter is conducted on complex biological samples including live mice or rats, which require the use of gradients and saturation pulses to select the voxel of interest. When MRS is used in human studies, the most commonly studied voxel size is 1–8 cm$^3$. Such voxels are larger than the entire rodent brain. For rodent studies, typical voxel sizes are 8–27 mm$^3$, approximately 1/100 to 1/1,000 the size of typical voxels in human MRS. The number of protons in such small voxels is several orders of magnitude less; therefore, the SNR is much lower under the same experimental circumstances. To overcome this, higher field strength and the averaging of hundreds of signals are needed along with other technical issues that include proper shimming. Although MR spectroscopy is gaining increasing popularity in human MS research, the number of publications utilizing in vivo spectroscopy in MS models is low. This is related to the above difficulties in small-animal MRS studies.

A study of MBP-induced marmoset EAE analyzed the relationship of changes between histology, T2-weighted imaging and MRS. The authors found that acutely fatal EAE lesions were large and monophasic as visualized by MRI, and increased choline (Cho)/creatinine (Cre) ratio was detected by MRS at disease onset. Cho is typically considered a marker of membrane turnover, and it can also be increased by cellular infiltration. Chronic EAE lesions in this model were preceded by multiple inflammatory attacks on T2-weighted imaging and were characterized by low levels of NAA (n-acetyl aspartate)/Cre, which were detectable even after the initial attack. NAA is a marker of neuronal and axonal integrity. Normal-appearing brain lesions were associated with low Cho/Cre ratio, although this did not reach significance [56].

In a study of acute EAE, an elevation in the ratio of choline-containing compounds to Cre was found. This was associated with an increase in choline, betaine, and a reduction in N-acetylaspartate (NAA), aspartate, N-acetylaspartatylglutamate and inositol when studied in vitro. Histological examination revealed inflammation without concomitant demyelination. The authors attribute the increased ratio of Cho:Cre to increased concentrations of phosphorylcholine, betaine, and choline in association with inflammation and not with demyelination. Dysfunctional neuronal metabolism may account for the reduction in NAA rather than actual neuronal or axonal loss [4].

In a TMEV-induced MS model, the presence of T1 hypointensities on imaging was associated with a decrease of the NAA/Cre peaks on single voxel MRS encompassing T1 hypointense lesions. As previously established histologically, these findings were associated with significant tissue damage in the areas of T1 black hole formation including neuronal loss [54].

The above studies highlight a role for MRS in small-animal models; however, the technical difficulties related to small voxel size and consequential low SNR are often difficult to overcome. Nevertheless, with the development of newer techniques including chemical shift imaging and with higher field strength systems, MRS and experimental NMR spectroscopy are emerging in the study of demyelinating disease models.

# 6  Cell-Specific Contrast Agents

While MRI is a very sensitive diagnostic modality, it does not provide cell-specific information about the visualized organs. The use of contrast agents like gadolinium-DTPA can increase the specificity of MR imaging, especially in the case of inflammatory diseases. However, as discussed above, contrast dye enhancement does not note whether cells actually have entered the inflamed organ, nor does it specify cell types. Ideally, intelligent contrast agents will be developed to allow visualization of arbitrary cell types to understand and characterize CNS inflammation and a broad range of other disease processes. Early approaches to target-seeking contrast material development include the use of conjugated gadolinium-DTPA or other agents such as europium, which is known to be taken up by macrophages. However, most early trials were unsuccessful; they either failed to provide adequate labeling specificity, or the labeling did not cross the BBB in sufficient amounts [59].

Another approach is to use non-proton MRI and label molecules or cells of interest with other nuclei capable of emitting NMR signal. An example is the use of fluor-based labeling of macrophages in adoptive transfer EAE. In this $^{19}$F MRI study, the early stages of lesion formation were associated with strong MRI signals, which decayed with time as the lesion turned more chronic and acellular. The problem with this approach is the need for special RF coils designed to match the frequency required for $^{19}$F imaging. Furthermore, anatomical details will not be readily visualized on $^{19}$F images; therefore, proton acquisition is still required for anatomical localization. This necessitates dual tuned ($^1$H and $^{19}$F) coils, further complicating the acquisition hardware and software requirements [46].

Most of the viable cell-specific imaging approaches utilize iron-based contrast materials, most commonly USPIO-s (ultrasmall superparamagnetic iron oxide). These contrast materials provide negative contrast or signal loss on T2*-weighted images. One example is the use of AMI-227 USPIO in an EAE model of MS. USPIO is readily taken up by macrophages, allowing for relatively easy visualization of this cell type. In this proof-of-principle study, the dosage and the scanning delay were investigated [8] (Fig. 7). A study utilizing iron-based contrast agents in chronic-relapsing EAE showed strong delineation of macrophage infiltrated areas by using MION-46L as contrast material. The lesions were shown on histology, and the presence of iron particles was visualized in lesions as small as 110 μm with the use of Prussian blue tissue stain [62]. In a study using both conventional gadolinium and USPIO-s, BBB leakage, as detected by gadolinium, always preceded USPIO-detected macrophage infiltration. The study also demonstrated the use of novel contrast agents to monitor the efficacy of therapeutic agents; for example, lovastatin reduced the observed signal changes in this model [11]. A study of the TMEV model of MS made novel use of commercially available paramagnetic antibodies as contrast materials. These antibodies are used for magnet-activated cell sorting, a routine procedure used to sort specific cell types based on their surface markers. When injected intravenously, they attach to the cell surface markers for which they are specific and allow the visualization of various different immune cell types. Since this contrast material is also based on susceptibility, the localization of antibodies is best detected on T2*-weighted

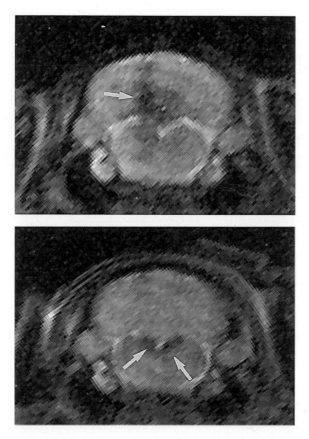

**Fig. 7** Cell-specific imaging with native USPIO-s. Coronal RARE T2-weighted images of two rat brains with clinical EAE 24 h after i.v. administration of AMI-227 at a dose of 300 mmol:kg Fe. Numerous sites with low signal intensities related to magnetic susceptibility effects (T2* hypointensities) due to iron-loaded macrophages are seen on the EAE rat brain parenchyma (*arrows*). Adopted from [8] with permission

images. However, they also cause faint but detectable signal increase on T1-weighted images. Therefore, combined use of T1 and T2* image sets will easily visualize the location of the labeled CD8 T cells [53] (Fig. 8). The same technique can also be used to study other immune cell types and biologically important macromolecules [50].

Cell-specific MRI techniques continue to evolve in both human and disease model applications. The techniques described above will be further refined and utilized in the study of MS models for years to come.

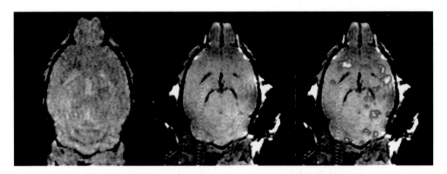

**Fig. 8** Cell-specific imaging utilizing commercially available MACS (magnet activated cell sorting) antibodies. *Left image*: T2\*-weighted gradient echo axial image of mouse brain, acquired 18 h after injection of CD8-specific superparamagnetic antibody. Note the areas of T2\* hypointensities depicting the location of CD8 T cells. *Middle image*: T1-weighted spin echo image; note slight T1 hyperintensities depicting the location of CD8 T cells. *Right image*: composite image. Using the T2\*- and T1-weighted images, a mask was generated by dividing the T1 image by the T2\* image using the image algebra tool in Analyze 6.2 (Mayo Clinic BIR, Rochester, MN, USA). Since the labeled lesions are bright (high number in matrix) on T1 and dark (low number in matrix) on T2\* images, the generated mask has very high numbers – thus very high intensity areas—corresponding to the labeled cells. The mask was color coded, a Gaussian filter was applied for edge smoothing, and finally it was superimposed on the original T1-weighted image. The composite image very clearly illustrates the location of the labeled CD8 lymphocytes

## 7   Imaging of Remyelination in MS Models

Toxin-induced models of demyelinating diseases may be the most suitable for monitoring remyelination by MRI. The advent of new therapeutic remyelination-inducing approaches makes this a critical tool. In the case of lysophosphatidylcholine-induced models, the toxin (a detergent) is injected in the CNS region (typically the spinal cord or the corpus callosum) where demyelinating lesions are to be induced. The injection results in focal inflammatory demyelination followed by remyelination. A sensitive MRI modality to follow this process is magnetization-transfer MRI, which shows that the initially decreased MTR (consistent with demyelination) normalizes over the course of weeks [7]. Another toxin-induced demyelinating model utilizes the copper chelator cuprizone. In this model, animals receive cuprizone every day, which results in demyelination of standard areas of the brain, including the corpus callosum, over weeks. Once chelator administration stops, slow and nearly complete remyelination follows. MRI, including T1- and T2-weighted imaging and MTI, allows for the visualization of remyelination. While MTR imaging is the most sensitive demonstrated treatment modality, changes detected on T1- and T2-weighted images also detect remyelination [37] (Fig. 9).

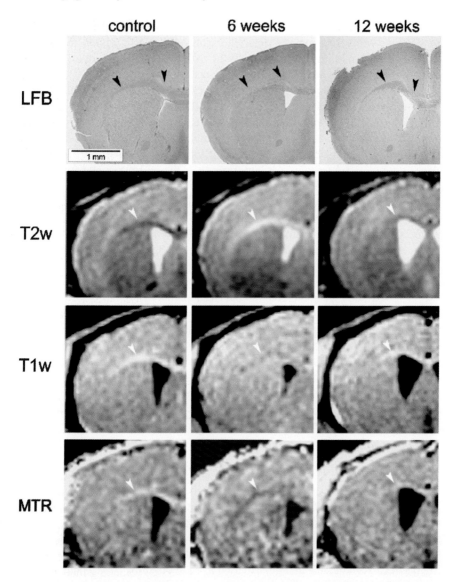

**Fig. 9** Light microscopy and MRI of the corpus callosum of mice treated with cuprizone. Six-week time point: demyelination; 12 weeks: remyelination. *LFB*, Luxol fast blue staining for myelin; *T2w*, T2-weighted images; *T1w*, T1-weighted images; *MTR*, magnetization transfer ratio of the brain of (*left*) controls, (*middle*) mice after 6 weeks of cuprizone treatment, and (*right*) after an additional 6 weeks on normal diet and withdrawal of the toxin (12 weeks). *Arrowheads* indicate corpus callosum. Note that the dark signal on MTR at 6 weeks is almost completely resolved by week 12. While less sensitive, T2- and T1-weighted images still demonstrate resolution of signal changes as remyelination occurs. Reprinted from [37] with permission

Diffusion-weighted imaging is another potentially useful imaging modality for studying remyelination. As detailed earlier, the classic dogma in diffusion imaging is that axonal damage results in axial diffusivity decrease, whereas demyelination results in radial diffusivity decrease. In the case of corpus callosum demyelination by cuprizone, the first changes seen are axonal changes, resulting in axial diffusivity problems, followed by radial diffusivity problems with the onset of demyelination. During the weeks of reversal, diffusivity returns nearly to normal values [61]. With the combined use of conventional imaging techniques and sophisticated postprocessing tools, texture analysis of the brain identified horizontal gray level nonuniformity as the best parameter for remyelination in a cuprizone-induced model [63].

In a serial spinal cord MRI study of a chronic progressive demyelinating disease model induced by TMEV, RARE-based T2-weighted sequences demonstrated sensitivity to remyelination induced by IgM class human antibodies. Five weeks after treatment with rHIgM22 antibody, the T2-weighted lesion load, as measured by 3D volumetry of the cervical and upper thoracic cords, was significantly decreased in most studied animals. The study also demonstrated that the rHIgM22 antibody is detectable in the cord parenchyma, utilizing molecular labeling methods described earlier. Some of the observed T2 hyperintense signal volume decrease may be related to the appearance of T2 hypointensities adjacent to the gray–white junction in cords while they undergo remyelination. As also demonstrated by Merkler et al. [37], T2-weighted images are not completely insensitive to remyelination. However, extrapolating from human observations at lower field strength, other modalities are possibly more suitable for detecting remyelination [2].

## 8 Conclusions and Future Directions

With increasing access to small-animal imaging systems at most universities and research centers, the importance of this noninvasive diagnostic modality will continue to grow. A key aspect of this growth is the capability to acquire full 3D data sets of the CNS with previously unprecedented details in vivo. Furthermore, as MRI is readily available and regularly used in the monitoring of MS patients, small animal MRI studies allow direct comparison of imaging features between MS models and the human disease. This is especially important as the MRI features accompanying MS cannot be readily dissected in the human disease itself. The advent of transgenic technology, with refined cell transfer techniques and pharmacological manipulation of the immune system, will allow comprehensive investigation of imaging findings in MS models. The last two decades have witnessed constant multilateral information exchange between the fields of experimental NMR, human MR imaging, and experimental small-animal MR imaging. This exciting interaction should grow in the coming years to allow for even more sophisticated noninvasive investigations of MS and its animal models.

# References

1. Ahrens ET, Laidlaw DH, Readhead C, Brosnan CF, Fraser SE, Jacobs RE (1998) Mr microscopy of transgenic mice that spontaneously acquire experimental allergic encephalomyelitis. Magn Reson Med 40:119–132
2. Barkhof F, Bruck W, De Groot CJ, Bergers E, Hulshof S, Geurts J, Polman CH, van der Valk P (2003) Remyelinated lesions in multiple sclerosis: magnetic resonance image appearance. Arch Neurol 60:1073–1081
3. Biton IE, Mayk A, Kidron D, Assaf Y, Cohen Y (2005) Improved detectability of experimental allergic encephalomyelitis in excised swine spinal cords by high b-value q-space DWI. Exp Neurol 195:437–446
4. Brenner RE, Munro PM, Williams SC, Bell JD, Barker GJ, Hawkins CP, Landon DN, McDonald WI (1993) The proton NMR spectrum in acute EAE: the significance of the change in the Cho:Cr ratio. Magn Reson Med 29:737–745
5. Cook LL, Foster PJ,Karlik SJ (2005) Pathology-guided MR analysis of acute and chronic experimental allergic encephalomyelitis spinal cord lesions at 1.5 T. J Magn Reson Imaging 22:180–188
6. Cook LL, Foster PJ, Mitchell JR, Karlik SJ (2004) In vivo 4.0-T magnetic resonance investigation of spinal cord inflammation, demyelination, and axonal damage in chronic-progressive experimental allergic encephalomyelitis. J Magn Reson Imaging 20:563–571
7. Deloire-Grassin MS, Brochet B, Quesson B, Delalande C, Dousset V, Canioni P, Petry KG (2000) In vivo evaluation of remyelination in rat brain by magnetization transfer imaging. J Neurol Sci 178:10–16
8. Dousset V, Gomez C, Petry KG, Delalande C, Caille JM (1999) Dose and scanning delay using USPIO for central nervous system macrophage imaging. Magma 8:185–189
9. Dousset V, Grossman RI, Ramer KN, Schnall MD, Young LH, Gonzalez-Scarano F, Lavi E, Cohen JA (1992) Experimental allergic encephalomyelitis and multiple sclerosis: lesion characterization with magnetization transfer imaging. Radiology 182:483–491
10. Duckers HJ, Muller HJ, Verhaagen J, Nicolay K, Gispen WH (1997) Longitudinal in vivo magnetic resonance imaging studies in experimental allergic encephalomyelitis: effect of a neurotrophic treatment on cortical lesion development. Neuroscience 77:1163–1173
11. Floris S, Blezer EL, Schreibelt G, Dopp E, van der Pol SM, Schadee-Eestermans IL, Nicolay K, Dijkstra CD, de Vries HE (2004) Blood–brain barrier permeability and monocyte infiltration in experimental allergic encephalomyelitis: a quantitative MRI study. Brain 127:616–627
12. Gareau PJ, Rutt BK, Karlik SJ, Mitchell JR (2000) Magnetization transfer and multicomponent t2 relaxation measurements with histopathologic correlation in an experimental model of MS. J Magn Reson Imaging 11:586–595
13. Gareau PJ, Wymore AC, Cofer GP, Johnson GA (2002) Imaging inflammation: direct visualization of perivascular cuffing in EAE by magnetic resonance microscopy. J Magn Reson Imaging 16:28–36
14. Genain CP, Lee-Parritz D, Nguyen MH, Massacesi L, Joshi N, Ferrante R, Hoffman K, Moseley M, Letvin NL, Hauser SL (1994) In healthy primates, circulating autoreactive t cells mediate autoimmune disease. J Clin Invest 94:1339–1345
15. Genain CP, Roberts T, Davis RL, Nguyen MH, Uccelli A, Faulds D, Li Y, Hedgpeth J, Hauser SL (1995) Prevention of autoimmune demyelination in non-human primates by a camp-specific phosphodiesterase inhibitor. Proc Natl Acad Sci U S A 92:3601–3605
16. Grossman RI, Lisak RP, Macchi PJ, Joseph PM (1987) MR of acute experimental allergic encephalomyelitis. AJNR Am J Neuroradiol 8:1045–1048
17. Guy J, Fitzsimmons J, Ellis EA, Beck B, Mancuso A (1992) Intraorbital optic nerve and experimental optic neuritis. Correlation of fat suppression magnetic resonance imaging and electron microscopy. Ophthalmology 99:720–725
18. Guy J, Fitzsimmons J, Ellis EA, Mancuso A (1990) Gadolinium-DTPA-enhanced magnetic resonance imaging in experimental optic neuritis. Ophthalmology 97:601–607

19. Guy J, McGorray S, Fitzsimmons J, Beck B, Mancuso A, Rao NA, Hamed L (1994) Reversals of blood–brain barrier disruption by catalase: a serial magnetic resonance imaging study of experimental optic neuritis. Invest Ophthalmol Vis Sci 35:3456–3465

20. Guy J, McGorray S, Qi X, Fitzsimmons J, Mancuso A, Rao N (1994) Conjugated deferoxamine reduces blood–brain barrier disruption in experimental optic neuritis. Ophthalmic Res 26:310–323

21. Hawkins CP, Mackenzie F, Tofts P, du Boulay EP, McDonald WI (1991) Patterns of blood–brain barrier breakdown in inflammatory demyelination. Brain 114:801–810

22. Hawkins CP, Munro PM, Landon DN, McDonald WI (1992) Metabolically dependent blood–brain barrier breakdown in chronic relapsing experimental allergic encephalomyelitis. Acta Neuropathol (Berl) 83:630–635

23. Hawkins CP, Munro PM, MacKenzie F, Kesselring J, Tofts PS, du Boulay EP, Landon DN, McDonald WI (1990) Duration and selectivity of blood–brain barrier breakdown in chronic relapsing experimental allergic encephalomyelitis studied by gadolinium-DTPA and protein markers. Brain 113:365–378

24. Heide AC, Richards TL, Alvord EC Jr, Peterson J, Rose LM (1993) Diffusion imaging of experimental allergic encephalomyelitis. Magn Reson Med 29:478–484

25. Karlik SJ, Grant EA, Lee D, Noseworthy JH (1993) Gadolinium enhancement in acute and chronic-progressive experimental allergic encephalomyelitis in the guinea pig. Magn Reson Med 30:326–331

26. Karlik SJ, Munoz D, St Louis J, Strejan G (1999) Correlation between MRI and clinico-pathological manifestations in Lewis rats protected from experimental allergic encephalomyelitis by acylated synthetic peptide of myelin basic protein. Magn Reson Imaging 17:731–737

27. Karlik SJ, Wong C, Gilbert JJ, Noseworthy JH (1989) NMR studies in the relapsing experimental allergic encephalomyelitis (EAE) model of multiple sclerosis in the strain 13 guinea pig. Magn Reson Imaging 7:463–473

28. Kim JH, Budde MD, Liang HF, Klein RS, Russell JH, Cross AH, Song SK (2006) Detecting axon damage in spinal cord from a mouse model of multiple sclerosis. Neurobiol Dis 21:626–632

29. Kuharik MA, Edwards MK, Farlow MR, Becker GJ, Azzarelli B, Klatte EC, Augustyn G, Dreesen RG (1988) Gd-enhanced MR imaging of acute and chronic experimental demyelinating lesions. AJNR Am J Neuroradiol 9:643–648

30. Lanens D, Van der Linden A, Gerrits PO, 's-Gravenmade EJ (1994) In vitro NMR microimaging of the spinal cord of chronic relapsing EAE rats. Magn Reson Imaging 12:469–475

31. Lassmann H, Ransohoff RM (2004) The CD4-th1 model for multiple sclerosis: A critical [correction of crucial] re-appraisal. Trends Immunol 25:132–137

32. Laule C, Vavasour IM, Moore GR, Oger J, Li DK, Paty DW, MacKay AL (2004) Water content and myelin water fraction in multiple sclerosis. A t2 relaxation study. J Neurol 251:284–293

33. Lennon VA, Wingerchuk DM, Kryzer TJ, Pittock SJ, Lucchinetti CF, Fujihara K, Nakashima I, Weinshenker BG (2004) A serum autoantibody marker of neuromyelitis optica: Distinction from multiple sclerosis. Lancet 364:2106–2112

34. Li DK, Li MJ, Traboulsee A, Zhao G, Riddehough A, Paty D (2006) The use of MRI as an outcome measure in clinical trials. Adv Neurol 98:203–226

35. McDonald WI, Compston A, Edan G, Goodkin D, Hartung HP, Lublin FD, McFarland HF, Paty DW, Polman CH, Reingold SC, Sandberg-Wollheim M, Sibley W, Thompson A, van den Noort S, Weinshenker BY, Wolinsky JS (2001) Recommended diagnostic criteria for multiple sclerosis: guidelines from the international panel on the diagnosis of multiple sclerosis. Ann Neurol 50:121–127

36. McFarland HI, Lobito AA, Johnson MM, Palardy GR, Yee CS, Jordan EK, Frank JA, Tresser N, Genain CP, Mueller JP, Matis LA, Lenardo MJ (2001) Effective antigen-specific immunotherapy in the marmoset model of multiple sclerosis. J Immunol 166:2116–2121

37. Merkler D, Boretius S, Stadelmann C, Ernsting T, Michaelis T, Frahm J, Bruck W (2005) Multicontrast MRI of remyelination in the central nervous system. NMR Biomed 18:395–403
38. Morrissey SP, Deichmann R, Syha J, Simonis C, Zettl U, Archelos JJ, Jung S, Stodal H, Lassmann H, Toyka KV, Haase A, Hartung HP (1996) Partial inhibition of AT-EAE by an antibody to icam-1: clinico-histological and MRI studies. J Neuroimmunol 69:85–93
39. Morrissey SP, Stodal H, Zettl U, Simonis C, Jung S, Kiefer R, Lassmann H, Hartung HP, Haase A, Toyka KV (1996) In vivo MRI and its histological correlates in acute adoptive transfer experimental allergic encephalomyelitis. Quantification of inflammation and oedema. Brain 119:239–248
40. Namer IJ, Steibel J, Klinguer C, Trifilieff E, Mohr M, Poulet P (1998) Magnetic resonance imaging of PLP-induced experimental allergic encephalomyelitis in Lewis rats. J Neuro-immunol 92:22–28
41. Namer IJ, Steibel J, Poulet P, Armspach JP, Mauss Y, Chambron J (1992) In vivo dynamic MR imaging of MBP-induced acute experimental allergic encephalomyelitis in Lewis rat. Magn Reson Med 24:325–334
42. Namer IJ, Steibel J, Poulet P, Armspach JP, Mohr M, Mauss Y, Chambron J (1993) Blood–brain barrier breakdown in MBP-specific t cell induced experimental allergic encephalomy-elitis. A quantitative in vivo MRI study. Brain 116:147–159
43. Nelson AL, Bieber AJ, Rodriguez M (2004) Contrasting murine models of MS. Int MS J 11:95–99
44. Noseworthy JH, Gilbert JJ, Vandervoort MK, Karlik SJ (1988) Postnatal NMR changes in guinea pig central nervous system: potential relevance to experimental allergic encephalomy-elitis. Magn Reson Med 6:199–211
45. Noseworthy JH, Lucchinetti C, Rodriguez M, Weinshenker BG (2000) Multiple sclerosis. N Engl J Med 343:938–952
46. Noth U, Morrissey SP, Deichmann R, Jung S, Adolf H, Haase A, Lutz J (1997) Perfluoro-15-crown-5-ether labelled macrophages in adoptive transfer experimental allergic encepha-lomyelitis. Artif Cells Blood Substit Immobil Biotechnol 25:243–254
47. O'Brien JT, Noseworthy JH, Gilbert JJ, Karlik SJ (1987) NMR changes in experimental allergic encephalomyelitis: NMR changes precede clinical and pathological events. Magn Reson Med 5:109–117
48. Peersman GV, Van de Vyver FL, Lohman JE, Lubke U, Gheuens J, Bellon E, Connelly A, Martin JJ (1988) High resolution nuclear magnetic resonance imaging of the spinal cord in experimental demyelinating disease. Acta Neuropathol (Berl) 76:628–632
49. Piraino PS, Yednock TA, Freedman SB, Messersmith EK, Pleiss MA, Karlik SJ (2005) Suppression of acute experimental allergic encephalomyelitis with a small molecule inhibitor of alpha4 integrin. Mult Scler 11:683–690
50. Pirko I, Ciric B, Gamez J, Bieber AJ, Warrington AE, Johnson AJ, Hanson DP, Pease LR, Macura SI, Rodriguez M (2004) A human antibody that promotes remyelination, enters the Cns and decreases lesion load as detected by T2-weighted spinal cord MRI in a virus-induced murine model of MS. FASEB J 18:1577–1579
51. Pirko I, Fricke ST, Johnson AJ, Rodriguez M, Macura SI (2005) Magnetic resonance imaging, microscopy, and spectroscopy of the central nervous system in experimental animals. NeuroRx 2:250–264
52. Pirko I, Gamez J, Johnson AJ, Macura SI, Rodriguez M (2004) Dynamics of MRI lesion development in an animal model of viral-induced acute progressive CNS demyelination. Neuroimage 21:576–582
53. Pirko I, Johnson A, Ciric B, Gamez J, Macura SI, Pease LR, Rodriguez M (2004) In vivo magnetic resonance imaging of immune cells in the central nervous system with superpara-magnetic antibodies. FASEB J 18:179–182
54. Pirko I, Johnson A, Gamez J, Macura SI, Rodriguez M (2004) Disappearing "t1 black holes" in an animal model of multiple sclerosis. Front Biosci 9:1222–1227

55. Polman CH, Reingold SC, Edan G, Filippi M, Hartung HP, Kappos L, Lublin FD, Metz LM, McFarland HF, O'Connor PW, Sandberg-Wollheim M, Thompson AJ, Weinshenker BG, Wolinsky JS (2005) Diagnostic criteria for multiple sclerosis: 2005 revisions to the "mcdonald criteria". Ann Neurol 58:840–846
56. Richards TL, Alvord EC Jr, Peterson J, Cosgrove S, Petersen R, Petersen K, Heide AC, Cluff J, Rose LM (1995) Experimental allergic encephalomyelitis in non-human primates: MRI and MRS may predict the type of brain damage. NMR Biomed 8:49–58
57. Rose LM, Richards TL, Peterson J, Petersen R, Alvord EC Jr (1997) Resolution of cns lesions following treatment of experimental allergic encephalomyelitis in macaques with monoclonal antibody to the cd18 leukocyte integrin. Mult Scler 2:259–266
58. Sriram S, Steiner I (2005) Experimental allergic encephalomyelitis: A misleading model of multiple sclerosis. Ann Neurol 58:939–945
59. Stavraky RT, Grant CW, Barber KR, Karlik SJ (1993) Baseline consideration of liposomal contrast agent. CNS transport by macrophages in experimental allergic encephalomyelitis. Magn Reson Imaging 11:685–689
60. Steinman L, Zamvil SS (2006) How to successfully apply animal studies in experimental allergic encephalomyelitis to research on multiple sclerosis. Ann Neurol 60:12–21
61. Sun SW, Liang HF, Trinkaus K, Cross AH, Armstrong RC, Song SK (2006) Noninvasive detection of cuprizone induced axonal damage and demyelination in the mouse corpus callosum. Magn Reson Med 55:302–308
62. Xu S, Jordan EK, Brocke S, Bulte JW, Quigley L, Tresser N, Ostuni JL, Yang Y, McFarland HF, Frank JA (1998) Study of relapsing remitting experimental allergic encephalomyelitis SJL mouse model using mion-46 l enhanced in vivo MRI: early histopathological correlation. J Neurosci Res 52:549–558
63. Yu O, Steibel J, Mauss Y, Guignard B, Eclancher B, Chambron J, Grucker D (2004) Remyelination assessment by MRI texture analysis in a cuprizone mouse model. Magn Reson Imaging 22:1139–1144
64. Zamaroczy D, Schluesener HJ, Jolesz FA, Sobel RA, Colucci VM, Weiner HL, Sandor T (1991) Differentiation of experimental white matter lesions using multiparametric magnetic resonance measurements. Invest Radiol 26:317–324
65. Zivadinov R, Bakshi R (2004) Role of MRI in multiple sclerosis I: inflammation and lesions. Front Biosci 9:665–683
66. Zivadinov R, Bakshi R (2004) Role of MRI in multiple sclerosis II: brain and spinal cord atrophy. Front Biosci 9:647–664

# Hormonal Influences in Multiple Sclerosis

**E.A. Shuster**

E.A. Shuster

Department of Neurology, Mayo Clinic College of Medicine, Rochester, MN 55905, USA

e-mail: shuster.elizabeth@mayo.edu

M. Rodriguez (ed.), *Advances in Multiple Sclerosis and Experimental
Demyelinating Diseases. Current Topics in Microbiology and Immunology 318.*
© Springer-Verlag Berlin Heidelberg 2008

**Abstract**  The function of hormones has expanded to include immunomodulation and neuroprotection in addition to their classic roles. The story of how hormones influence inflammation and neuron and glial function is being slowly unraveled. There is increasing evidence that estrogen, progesterone, and testosterone contain immune responses and influence damage repair in the nervous system. Hormones such as prolactin and vitamin D are being explored as immunomodulators and may influence diseases such as multiple sclerosis (MS) or may be used therapeutically to modulate the immune response. More recently identified hormones, such as leptin and gherlin, may also influence the course of disease. This chapter reviews some of the evidence that supports a role for hormones in MS.

# 1   Introduction

The classic role of hormones is to promote normal growth, metabolism, and reproduction. Hormones are able to initiate a cascade of responses in their target tissues that is often followed by a feedback loop to bring physiological systems back to equilibrium. They come in five major classes: steroids, amino acid derivatives, small neuropeptides, large proteins, and vitamin derivatives. Two major observations led to the hypothesis that hormones influence autoimmune diseases. First, corticosteroids influence inflammation, and many autoimmune disorders respond to corticosteroids. Second, most autoimmune diseases have a gender bias and are more common in women. In addition, some autoimmune disorders improve, while others worsen, during periods of significant hormonal change such as pregnancy. While MS may not be an autoimmune disease, it has many features in common with autoimmune diseases including the gender bias and tendency to relapse and remit, and immunomodulation appears to be at least somewhat effective in containing the inflammatory component of the disease process.

Research exploring how hormones influence the immune system began in the 1950s and 1960s [117]. These studies have unquestionably changed our thinking about hormone action. In the last decade, there has been a tremendous growth in our understanding of the nonclassical immunomodulating role of hormones. Their cytokine-like effects on the cells of the immune system and their cytoprotective or cytotoxic effects on cells of the nervous system are particularly relevant to MS. Recent studies have revealed that some hormones can be produced in immune cells themselves. Hormone receptors exist on or in immune cells as well as in cells of the CNS. Many hormones have an expansive effect on a wide variety of cells. The tools are now in place to study the actual mechanisms of action.

The idea of hormone therapy is very appealing because hormones are considered natural and the side effects are understood. Corticosteroids have been the mainstay of MS treatment since the 1980s. We are learning more about their actions and, hopefully, will be able to utilize them more effectively in the future. We may be on the verge of using other hormones, as well as designer versions of them, to manipulate the immune system and nervous system repair. Investigators have already done pilot clinical trials of estrogen and testosterone, progesterone, and vitamin D for the treatment of MS.

This chapter reviews hypotheses about how hormones influence MS and its experimental animal model, experimental autoimmune encephalomyelitis (EAE). While we must address many more questions before hormone therapy becomes standard clinical practice, the momentum is rushing forward.

# 2 Glucocorticoids

## 2.1 Background

The first reports by Hench et al. in 1949 ushered in the therapeutic use of the anti-inflammatory and immunosuppressive properties of glucocorticoids [99]. One could argue that no hormones have had more relevance to MS patients than the glucocorticoids. Corticotrophin (ACTH), along with the newer synthetic glucocorticoids (methylprednisolone and dexamethasone), has been the mainstay of treatment for MS clinical attacks since the 1960s. A recent textbook [158] reviews the evidence for a positive short-term effect.

The communications networks between the neurological, immunological, and endocrine systems are highly influenced by glucocorticoids and vice versa [151]. Much interest focuses on how control of endogenous cortisol production and immune cell responses influences susceptibility to disease onset, relapse, and glucocorticoid-receptor (GR) regulation of gene transcription. GR monomers also bind to nuclear factor-κB, adaptor protein 1, and other transcription factors. In addition, they exert their influence by nongenomic means mediated by receptor-like proteins on cell membranes; this latter pathway may be one of the most important anti-inflammatory and immunomodulating effects of exogenous pulse therapy with glucocorticoids [45]. Different forms of the enzyme 11-β-hydroxysteroid dehydrogenase in different tissues determine how much active cortisol is present at a given time. In turn, immune cell glucocorticoid resistance has several mechanisms induced by glucocorticoids themselves, by chronic inflammation, and by stress [151].

Relevant to our current understanding of the immunology of MS, tumor necrosis factor alpha (TNF-α), interleukin-1 (IL-1), and interleukin-6 (IL-6), the prototypical pro-inflammatory cytokines, activate both the hypothalamic pituitary axis and the intimately related sympathetic nervous system (SNS) [24, 35]. IL-1β may be a crucial cytokine in the neuro-immuno-endocrine response [26, 53, 102, 201]. Multiple factors affect the response of the hypothalamic pituitary adrenal (HPA) axis and the intimately related sympathetic nervous system to inflammation or other stressful stimuli with the goal of bringing the organism back to health. Optimal versus suboptimal functioning of the hypothalamic–pituitary–adrenal axis could influence resistance to and/or modify the course of inflammatory diseases. In turn, the multifocal nature of MS may upset the sophisticated neural communication networks and feedback loops of both the hypothalamic pituitary adrenal system and the SNS [36]. We are progressing in our understanding of these communication networks, which will hopefully improve our ability to utilize glucocorticoids more effectively in the clinically setting.

## 2.2 The Hypothalamic Pituitary Adrenal Axis Function in EAE and MS

In 1980, Levine and colleagues showed that Lewis rats had a dramatic increase in serum corticosterone levels during the acute phase of EAE [131]. While high versus low hypothalamic–pituitary–adrenal axis response alone does not explain increased susceptibility [143, 200, 201], several EAE models have shown that the degree of HPA response plays a role. In 1990, Mason showed that a resistant rat strain could be made susceptible by removal of the adrenal glands and that recovery occurred when corticosterone was given at doses that achieved the acute phase levels in the susceptible Lewis rat [143]. Lower levels of endogenous cortisone production to the initial inflammatory phase were linked to increased susceptibility and more severe course. Continuous dexamethasone treatment completely blocks EAE in a susceptible rat model, while sudden withdrawal of dexamethasone triggers severe exacerbation [178]. In a model resembling human MS, failure to produce an adequate level of cortisone with the first attack of EAE results in failure to resolve the acute inflammation and leads to chronic progressive EAE [26, 201]. The second relapse is not associated with as high a rise in cortisone as was seen in the first phase, and the HPA axis is hyporesponsive to injection of IL-1β. In the second phase, associated with demyelination, macrophage production of IL-1β is reduced compared to the primary phase, reducing the stimulus for cortisone production as well. Cortisone implants suppress this second demyelinating phase of the disease [201]. These studies suggest that an appropriately strong hypothalamic–pituitary–adrenal axis response to the induction of EAE is necessary for recovery from the initial phase of the disease and that subsequent phases are associated with less inflammatory cytokine stimulus and lower glucocorticoid response. Exogenous steroid can replace endogenous steroid in preventing or limiting the disease.

MS disease onset is not as clearly defined as in EAE. No studies exist of the HPA axis response specifically targeting the early group of patients with clinically isolated syndrome. The delay of the second, MS-defining attack in optic neuritis patients treated with high-dose intravenous methylprednisolone suggests that a robust glucocorticoid response affects subsequent disease in humans as well. Several studies have evaluated the HPA axis of patients with established disease. Although they conflict at times, these studies generally indicate that chronic activation of the central HPA occurs with progressive disease.

Reder et al. studied 19 patients during acute exacerbations of progressive MS (mean age ,36.6 years ± 2.6) [177]. All MS patients had normal baseline cortisol levels and normal circadian fluctuation; 9 of 19 did not have normal dexamethasone-suppression tests. In this study, the MS patients had lower dexamethasone blood levels, suggesting that the lack of suppression was due, at least in part, to more rapid metabolism of dexamethasone, poor absorption or both. In 1994, Reder et al. reported adrenal gland weight to be increased in ten patients with MS when compared to 13 with ALS and 14 with acute myocardial infarction [178]. None of the patients had depression nor had they been treated with glucocorticoids or corticotrophin within the year prior to death. The adrenal medulla was normal in all patients; cortical hypertrophy was specifically noted in five. They hypothesized that the increased size was due to chronic excessive stimulation of the HPA axis by elevated ACTH.

Michelson reported elevated basal corticotropin (ACTH) and cortisol levels and an abnormally low ACTH to cortisol ratio [148]. Using the more sensitive combined dexamethasone-corticotropin releasing hormone (CRH) test, Grasser et al. found a normal ACTH response but a higher mean plasma cortisol response in 19 MS patients in acute relapse compared to age-matched controls. Six of the 19 had an excessive release of cortisol; four did not respond at all [89]. Wei and Lightman studied 21 patients with definite MS, most within 1 month of clinical relapse [227]. Cortisol levels were comparable to controls with other neurological disorders. The cortisol diurnal rhythm was preserved, but there was a trend of lower amplitudes of the diurnal curves in those with primary progressive MS (PPMS) and secondary progressive MS (SPMS) compared to controls with other neurological disorders ($p < 0.06$ and 0.07, respectively) [227]. Baseline ACTH levels (data only in patients with MS, no controls) did not differ between the different types of MS. The time-integrated cortisol response to corticotrophin-releasing hormone showed normal patterns of cortisol response, but the mean total cortisol response was lower in patients with SPMS than in those with PPMS and controls. The ACTH levels in response to CRH was significantly greater in patients with enhancing lesions than in those without, while the cortisol response to synthetic ACTH was lower, suggesting either reduced adrenal sensitivity or reduced adrenal reserve. Ten patients had the dexamethasone suppression test, and all ten suppressed. Two patients with gadolinium-enhancing lesions on MRI had undetectable postdexamethasone cortisol levels. The authors concluded that the extent of the activation of the HPA axis (as measured by cortisol output) is up 2.5-fold in MS patients compared to normal controls. This is comparable to the levels seen in rheumatoid arthritis patients and in nonrheumatoid arthritis patients undergoing major hip surgery; it is considerably less, however, than the sixfold rise in acute EAE. The central HPA axis upregulated, but the cortisol response at the adrenal level was lower in some patients. Patients with secondary progressive MS had a decreased cumulative HPA response to stress, but the degree of impairment was modest. The investigators concluded that the HPA axis had only a minor role in the initial pathogenesis of MS or disease evolution.

Fassbender et al. reported in 1998 that MS patients failed to suppress with dexamethasone and that this was associated with depression and anxiety [71]. Cerebrospinal fluid (CSF) cell counts correlated with stronger HPA responsiveness. Heesen also found HPA hyperactivity, particularly in the area under the curve for ACTH responses in the dexamethasone-CRH test; this related to the degree of cognitive impairment and progression [98].

Then Bergh et al. studied a group of 60 MS patients. They found that MS patients have hyperactivity of the HPA as measured by the dexamethasone-CRH test. The degree correlated with the severity of the disease (as measured by neurological disability) and not duration, previous relapses, treatments with ACTH or glucocorticoids, or depression. Patients with RRMS had a moderate degree of hyperactivity; those with SPMS, intermediate; and those with primary progressive, the highest [205]. Schumann et al. studied 53 patients and found fewer gadolinium-enhancing lesions in patients with HPA axis hyperactivity as measured by cortisol production in the dexamethasone-CRH test [189]. They found a positive correlation between the cortisol production (area under the curve) and brain atrophy as measured by ventricular volume; the correlation held for RRMS patients as well as for those with progressive disease, even though brain atrophy was also significantly affected by age. When RRMS patients were treated with reversible monoamine oxidase (MOA) inhibitors, moclobemide and oral fluocortolone, during an acute exacerbation, the HPA response normalized when compared to patients treated with fluocortolone alone, supporting a role for SNS in the level of HPA response [206].

From this body of evidence, one might infer that the early ability of the HPA axis to activate in response to MS inflammation modulates the recovery from attacks or disease severity. However, the evidence suggests that chronic hyperactivity of the HPA axis may be more a marker for neurodegeneration than for inflammation. It will be important to determine whether the increased HPA activation seen in patients with progressive disease represents a protective response that evolves with relentless progression of the disease or, possibly, the detrimental effect due to damage of the neuroendocrine communication system, which could be therapeutically manipulated to prevent later progression. A longitudinal study by Gold et al. linked hyperactivity of the HPA axis to more progression and cognitive impairment 3 years later and suggested it as a marker for a subgroup of MS patients destined to progress early [85].

## 2.3  Hypothalamic Lesions in Patients with MS

Lesions in strategic regions of the brain potentially affect the neuroendocrine networks, further leading to disruption of adaptive HPA responses of individuals with

MS. Huitinga et al. systematically reviewed the brains of 17 MS patients (disease duration, mean of 21 years; age range, 33–81 years) for hypothalamic lesions and found 16 of 17 to have demyelinating lesions in the hypothalamus [103]. Sixty percent of the lesions were considered active (containing activated macrophages); 12 of 16 brains had both active and chronic inactive lesions, which suggested that hypothalamic involvement was not only common but ongoing over time. The active lesion score correlated negatively with disease duration and the degree of activation of CRH neurons [103]. In another study, the number of CRH/vasopressin (VP) immunoreactive neurons increased 2.7-fold in MS patients compared to controls, and the CRH mRNA expression increased twofold in the MS patients. More active lesions in the hypothalamus correlated to a lower number of CRH/VP neurons, and a higher active lesion score correlated with a shorter duration of disease until death. This indicates that patients with severe disease have more impaired CRH/VP neurons; these patients also had more lesions elsewhere in the CNS [105]. Erkut et al. reported in 1995 that the CRH cell populations became more activated with age in both MS patients and controls, beginning at age 40; the CRH neurons showed a higher level of activation in the MS patients, and more cells co-expressed both CRH and vasopressin [70].

Hypothalamic lesions have also been described in neuromyelitis optica (NMO). The investigators localized the lesions to sites of high aquaporin-4 expression, the target of their NMO IgG antibody [171].

## 2.4   Glucocorticoid Responsiveness in MS

Glucocorticoid responsiveness can be altered in MS. In spite of an activated HPA axis in patients with MS, the HPA response in MS patients who died of sepsis shows more impairment than the response of non-MS patients who died of sepsis. The CSF IL-6 levels do not correlate with the CSF or serum cortisol levels of MS patients; IL-6 levels do correlate with increased cortisol levels in controls with sepsis, who had a significantly greater cortisol response to sepsis than the patients with MS [104]. Blood from MS patients treated with dexamethasone has impaired inhibition of IL-6 production to lipopolysaccharide stimulation in vitro [55]. Use of steroids in the 3 months prior to the study or use of anti-inflammatory drugs does not affect steroid insensitivity. MS patients, as a whole, show greater variability than controls. When the test is repeated over time, however, there is little variability among individuals.

Although not originally intended as a prospective long-term follow-up study, investigators did obtain follow-up examination data, for 16 of 24 patients. Among these 16, they did find a trend toward a negative correlation (18%) between dexamethasone insensitivity and severity of disease. In a similar study, blood from MS patients treated with dexamethasone failed to suppress TNF-$\alpha$ production to lipopolysaccharide stimulation [215]. An in vitro study of GR binding in lymphocytes of MS patients found no difference from controls, but the usual dependence of binding of lymphocyte GR to the hypothalamic GR was abnormal [205].

There is also limited evidence that early high-dose exogenous corticosteroids provide some resistance to future attacks of MS and to a slower rate of change in brain volume. The results of the human optic neuritis treatment trial showed that patients treated with high-dose intravenous methylprednisolone (IVMP) for 3 days within 14 days of the onset of symptoms had delayed onset of a second, MS-defining episode by 2 years [19, 20]. Regular pulsed IVMP treatment given to patients with RRMS for 5 years showed a statistically significant difference in mean change in brain MRI -T1 black hole volume and brain parenchymal volume. Expanded disability scale scores (EDSS) changed more in controls treated only with relapses. There was no change in brain MRI T2 volume or in clinical relapse rate [235].

## 2.5   Mechanism

The body of evidence indicates that MS patients may not achieve an adequate endogenous glucocorticoid response to suppress inflammation and allow subsequent recovery. Exogenous glucocorticoids may supplement the beneficial effects of endogenous glucocorticoids, many of which are applicable to MS [45]. Glucocorticoids act via genomic and nongenomic mechanisms; with high-pulse doses, the nongenomic effects may account for the early and sometimes dramatic responses. Nongenomic responses can work via the GR, nonclassical receptors, or through direct interaction with cell membranes.

Glucocorticoids counteract the inflammatory effects on the microcirculation [168]. They induce apoptosis of T cell subsets [130]. They suppress production or receptor expression for many cytokines believed to promote inflammation in MS, including IL-2, TNF-$\alpha$, IFN-$\gamma$, IL-12 production by antigen-presenting cells (APCs), andexpression of IL-12 receptors on T and natural killer (NK) cells [36]. In addition, while they do not affect production of IL-10 by monocytes, treatment of MS patients with corticosteroids increases IL-10 production, possibly due to disinhibition [80]. Finally, glucocorticoids might induce differentiation of $T_{reg}$ 1 cells and upregulate the transforming growth factor (TGF) $\beta$ receptors on lymphocytes, which may, in turn, enhance $T_{reg}$ function [15].

In general, corticosteroids seem to have desirable effects in the setting of acute inflammation associated with MS. There may, however, be specific local responses that are not favorable. TGF-$\beta$ production by glial cells are suppressed by glucocorticoids, which could have a negative effect on MS [16]. Exogenous glucocorticoids can also be potentially neurotoxic. Diem et al. reported that methylprednisolone increased apoptosis of retinal ganglion cells in a rat model of optic neuritis [56]. Brunner et al. reported transient negative effects on long-term memory in MS patients [30]. The systemic side effects to bone, muscle, and other organs are well known.

The commonly prescribed synthetic glucocorticoids, methylprednisolone and dexamethasone, likely work in both the periphery and in the central nervous system in MS, where the blood–brain barrier (BBB) is not likely to be intact during acute episodes of inflammation. With an intact BBB, however, the multi-drug efflux transporter prevents uptake into most brain regions, the pituitary being an exception [118]. Drugs that also use the same transporter could potentiate uptake of prednisolone into the brain, e.g., anthracyclines such as mitoxantrone. As BBB-stabilizing drugs are introduced into the armamentarium of MS treatments, synthetic corticosteroids that do not have both the 17-hydroxyl and 11-hydroxyl groups and do not utilize this transporter might be a better choice to treat inflammation in the CNS.

It will be important to define the specific role for corticosteroids in a given individual or subgroup of persons with MS. Understanding the role of endogenous and exogenous glucocorticoids in modulating inflammatory and neuronal activity will target specific actions to ameliorate the course of the disease with designer steroids that have fewer undesirable effects. Resistance to the anti-inflammatory and immunosuppressive influences of glucocorticoids, which can be conveyed through multiple mechanisms, continues to be a barrier to optimal use of glucocorticoids in MS. Understanding their interactions with other immunomodulating therapies for MS will also enhance their value.

# 3   Female Hormones of Reproduction and MS

## 3.1   Background

The female gender bias for MS has provoked interest in the role of the female reproductive hormones in the development and course of MS. The gender bias of MS has been shown with convincing epidemiological studies since the 1970s and may be increasing [161]. The traditional female reproduction hormones include estrogen, progesterone, and prolactin. Receptors for these hormones are present on a wide spectrum of cells, including nervous tissue and immune cells of both genders. Gender differences in the morphological development of nervous tissue and immune tissue influence the physiologic function of the female and male sex hormones. These, in turn, make it especially difficult to sort out the role of a specific hormone in influencing MS. It is also important to understand that hormone influence does not account for all gender imbalances in MS. Male Lewis rats, for example, are more susceptible to EAE; removal of testes makes no obvious difference in that susceptibility. Removal of the ovaries, however, increases female susceptibility [211]. A set of recent series of experiments in mice demonstrated that the XX chromosome complement, even in oophorectomized animals, conferred greater risk of disease [195]. Finally, a recent human genetic study showed men with MS to be 2.21 times more likely to transmit the disease to their children than women, indicating that more than sex hormones are relevant in the gender bias [115].

Bouman et al., in their review of the literature on sex hormones and the immune system, concluded that males have lower lymphocyte numbers, possibly related to testosterone enhancing T lymph apoptosis. However, T cell cytokine production or function exhibited no obvious differences between males and females or during different phases of the female menstrual cycle [28]. Estrogen likely decreases peripheral NK cell numbers. In vitro, low dose and short exposure to estrogen does not affect NK activation; high-dose prolonged exposure increases activation. During pregnancy, stimulated NK cells produce less IFN-γ, but sex hormones do not appear to mediate this. Menopause is associated with significant decrease in the B2 subset cell numbers, and prolonged hormone replacement therapy (hRT) induces a significant increase. Estrogen increases B cell progenitor cells, B cell development and autoreactive B cell survival. Estrogen increases and testosterone decreases antibody production.

Males and postmenopausal women have increased monocytes; estrogen, and possibly progesterone, may decrease monocyte numbers, although monocyte numbers increase in pregnancy, possibly due to estrogen-induced release from the bone marrow. Estrogens appear to decrease monocyte IL-6 cytokine production. Stimulated TNF-α and IL-1β production increases in males; it also increases in females during the luteal phase, compared to the follicular phase, of the menstrual cycle. Whether these differences are regulated by sex steroid hormones is still unclear. Estradiol seems to have an anti-inflammatory effect on neutrophils while progesterone may have a pro-inflammatory effect. The inducible transcription factor, nuclear factor-κB, may mediate the sex steroid effects on cytokine production. The ER receptors may be important in mediating the effect in monocytes. Pregnancy induces the appearance of progesterone receptors on peripheral blood lymphocytes, and this may, in turn, induce production of pregnancy-blocking factor, which may control NK activity as well as promote a Th2 bias [28].

We are fortunate to be able to study the complex contributions and interactions between gender and sex hormones in animals. Estrogens, progesterones, prolactin, and androgens can be given to male and female animals, both neutered and intact; it is, of course, not possible to do similar studies in humans. Animal studies are very useful in reaching a basic understanding of the influences of each sex hormone. The hope is that designer sex hormones may be developed to use for immunomodulation in both males and females without causing gender behavior and reproductive disturbance.

## 3.2   Pregnancy and MS

There is convincing evidence that MS exacerbations diminish during the later stages of pregnancy and increase in the early postpartum period [41]. All of the known studies of pregnancy and MS have limitations. Early studies had uncertain diagnostic criteria, enrolled few patients, and were often retrospective. The many confounding factors in the design of studies of pregnancy and MS have been reviewed [48]. The most uncontrollable factor of all is each woman's decision to become pregnant; MS is only one of many factors on which the decision may be based. In spite of these limitations, however, convincing evidence exists that pregnancy ameliorates MS. Pregnancy also suppresses EAE [1, 119], and the EAE model has led the way in evaluating the role of the hormonal influence on MS. A reasonable inference is that the hormonal milieu of pregnancy ameliorates MS by modulating the immune system. Protein and glycoprotein hormones, steroid hormones, growth factors, and cytokines are all elaborated by the human fetoplacental unit; in fact, the secretory repertoire of the fetoplacental unit surpasses that of all other endocrine tissues [165].

Estrogens have received much attention. Preliminary evidence indicates estriol, the major estrogen produced during pregnancy, as one of the major factors influencing pregnancy-related immunological changes. Preliminary estriol trials in humans have generated enough support to justify a clinical trial. Progesterone is also a candidate hormone, leading to an ongoing clinical trial of progesterone in the postpartum period. Glucocorticoids rise in pregnancy to levels that result in mild Cushing's syndrome [37]. Cortisol, 1,25 hydroxyvitamin D3-induced inhibition and subsequent rebound of IL-12 and TNF-$\alpha$ production may be mechanisms by which pregnancy suppresses MS [67]. Undoubtedly, it is the combination of hormonal changes that contributes to the amelioration of attacks during pregnancy.

### 3.2.1 Selected Studies

Two studies of pregnancy's effect on MS disease activity are notable for their size and design, and they illustrate that pregnancy's ameliorating effect on MS exacerbations is present even when there is a marked difference of MS activity in the populations studied. Korn-Lubetzki et al. were the first to include consistent definitions for both MS diagnosis and relapse [125]. They studied 338 women in Israel who had been diagnosed with MS since 1960. Of the 338, 36 (10%) had onset of the disease during pregnancy. Eighty-five relapses occurred in relationship to 199 pregnancies; 20 occurred during the pregnancy and 65, in the 6 months postpartum, the majority of these in the first 3 months. When comparing the rate of relapse during pregnancy (0.13) to an external control average relapse rate of women of similar age and disease duration (0.28), they found a statistically significant reduction of relapses in the third trimester. In the 6 months postpartum, the rate increased to 0.82, nearly three times higher than that of their controls in the first 3 months postpartum [125].

Confavreux et al. reported on the PRIMS (Pregnancy-Related Relapse In Multiple Sclerosis) study of 256 pregnancies of 241 European women with MS whose disease began prior to the evaluated pregnancies [41]. Patients were recruited when pregnant for at least 4 weeks. Recruitment began in January 1993 and ended in July 1995. Patients enrolled early in their pregnancy were examined at 20 and 28 weeks; all patients were examined at 36 weeks, 3, 6, and 12 months postpartum. The effect of pregnancy, both on relapses and on the level of disability, was measured by Kurtze score. Only first pregnancies resulting in a live birth were included in their analysis (227 pregnancies). Patients served as their own controls. The relapse rate (0.72) 1 year prior to pregnancy was compared to relapses rates in the three trimesters of pregnancy (0.5, 0.6, and 0.2 in the first, second, and third trimesters, respectively). They found a decrease in relapses during the second and, especially, the third trimester of pregnancy and an increase in relapses in the first 3 months postpartum. The risk of relapse in the postpartum period was not affected by epidural anesthesia or by breast feeding. There was a steady worsening of the Kurtze score during the 33-month study period (0.7 points, mean $1.3 \pm 1.4$ at onset of pregnancy to $1.8 \pm 1.6$ at 1 year postpartum). Of the women studied, 72 percent did not experience any relapse during the postpartum period [223]. A higher relapse rate prior to pregnancy, greater disability, and relapse during pregnancy correlated with increased risk of postpartum relapse, but their multivariate model was unable to predict with more than 72% accuracy.

There is only a single report of MRI imaging of MS patients during pregnancy [214]. In that study, two women with RRMS followed in a longitudinal MRI study became pregnant and continued in the study during pregnancy; one was scanned monthly and one every 3 months. Both had a decrease in the number of new or enlarging T2 lesions during the second half of the pregnancy. While extremely limited in size, this paper provides limited supportive evidence that MS becomes less during pregnancy due to a reduced inflammatory component. (Gadolinium-contrasted MRI, the standard often used to show active inflammation in clinical trials, cannot be performed during pregnancy because of potential gadolinium toxicity for the fetus).

### 3.2.2 Mechanism for Pregnancy Modulation of MS

Pregnancy is characterized by local immunosuppression and a heightened state of maternal immunocompetence [48]. Explanations for the increased postpartum exacerbation rate include loss of the placenta and its many hormonal factors, particularly a dramatic drop in estriol and progesterone levels, increase in prolactin, and possible change in thyroid hormone level, particularly in women who have autoimmune thyroid disease [181]. While many changes occur during pregnancy, most studies have focused on estrogen, progesterone, and prolactin. Other candidate hormones for immunomodulation during the third trimester, however, include inhibins, activins, and follistatin, which are glycoproteins belonging to the transforming growth factor $\beta$ family; chorionic somatomammotropin, which may increase levels of insulin-like growth factor 1; leptin; and calcitriol (activated vitamin D) [165]. Cortisol and 1,25 hydroxyvitamin D3 induce inhibition, and the subsequent rebound of IL-12 and TNF-$\alpha$ production may be the mechanism by which pregnancy suppresses MS [67]. Comments on some of these other hormones are found in other parts of this chapter.

Elenkov et al. studied 18 women with normal pregnancies in their third trimester and early postpartum period [67]. IL-12 production was threefold higher and TNF-$\alpha$ production nearly 40% lower than postpartum values. They attributed this to cortisol, norepinephrine, and 1,25 dihydroxyvitamin D-induced inhibition [67]. Al-Shammri et al. studied eight women during pregnancy and found a shift from Th1 cytokine profile to Th2 profile in six as measured by in vitro mitogen stimulation and measurement of IFN-$\gamma$, TNF-$\alpha$, IL-4, and IL-10 [5]. Gilmore et al. compared the in vitro production of cytokines from peripheral blood mononuclear cells taken during the third trimester and postpartum and found an increase in IL-10 in the third trimester and an increase in interferon $\gamma$ postpartum [82]. Lopez et al. recently characterized the third trimester as notable for decreased CXCR 3 expression by CD4[+] and CD 8[+] T cells, increased expression of chemokine receptor CXCR4 and increased mRNA expression of IL-10/ IFN-$\gamma$ ratio [138].

In a study of 13 pregnant MS patients, 21 healthy pregnant women, and 16 non-pregnant healthy controls, Sanches-Ramone et al. found a progressive increase in the percentage of regulatory T cells (CD4[+]CD25[+]) in the pregnant women compared to nonpregnant women and a higher percentage of CD4[+]CD25[hi+] regulatory T cells. There was no difference in total lymphocytes, CD4[+] T lymphocytes or activated CD4[+] lymphocytes between pregnant and nonpregnant women. Pregnant women with MS had higher percentages than healthy pregnant women of both activated T lymphocytes (CD4[+]HLA-DR[+]CD38[+]) and higher CD4[+]CD25[+] [185]. The MS women showed a postpartum decrease in the CD4[+]CD25[+] $T_{reg}$ subset (also seen in healthy pregnant women) and a significant increase in the CD4[+]CD 25[hi+] T lymphocytes (which have previously been shown to also increase during relapses) compared to the third trimester. The regulatory T cells could suppress autologous CD4[+]CD25[-] T lymphocytes in CD3-stimulated and allogeneic mixed lymphocyte reaction. Bebo et al. have proposed that pregnancy-specific glycoproteins regulate T cell function during pregnancy [17]. There was no evidence of increased $T_{reg}$ cells during pregnancy.

### 3.2.3    Treatment of MS During Pregnancy

In general, methylprednisolone is considered safe during the second and third trimesters of pregnancy when given 0.5–1 g/day for up to 7 days [73, 140]. Sixteen patients received steroids in the Confavreux et al. cohort [41]. DeSeze et al. studied monthly 1-g intravenous solumedrol pulse therapy for 6 months postpartum in 20 women and found their rate postpartum relapse rate to be lower than 22 patients followed earlier who were not treated ($p = 0.018$) [52]. Shah et al. used 7 days of IV methylprednisolone to treat a 31-year-old ADEM patient who was 32 weeks pregnant; labor was induced prior to treating with plasma exchange [192].

Achiron et al. retrospectively studied 108 pregnancies of women with MS; 39 were untreated during the pregnancy, 41 were treated with intravenous immunoglobulins (IVIG) after delivery, and 28 were treated from 6 to 8 weeks' gestation through the postpartum period [3]. The study was open, and the patients were not randomized. They found no adverse effects, and the women treated during pregnancy and postpartum had lower relapse rates in all trimesters as well as postpartum [3]. This group had earlier reported a pilot trial of IVIG to prevent postpartum relapses [4]. Nine patients were treated with 0.4 g/kg per day for 5 consecutive days during the 1st week postpartum and at 6 and 12 weeks. None relapsed in the first 6 months postpartum. Haas recommended using 60 g IVIG within 3 days of delivery and 10 g monthly in patients considered high risk for postpartum relapse [92].

## 3.3 Menstrual Cycle and MS

A characteristic of the female hormones of reproduction, estrogen and progesterone, is their cyclic release from puberty until menopause. There have been limited reports of MS symptoms that vary depending on phase of the menstrual cycle, and emerging MRI data support those reports. Smith and Studd reported 82% of premenopausal MS women experienced worsening symptoms in the premenstrual phase of their cycle; 18% reported an improvement [196]. Zorgdrager and DeKeyser reported that 43% of 60 women with RRMS experienced worsening of their symptoms just prior to onset of their menstrual flow, especially worsening spasticity and weakness or trouble walking [236]. Twelve patients on oral contraceptives reported less worsening in that study. Patients with progressive MS reported worsening. Of 56 women with MS, ten reported onset of all exacerbations in the premenstrual period. Twelve women reported exacerbations that started during the premenstrual period as well as other times in their cycle, but the proportion of attacks starting premenstrually was greater than expected. Oral contraceptive use did not seem to have any effect [237]. Wingerchuk and Rodriguez reported that aspirin prevented stereotypical luteal phase pseudo-attacks in three patients [233]. Holmqvist et al. reported on 18 premenopausal women, of whom 39.1% had regular menstruation. Symptom changes were reported in 38.9% of patients with respect to the menstrual cycle [101].

Pozzilli and colleagues examined eight women with RRMS, ages 27–40, by serial MRI done with triple dose gadolinium, delayed postcontrast scanning during four consecutive menstrual cycles [174]. Levels of 17β-estradiol (E2), FSH, LH, and progesterone (P4) were all measured on the same day as the MRI; similar blood levels were done on eight healthy age-matched control women. There was no difference in the frequency of enhancing lesions during follicular (day 3–9) or luteal (day 21–28) phase of the menstrual cycles, nor between the number and volume of gadolinium-enhancing lesions and levels of a single hormone, but there was a significant relationship ($R = 0.7$, $p = 0.009$) between the number and volume of enhancing lesions and the ratio of progesterone/E2, with higher levels corresponding to more MRI activity.

Bansil, et al. studied 30 premenopausal women with clinically definite or laboratory supported MS [14]. Because they found that estrogen levels did not correspond to the time of the cycle in some patients, they correlated MRI imaging to three separate ratios: Group 1 had low E2 and low P4 (early follicular), Group 2 had high E2 and low P4 (late follicular), and Group 3 had high P4 with variable E2 (luteal). They found the number of gadolinium-enhancing lesions to be significantly higher ($p = 0.04$) in those patients with high E2 and low P4 than in the group with low E2 and low P4. This would indicate a pro-inflammatory effect caused by high estrogen combined with low progesterone. Patients with both high estrogen and high progesterone had less activity than those with high estrogen and low progesterone, supporting a protective effect for combined high levels of progesterone and estrogen. More Group 2 patients had relapsing progressive MS; one patient had a high number of gadolinium-enhancing lesions that may have skewed the results, which used mean number of gadolinium-enhancing lesions in their comparisons. Wei and Lightman found low estradiol levels in 4 out of 16 premenopausal women with MS [227]. There is no evidence, however, for infertility among women with MS.

Surprisingly little is known about how menopause affects MS. Holmqvist et al. reported that 39% of 72 postmenopausal women reported worsening of symptoms after menopause, while 5% reported a decrease. Although 54.7% of the women had used or were using hormone replacement, only a minority (12 women) reported changes in their symptoms [101]. Smith and Studd gave questionnaires to women with MS at an annual meeting for MS patients, and 54% of 19 postmenopausal women who returned the questionnaires reported worsening symptoms with menopause. Of these, 75% had tried hormone replacement and noted improvement.[196]. Wei and Lightman found that one of six postmenopausal women with RRMS had an inappropriately low level of FSH [227].

## 3.4   Oral Contraception and MS

In 1960, the first birth control pill was introduced in the United States. It was a mixture of 150 μg mestranol and 9.5 mg norethynodrel. It was effective but plagued with serious thrombogenic side effects that led to refinement in the subsequent preparations. Since 1970, the main component of oral contraceptives has been the synthetic estrogen, ethinyl estradiol. Doses are low, 20 to 35 μg, with the new transdermal patch providing a higher blood level than most oral formulations. Numerous formulations also contain progestins. A novel progestin, drospirenone, was introduced in 2001; it blocks testosterone binding to androgen receptors [49].

Poser et al. were among the first to report on oral contraception in patients with MS. They reported that of 46 patients who used oral contraception for at least 3 months, nine reported improvement and three showed deterioration in their disease during the use [172]. None had had an acute deterioration within 1 month after stopping. Villard-MacKintosh et al. studied a large group of women from 17 clinics in Britain and found a slightly lower rate of onset of MS in oral contraceptive users vs nonusers [222].

Thorogood and Hannaford, reporting on a larger cohort of British women, did not show a significant risk in uses of low-dose pills but suggested an increased risk of developing MS for users of high-dose pills (>50 μg of estrogen) [208]. Using the power of two large cohorts of US women, the Nurses' Health Study and Nurses' Health Study II, Hernan et al. 2000 found no protection from, or risk for, developing MS following use of oral contraception [100]. Sena et al. reported at the 2006 AAN on their retrospective study of 70 women with MS for an average of 7 years. Half had used oral contraception for at least 3 years; the other half had never used them. Those who took oral contraceptives had lower disability scores even prior to going on INFβ-1b or -1a [191]. Animal studies of ethinyl estradiol, the synthetic estrogen found in many oral contraceptives, showed reduced development of EAE in rat (see discussion of animal studies).

Progestin-only based contraception, i.e., medroxyprogesterone, suppresses estrogen concentration [11]. Little evidence is available for its impact on MS. It remains to be determined whether newer, selective progestins will have any impact on MS. These include levonorgestrel, norelgestromin, drospirenone, and etonogestrel, which are used in the newer generation of combinations of oral, injectable, vaginal, intrauterine, transdermal and implantable contraceptives.


## 3.5  Estrogen

Kappas et al. reported in 1963 that estrone (E3) did not influence the incidence of EAE in a single experiment using groups of six rats (control and treated) [116]. Numerous subsequent experiments have shown that the synthetic estrogen ethinyl estradiol as well as two natural estrogens, estradiol and estriol, suppress EAE. Arnason and Richman treated young adult female rats with human oral contraceptives then available and found that estrogens alone, or a combination with high estrogen to progestin ratios, suppressed EAE; the progestin alone did not do so [11]. The doses they used were 40-fold higher than those used for human contraception at that time and were similar to the doses seen in the later months of pregnancy. They proposed that estrogen treatment in the immediate postpartum period reduced the risk of relapse. Trooster et al. reported that $17\alpha$ ethinyl estradiol partially suppressed EAE in female Lewis rats and caused changes in the peripheral blood leukocyte subpopulations; the important factor in the amelioration of EAE, however, appeared to be a local action at the site of the lesion [212]. Subramanian et al. showed that oral feeding with ethinyl estradiol suppressed EAE in the SJL mouse. Furthermore, it reduced the clinical severity if given before or after the onset of signs [202]. It decreased cytokines IFN-$\gamma$, TNF-$\alpha$, and IL-6 (proinflammatory) and expressed TGF$\beta$3 in the CNS. There was no CNS infiltration by lymphocytes, and matrix metalloproteinase was suppressed.

Jansson et al. (1994) treated mice with implanted $17\beta$ estradiol (E2) at doses mimicking estrogen levels in late pregnancy; the treatment delayed the onset of the disease. Estriol (E3) had similar effects at a much lower dose [110]. Bebo et al. showed that low-dose (one-fifth pregnancy levels) estradiol subcutaneous time release pellets given at the time of EAE induction suppressed disease in two mouse models, but it was not effective if given after onset [18]. Estradiol treatment profoundly downregulated TNF-$\alpha$ production but did not shift the T helper profile [109].

Kim et al. treated SJL mice with estriol pellets, and the treated animals showed dramatic reduction of severity of EAE; again, progesterone had no effect [120]. Estriol treatment resulted in increased production of IL-10 and IgG1 specific for MBP by cultured splenocytes, consistent with a shift in response from TH 1 toTh2. There were no significant changes in IFN-$\gamma$, IL-4, IL-5, IL-2, and IL-12. Doses equal to or greater than the levels seen with late pregnancy were most effective. Progesterone and cortisol levels were unchanged. They hypothesized that the effect was mediated through the ER-$\beta$ receptor, which has a higher affinity for estriol and which had been identified in lymphoid tissue [126]. They also observed no progesterone effect. They believed the increase in IL-10 influenced how estriol mediated the reduction of EAE. A study by Morales et al., however, showed that treatment with an ER-α ligand caused the anti-inflammatory effect [150].

Collectively, studies show a multitude of estrogen-influenced processes in both the immune and nervous systems. With respect to our current autoimmune paradigm for MS, the ability of estrogen to drive a Th1 to Th2 shift in cytokine profile may be the most relevant. While the paradigm has, in part, driven animal tests and human trials, this shift in cytokine profile is not estrogen's only effect and, indeed, may not be its predominant influence. Evidence from EAE and other inflammatory neurological disorders, such as stroke, have increased understanding of the other mechanisms behind estrogen's influence. Perhaps equally important to MS is estrogen's ability to impair cell adhesion and movement into the CNS [187] and to downregulate microglial activation within the brain and spinal cord [173, 218, 219]. Both the ER-α and ER-β receptors may mediate these actions with the possible involvement of genomic and nongenomic factors according to several recent excellent reviews [61, 173]. Estrogen appears to interfere with early events in inflammatory cell activation by controlling the NF-κB intracellular localization [81]. This novel cytoplasmic mechanism may lend itself to therapeutic intervention [173].

Kalman et al. gave 17β estradiol to male patients with MS and male blood donors and measured the IgG-, IgA-, and IgM-producing cells in culture; alone, there was no effect, but the cells producing IgG and IgA increased when stimulated with pokeweed mitogen [113]. Sicotte et al. reported on a small trial of estriol treatment in women (six with RRMS and six with SPMS) in 2002 [193]. They used oral estriol, 8 mg per day, which compares to endogenous levels seen in the 6th month of pregnancy. Delayed-type hypersensitivity to tetanus was decreased after patients had been on estriol for 6 months; IFN-γ levels were variably decreased after 3 months on treatment in the RRMS patients only. The total number and volume of gadolinium-enhancing lesions on MRI decreased for all patients during treatment. This effect started by 3 months in the RRMS patients. There did not appear to be a rebound increase in enhancing lesions upon withdrawal, but scans returned to baseline activity levels by 6 months. Three patients underwent endometrial biopsies for abnormal bleeding, but all were benign. Another patient had an enlarged fibroid during treatment [194].

There is limited evidence from the studies of pregnant women and the women in the small pilot estriol trial [193]. Cytokine analyses of the blood of patients in the estriol trial revealed increased IL-10 and IL-5 and decreased TNF-α during treatment, consistent with a partial Th1-to-Th 2 shift in the peripheral blood [199]. The increased IL-10 was primarily due to increased CD 64$^+$ monocytes/macrophages. Subpopulations of circulating immune cells were also altered; CD4$^+$ and CD8$^+$ cells decreased and B cells increased. There was a decrease in memory T cells (CD4$^+$CD45Ro$^+$) and an increase in naïve T cells (CD4$^+$CD45Ra$^+$). The mean volume of enhancing MRI lesions in the RRMS group correlated with the cytokine profile shift.

Estrogen also appears to promote neuronal survival by interfering with apoptosis. Evidence for estrogen as a neuroprotectant comes largely from diseases other than MS. A full discussion is outside of the scope of this chapter but has been recently reviewed [173]. Estrogen appears to promote neuroprotection in the face of oxidative stress, β-amyloid formation, and excessive excitatory neurotransmitters, and it reduces neuronal death from apoptosis [21, 77, 88, 169].

## 3.6 Progesterone

Progesterone's immunomodulatory role is suggested by markedly decreased MS exacerbations during late pregnancy, when progesterone levels are highest. While progesterone receptors are not present in resting lymphocytes, pregnancy induces the appearance of progesterone receptors on peripheral blood lymphocytes. Its effects also include the ability to induce production of progesterone-induced blocking factor (PIBF) which may, in turn, control natural killer cell activity as well as promote a Th2 bias [28]. PIBF suppresses production of IFN-γ and stimulates secretion of IL-4 and IL-10 in activated T cells [162].

More importantly, progesterone may play an essential role in maintaining neuron and oligodendroycte survival and myelin production. In trauma and ischemic injury models, progesterone has been associated with decreased edema [111, 182, 207]. In the Wobbler mouse, a model for motor neuron degeneration, treatment with progesterone for 15 days had beneficial effects on survival and muscle strength [87]. Longitudinal MS studies have documented relentless aging-related decline of function [42]. Myelin aging and diminished myelin repair are likely significant factors contributing to the disability of MS. Chronic MS lesions have fewer oligodendrocytes and less remyelination than earlier lesions [128]. There is now evidence that human CNS cells can make progesterone and that genes regulating repair may become hormone-sensitive after injury. Receptors in addition to the classic progesterone receptors may be more important to mediating the CNS effect [188]. Emerging knowledge of progesterone's role in protecting oligodendrocytes may prove important to treatment of MS [76].

In the aging rat, there is a dramatic reduction in the expression of all three genes related to myelin, MBP, PLP, and Gtx. Both progesterone metabolites, tetrahydroprogesterone (THP) and dihydro-progesterone (DHP), induce slight but significant increases in MBP mRNA expression. In a toxic model of demyelination, rats less than 3 months of age remyelinate fully in 4 weeks, while rats older than 9 months take 9 weeks. Progesterone treatment does not impair remyelination in the young animals. When older rats were demyelinated using a toxin model of demyelination, treatment with progesterone doubled the amount of oligodendrocyte remyelination from 10% to 20% [106].

Fewer studies exist on progesterone treatment of EAE, and the results have been inconclusive. In female rats, melegestrol delays onset of EAE at low dose and completely inhibits it at high dose. Very high doses show some reversal of disease already manifest [91]. Elliott et al. observed a 50% reduction in motor deficit in rats given medroxyprogesterone acetate 2 weeks after EAE [68]. However, Arnason and Richman did not find that medroxyprogesterone inhibited EAE in their model [11]. Using oligodendrocytes cultures in vitro, Demerens et al. showed myelination reduced by a factor of 3.5 in a progesterone-depleted medium [54].

## 3.7  Prolactin

Prolactin may have immunomodulating effects. Elevated levels of prolactin may account for increased MS exacerbations in the early postpartum period. Bernton et al. described suppression of macrophage and T cell activation in hypoprolactinemia mice in 1988 [23]. Prolactin receptors are expressed on all immune and hematopoietic cells. Prolactin may be an immuno-expanding agent and stimulator of Th2 lymphocytes, yet it also increases the production of Th 1 cytokines such as IFN-γ. It induces the expression of IL-2 receptors and increases the effect of IL-2 on lymphocytes. Prolactin may counterbalance the immunosuppressive influence of glucocorticoids [50]. All these effects could be relevant to MS. Draca and Levic hypothesized in 1996 that prolactin is a factor in MS pathogenesis [60].

Riskind et al. reported that prolactin levels rise on day 4 after immunization in a rat model of EAE and remain elevated on day 10, before neurological symptoms start [179]. Bromocriptine reduces prolactin levels and is protective if initiated 1 week after immunization. It also suppresses late disease. Dijkstra et al. found bromocriptine to reduce the severity and duration of acute EAE and, in a chronic relapsing model, reduce the duration of the second attack [57]. Nagy et al. reported that treatment of rats with bromocriptine prevents EAE [154].

Azar and Yamout reported elevated baseline prolactin levels in 12 patients with MS, and their prolactin levels post-TRH stimulation remained higher than in patients without MS [12]. Kira et al. also found elevated prolactin levels in eight of 27 patients with MS; four of the eight had diencephalic hypothalamic lesions [121]. All of the patients with elevated prolactin levels had a rise in prolactin levels in the acute stage of relapses. In a case-controlled study by Harirchian and colleagues, there was no difference in baseline levels between 43 cases of MS and 43 controls nor in the relationship between prolactin levels and clinical disease activity, duration or EDSS [94].

The largest study (132 patients with MS) found no association between prolactin levels and disease course or activity and concluded that prolactin could not be used as a disease marker; they considered the possibility that pathological, rather than clinical, subtypes are more relevant to prolactin's possible role in immune dysfunction [97]. Reder and Lowy found normal baseline prolactin levels in 35 patients with chronic progressive MS and in 19 with acute relapses [176].

Bissay et al. treated 18 patients with bromocriptine, 2.5 mg twice a day, in an open label pilot study. Of 15 patients who completed one year of the study, 14 showed disease progression by one or more measurements including EDSS score, relapses, new MRI lesions, or increased latency of visual or auditory evoked responses [25]. In a study correlating monthly gadolinium-enhanced lesions to prolactin levels in patients treated with monthly pulses of 500 mg of IV MP, Bergh found a parallel decline [206]. Recently, Gregg et al. showed that prolactin regulates oligodendrocytes precursor proliferation and increases the generation of myelin-forming oligodendrocytes in the mouse [90].

## 3.8   Clinical Relevance

The role for the female sex hormones in the treatment of MS will not be easy to elucidate. However, it is important to determine if the roles of the hormones, alone or in combination, are significant enough to justify the risk of long-term use, which, in the case of estrogen combined with progesterone, arguably approaches 1% over 10 years of use in postmenopausal women [7, 183, 225]. As more selective hormone-receptor ligands become available, specific interventions may be possible without disruption of the reproductive and other normal physiological roles and without the thrombotic and cancer risks of current preparations.

A Phase II study of estriol therapy combined with glatiramer is now recruiting 130 patients [157]. A human study using a combination of a progestin and estriol, POPART'MUS, launched in late spring 2005, aims to test whether progestin given at high doses similar to pregnancy, combined with low-dose estriol, reduces postpartum relapses of MS [66].

Some drugs currently used to treat MS, such as mitoxantrone and Cytoxan, can precipitate premature gonadal failure, even in young women and men. While short-term control of inflammatory disease may be attained, long-term loss of the possible neuroprotective role of estrogen may cause later acceleration of the disease. High-dose estrogen-containing oral contraception has been recommended to prevent ovarian failure in menstruating women treated with cytotoxic drugs such as mitoxantrone [136]. This treatment might be appropriate for women several years away from natural menopause, even if they are not planning to have more children.

## 4   Testosterone and DHEA

### 4.1   Background

While males are typically less susceptible to MS, affected males do have a more severe and progressive course [43, 95, 228]. Males have fewer active lesions and less accumulation of T2 lesion burden than women [132, 226]. Men may be less responsive to interferon [95]. This has been corroborated by MRI evidence [175].

Gender bias raises the possibility that testosterone plays a role in the susceptibility and the clinical course of MS. Men have a generally steady release of testosterone that begins to decline late in the third decade. The decline often correlates to co-morbid health conditions including obesity [6]. Lower testosterone levels were reported in 24% of males with MS [227]. There is no convincing evidence, however, that male MS patients with lower testosterone levels do worse.

Androgens have a potential immunomodulating role; they upregulate expression of TGF-β mRNA and protein levels and downregulate IFN-γ. They shift an autoantigen-specific T cell response toward the Th 2 phenotype, but they also have immunosuppressive actions in Th 2-linked disorders [159]. The balance of androgen levels compared to estrogen levels may determine testosterone's impact, perhaps even in women. Klinefelter syndrome, a chromosomal disorder (classic form has karyotype XXY), is a naturally occurring situation that may reflect the importance of the testosterone-to-estrogen balance. Klineflelter syndrome has been linked to increased risk of autoimmune disorders such as rheumatoid arthritis, SLE, and thyroid autoimmune diseases. Men with the disorder have low androgens, increased gonadotropins, and strengthened estrogenic effects [10]. Klinefelter syndrome is also associated with brain morphological changes [166]. No cases, however, of Klinefelter syndrome and MS have been reported to date.

## 4.2 Testosterone as an Immunomodulatory and Neuroprotective Hormone

The present evidence supports androgens' influence on immune response and inflammation via a pathway similar to glucocorticoids. Androgens may also have distinct influences via downstream targets [159]. Endogenous testosterone is disease-protective in the SJL mouse model of EAE; castration removes this protection. Exogenous androgen treatment confers protection. In the C57BL/6 mice, where endogenous testosterone does not appear to confer protection, exogenous testosterone at supraphysiologic doses does. The protective effect is mediated by 5α-dihydroxytestosterone, which cannot be converted to estradiol in vivo [163]. Dalal et al. reported that testosterone therapy ameliorated EAE and induced a Th 2 bias, as demonstrated by significantly higher levels of IL-10 production by MBP-specific cells, after induction in normal males; a similar finding was reported in females treated with dihydrotestosterone pellets [47].

Earlier studies found that endogenous IL-12 production was related to decreased encephalitogenic response in male SJL mice; administering IL-12 enhanced the response [120]. Testosterone treatment in female mice enhanced IL-10 production by CD4+ T lymphocytes while decreasing IL-12 production [137].

Tomassini et al. could not show correlation between endogenous testosterone levels in men with MS and gadolinium-enhancing lesions or T1 hypodense lesions, but estradiol levels correlated with both T2 lesion load and T1 lesion load in men [209]. Interestingly, the MS women with testosterone levels lower than 2 SD below the mean level for controls had a significantly greater number of gadolinium-enhancing lesions than did the MS women with normal testosterone levels. Women with higher testosterone levels had a greater likelihood of T1 hypodense lesions. Palaszynski et al. ran a series of experiments to try to separate the effects of gonadal hormone influence and chromosome complement influence [164]. They found lymph node cells from intact gonadal female (XX) SJL mice produced higher levels of TNF-$\alpha$, IFN-$\gamma$, and IL-10 in response to myelin basic protein immunization compared to intact gonadal males (XY). The difference was less in castrated females compared to castrated males; the castrated males had increased response, while castrated females had no significant change. Using mice in which gonadal development and the chromosome complement were either congruent or discongruent, they found that gonadal type determined the immune response. However, when the gonadal hormone influence was removed, they found higher responses in oophorectomized XY mice than in oophorectomized XX mice. In gonadal male mice, castrated XY animals had a greater immune response than XX animals.

Gold et al. reported the results of a small exploratory clinical trial of 1% testosterone gel treatment of men with MS [84]. Ten men with RRMS, average age 46, were studied. Monthly MRIs during 12 months of treatment were compared to scans in the 6 months prior to treatment. No effect of testosterone treatment was found on gadolinium-enhancing lesions; enhancing activity overall was low. One patient with gadolinium-enhancing lesions prior to treatment showed a significant decrease during treatment, while another showed a flare while on treatment. Brain volume loss stabilized. The delayed-type hypersensitivity skin response to tetanus was reduced. In vitro PBMCs showed reduced IL-2 production and increased production of BDNF and PDGF. Neurocognitive tests showed improvement by month 12. Sicotte et al. reported that the subjects had improved performance on PASAT and spatial memory tasks and reported higher quality of life measure related to physical activity [193].

Caruso et al. studied the role of testosterone on excitotoxic death of oligodendrocytes. Using pure fresh rat oligodendrocyte cultures, they triggered excitotoxicity by stimulating AMPA/kainite receptors with kainate or AMPA+cyclothiazide [34]. In both cases, testosterone promoted the effect by amplifying all gene targets of p53, including mdm-2, bax, GADD45, and growth- arresting factor, p21$^{cip/kip}$; it also induced expression of c-fos, grp 78, and jun kinase kinase 1 (JNKK1). It also potentiated the stimulation of 45Ca2+ influx, an indictor of AMPA or kainite receptor activation. Even tested alone, testosterone was slightly toxic, suggesting that it enables the potential toxicity of endogenously activated AMPA/kainite receptors. These effects were mediated by the androgen receptors and were resistant to aromatase inhibitors. Testosterone did not induce any change in the AMPA or kainite receptors. This finding of testosterone promoting oligodendrocyte excitotoxic injury contrasts to its effects on neurons. Testosterone is generally neuroprotective of human neurons in vitro [93]. Taken with the finding by Pozzilli et al. that males with MS have more MRI evidence for atrophy and tissue loss, this suggests that axonal loss in MS is, at least in part, secondary to demyelination and oligodendrocyte loss and that the neuronal neuroprotective effects are either overcome or less active in the setting of MS [175].

## 4.3    Dehydroepiandrosterone (DHEA)

Dehydroepiandrosterone (DHEA) is an adrenal steroid that abounds in serum; it is precursor to both androgens and estrogens. Kumpfel et al. reported decreased DHEA and increased cortisol in response to the ACTH and DEX-CRH tests in 24 male and female patients with MS; there was a positive correlation between the EDSS and the maximum cortisol to DHEA ratio [127]. Du et al. reported that DHEA treatment suppressed EAE in the SJL/J mouse model by decreasing T cell proliferation and inflammatory cytokine production and by decreasing activation and translocation of the nuclear transcription factor, NK-κB [62].

   Limone et al. found normal levels of DHEA and DHEAs in ten RRMS patients prior to and during IFN-β treatment [134]. Tellez et al. reported on 73 patients with progressive MS followed longitudinally and found that fatigued patients had lower levels of DHEA and DHEAs [204].

## 4.4    Clinical Relevance

Several mechanisms of testosterone could be amenable to therapeutic intervention; for example, its effect on the AMPA/kainite receptor activation [34]. In addition to the possible immunomodulatory and neuroprotective roles, testosterone might also promote muscle strength and sexual function in men with MS; sexual dysfunction among men with MS, even with normal testosterone levels, is common [147]. The role for testosterone in MS remains to be substantiated before it should be used clinically.

# 5    Vitamin D

## 5.1    Background

The structures of vitamin D2 and D3 were identified in 1928 by Windaus, a German chemist [231] who won the Nobel Prize in chemistry for this contribution. Vitamin D2, ergocalciferol, is found in vegetables and vitamin D3, cholecalciferol, from animal sources; vitamin D3 is also produced in human skin from 7-dehydrocholesterol after exposure to UV-B. Humans store vitamin D3 in fat. It is converted to 25 hydroxyvitamin D3, which is then stored in the liver. 25 hydroxyvitamin D3 levels are used to monitor vitamin D status, but it is not the active form. 25 Hydroxyvitamin D3 has to be activated in the kidney and many other cell types, including neurons, microglial cells, and activated macrophages, to 1,25 dihydroxyvitamin D3 (calci-triol), the metabolically active form [27, 216]. A daily supplement of 1,000 IU of vitamin D3 has been recommended for adults [220, 221]. The tolerable upper intake level for adults is 2,000 IU/day, set by the Food and Nutrition Board of the Institute of Medicine (USA) [107].

Most cells, including many immune cells relevant to MS, have receptors for vitamin D. Activated T lymphocytes and macrophages respond to vitamin D with decreases in IL-12, IFN-γ, and IL-2. Oligodendrocytes, neurons, astrocytes, and microglia all have the vitamin D receptor and respond to the hormone [216]. Vitamin D can cross the BBB and be produced locally in the CNS [79]. The immunomodulatory and possible neuroprotective roles for vitamin D have been a focus of MS research.

## 5.2  Sunlight, Vitamin D, and Susceptibility to MS

The geographic distribution of MS links sun exposure to the prevalence of MS. In the report of the Proceedings of the Association for Research in Nervous and Mental Diseases held in December 1948, Charles Limburg presented crude death rates for MS with countries arranged by mean annual temperature. "For the most part, there is an inverse and rather striking relationship between reported mortality due to MS and mean annual temperature" [133]. Over the next two decades, the north–south gradient of MS incidence was hypothesized to be secondary to sunlight exposure and, subsequently, to vitamin D levels. Subsequent multiple studies have reinforced the link between sun exposure, vitamin D levels, and MS [216].

A recent study used blood samples collected an average of 5.3 years prior to the first symptoms of MS [152]. In this study of United States veterans, only white veterans with the highest quartile of 25-hydroxyvitamin D levels (over 99.1 nmol/l) were significantly less likely to develop MS (odds ratio, 0.38; 95%CI, 0.19–0.75). Although blacks had significantly lower levels of vitamin D than whites, their risk of developing MS did not correlate with their 25-hydroxyvitamin vitamin D levels, most of which were less than 75 nmol/l. If vitamin D has a protective effect only above a certain high level, then blacks are unlikely to benefit, even though their overall risk of developing MS is lower than that of whites. Soilu-Hanninen et al. studied patients with early MS in Finland and found lower vitamin D levels during MS relapses, but there was no correlation with the EDSS, the magnitude of elevation of the CSF IgG index, oligoclonal bands, or gadolinium-enhancing MRI lesions in brain or spinal cord [198]. Embry and colleagues reported an inverse relationship between gadolinium-enhancing lesions on MRI and vitamin D levels [69].

The mechanisms for vitamin D protection against MS are unclear. Several seem plausible given our current knowledge of MS pathogenesis. The two with the most support are a decrease in IL-12 production by APCs and an increase in TGF-β. Vitamin D is produced by activated macrophages and is a potent inhibitor of T cell proliferation and of Th1 cytokine production. Also, 1,25 (OH2) vitamin D3 suppresses APC production of IL-12 and inhibits both IFN-γ and IL-2 secretion. It promotes Th 2 activity and enhances IL-10 production [36, 46, 129, 181]. The doses of oral vitamin D needed to change cytokine levels was found to be 1,000 IU daily for 6 months; increased TGF β was found without changes in other cytokines, TNF-β, or IFN-γ [141].

## 5.3   Therapeutic Trials of Vitamin D in EAE

Several studies have shown that vitamin D ameliorates EAE in rat and mouse models [31, 78, 155]. Treatment influences both the severity of the first paralytic attack and the earlier occurrence of a less severe second attack. The mechanism of action was not consistent: vitamin D treatment increased TGF-β in one model, while it drastically reduced the nitric oxide synthase II expression and downregulated MHC II and CD4 expression in another.

Mattner and colleagues showed that 1,25 dihydroxyvitamin D3 and an analog of vitamin D3, Ro 63-2023, inhibits EAE; both potently inhibited IL-12 production, and the analog provided long-term protection [146]. Muthian et al. reported that 1,25 dihydroxyvitamin D3 ameliorates EAE and is associated with inhibition of IL-12 production and neural antigen-specific Th 1 response [153]. In vitro, they found it modulates the JAK-STAT pathway in the IL-12/IFN-γ axis.

A combination study by Van Etten et al. showed synergistic protection from EAE in SJL mice treated with IFN-β and a vitamin D analog, TX527 [217]. They combined TX 527 with IFN-β in an SJL mouse EAE model and found the combination superior to either treatment separately. They also tested a combination of interferon with cyclosporine A and found it aggravated the disease. However, the triple combination protected the mice from paralysis.

## 5.4   Vitamin D Trials in Humans

Goldberg published an early study treating MS with dietary supplements of calcium, magnesium and vitamin D [86]. This study showed decreased frequency in exacerbations, and the investigators concluded that calcium and magnesium helped stabilize myelin, assuming that vitamin D was acting through its role in calcium metabolism. At that time, only vitamin D's role as a hormone for bone development and remodeling was well established.

Fleming et al. conducted a pilot trial of an analog, 19-nor-1,25-dihydroxyvitamin D2, which was tested for safety in 11 patients with early RRMS. They presented the results in a poster at the 2000 AAN [74]. There was no significant impact on gadolinium-enhancing lesion formation or on clinical symptoms. Wingerchuk et al. performed a 48-week pilot trial of calcitriol in 15 patients with RRMS. Two patients withdrew due to hypercalcemia from dietary indiscretion, and two more required temporary dose adjustments due to mild asymptomatic hypercalcemia. Four patients experienced a relapse during treatment; four worsened by at least one EDSS point. Nine exacerbations occurred in seven of 14 patients during the mean follow-up of

10 months; EDSS scores increased by at least 1 in eight patients during follow-up. MRI done during the trial showed new T2 lesions in 43% of scans at 24 weeks and 29% at 48 weeks; gadolinium-enhancing lesions were present in 33% of baseline scans and 29% at each follow-up [232]. Mahon et al. reported on 39 patients (part of a larger study), who were randomized to receive 800 mg calcium (22 patients) or calcium plus 1,000 IU vitamin D (17 patients). All had baseline and 6 months' follow-up. The patients who received vitamin D plus calcium had increased TGF-β; TNF-α, IFN-γ, and IL-13 were unaffected. Both groups had decreased IL −2 mRNA in [141]. Achiron et al. reported safety of alfacalcidol in five patients treated [2].

A recent report by Obradovic and colleagues showed a role for vitamin D3 in protecting hippocampal neurons in vitro from dexamethasone-induced apoptosis [160]. Pretreatment for 24 h with even low doses of vitamin D3 were protective.


## 5.5   Clinical Relevance

Vitamin D as an adjunct treatment for MS is an attractive approach and one that many patients are likely already utilizing for bone preservation. It is reassuring that the combination of IFN-β and vitamin D in the mouse EAE model appears to be safe and synergistic, although projecting these results to human MS is premature. The recent US veterans' study by Munger et al. is particularly important to planning clinical trials of vitamin D in MS. In the study by Mahon, a dose of 1,000 IU/day achieved levels up to 70, below what appeared to be the protective levels found by Munger [141]. The early study by Goldberg used much higher doses (5,000 IU, given as cod liver oil) and showed reduced exacerbations, but this study was limited (six of 16 dropped out) [86, 141]. Unfortunately, high doses of natural vitamin D cannot be used for long periods of time due to risk of hypercalcemia and toxicity to bone. Synthetic analogs will be more appropriate for long-term study [213].

In addition to its adjunctive immunomodulatory potential, vitamin D has a mood-elevating effect that may be useful in MS patients, who often suffer from depression. It may also have a possible neuroprotective effect on memory [114].


## 6   Thyroid Hormone

### 6.1   Background

Kendall isolated thyroid hormone on Christmas Day 1914 [230]. Thyroid hormone has an essential role in normal differentiation of oligodendrocytes and successful myelination in the developing CNS [180]. Not surprisingly, thyroid hormone's role in remyelination is now being studied with potential implications for MS.

Hypothyroidism and MS have many overlapping symptoms including fatigue, poor cognitive functioning, anxiety and depression, numbness and paresthesias, ataxia, stiff muscles, easy fatigability of muscles, cramps, and weakness. Hypothyroidism, especially subclinical hypothyroidism, is common, with a strong female predominance. Autoimmune thyroid disease is the most common cause [230]. Hyperthyroidism is associated with heat intolerance, anxiety and tremors, which are also common MS symptoms.

Treatment of MS exacerbations with glucocorticoid may affect thyroid function transiently. Glucocorticoids reduce the conversion of T4 to T3, which may cause a transient hypothyroid state. Brinar et al. recently reported a case of Hashimoto's thyroiditis that presented with isolated retrobulbar neuritis and another with left hemifacial spasm, paresthesiae of the face and leg with demyelinating lesions on MRI [29]. This report is of particular interest because treatments for MS have also been associated with autoimmune thyroid disease. The association of autoimmune thyroid disease with MS-immunomodulating therapies (alemtuzumab in particular) has raised recent interest in thyroid hormone function and MS.

## 6.2   Thyroid Hormone and EAE

Using both the Lewis rat model and the Dark Agouti rat model of EAE, the latter of which develops a severe, protracted and relapsing encephalitis with demyelination, Fernandez et al. studied T4 treatment, either during the acute (first relapse, days 11, 13, or 15 after immunization) or during second relapse (days 21, 23, 25). Animals treated in the acute phase had an increased number of oligoprogenitor cells expressing platelet-derived growth factor; myelin sheath thickness and organization as well as myelin basic protein levels were restored to control values (as measured at 55 days after injection) [72]. They also found increased axonal diameters in the spinal cords of the treated animals. There was a slight but significant effect on the clinical scores of the animals in the Lewis, but not Dark Agouti, rats. While perhaps disappointing, the motor deficit in this rat model of EAE may not be due to the demyelination primarily.

## 6.3   Evidence for Thyroid Dysfunction and Autoimmune Thyroiditis

Completely evaluating thyroid function is not as simple as one would expect. Serum thyroid stimulating hormone (TSH) is a commonly used laboratory test to screen for hypothyroidism, but TSH alone may not be adequate to determine the peripheral state of hypothyroidism. Which tests best reflect thyroid status depend on whether the hypothalamic–pituitary–thyroid axis is intact, among other factors.

In general, combined free T4 and TSH are better than either alone [229]. Central hypothyroidism seems to be rare in the general population (0.005%). The TRH test for TSH response is useful in evaluating the central components of the axis, but it does not clearly distinguish between hypothalamic and pituitary dysfunction [230]. Central hypothyroidism can be associated with low, but also normal or even slightly elevated TSH, the latter being a paradox explained by reduced biological activity of TSH. Loss of the usual nocturnal TSH surge is characteristic.

While hypothalamic involvement of MS is a risk for central thyroid axis dysfunction, there is no convincing evidence for inherent dysfunction of the axis in patients with MS. In a study by Wei and Lightman, 52 patients with MS had baseline TSH, free T3, free T4 measured, and all were normal compared to controls. TRH stimulation testing showed no difference in TSH or prolactin responses [227]. After eliminating study candidates with overt thyroid disease (number not reported), Durelli et al. [65] investigated 152 RRMS pre-interferon-treated patients compared to 437 controls. They showed no increased TSH, but the men in the study demonstrated a trend of increased subclinical hypothyroidism and anti-TMA autoAb positivity. In a study done prior to the introduction of the current MS-immunomodulating drugs, circulating thyroid antibodies were described in 19 of 63 (30.1%) MS patients [108]; this was significant compared to the incidence in control females of 5.9%. Niederwieser et al. studied 353 consecutive MS patients and 308 controls with back pain or headache and found a higher prevalence of autoimmune thyroid antibodies in men with MS than controls (9.4% vs 1.9%) but not females (8.7% vs 9.2%). Hypothyroidism tended to be more frequent and more severe in the MS patients than in controls [156].

Evidence for autoimmune thyroid disease has appeared in patients taking immunomodulatory drugs for MS [63, 64, 96, 142, 149, 184, 190]. The incidence may be increased in women and in those with positive thyroperoxidase antibodies (TPO) prior to initiation of therapy. One study [65] did not find increased incidence in patients on IFN-β. No correlation between disease severity or progression and the development of thyroid antibodies appeared in any of these reports.

The immune mechanism behind the appearance of autoimmune thyroid disease in MS is an inviting area for more research. In rats, lymphocyte depletion by thymectomy or irradiation is associated with autoimmune thyroiditis [167]. An interesting similar situation occurs in humans, specifically the association of autoimmune thyroid disease appearing in patients with MS treated with alemtuzumab, which markedly and nearly immediately depletes lymphocytes. Nine of 27 patients treated in a study protocol and three of 19 patients treated off study developed Graves' disease [39]. This complication of treatment was considered to be unique to MS patients. Recently, however, in a published report of this association in renal transplant patients, a woman received a dose of alemtuzumab two to four times higher than that usually used in transplant immunosuppression and similar to the dose used in the MS trial [122]. A recent update of the use of alemtuzumab to treat MS showed that 27% of 57 treated patients developed Graves and one, autoimmune hypothyroidism [38]. The alemtuzumab vs IFN-β-1a study was recently halted due to serious and life-threatening idiopathic thrombocytopenic purpura;

11.1% of patients in the study receiving alemtuzumab developed autoimmune thyroid problems [40]. Unfortunately, the drug seems to be markedly effective in treating MS as measured by reduction of MRI lesion formation and relapse rate.

It is unclear if patients with autoimmune thyroid disease have a different MS course from those who do not; Annunziata et al. found an inverse correlation between the presence of antithyroglobulin antibody titers and EDSS score in 11 of 129 patients with these antibodies [9]. No correlation was found between the presence of anti-thyroglobulin and MRI T2-weighted lesions, but none of the patients with antibodies had gadolinium-enhancing lesions. Petek-Balci and colleagues reported two cases of patients who had thyroid disease approximately 7 years prior to developing MS symptoms [170]. Presumably, the mere presence of thyroid antibodies does not prevent the development of MS, but their presence should be studied more thoroughly with respect to implications for the type or course of MS. It is intriguing to hypothesize that thyroid antibody, but not thyroid hormone per se, is a biomarker reflecting either more benign course or successful modulation of the disease by treatment. Their presence may reflect a shift to higher B cell activity similar to the way estriol shifts the immune system during pregnancy.

Autoimmune thyroid disease has been associated with recombinant IFN-α treatment of hepatitis C and was not always reversible [32]. IL-2α treatment and IFN-α treatment for cancer have also been associated with autoimmune thyroid disease. In the case of IFN-α treatment for melanoma, it appears to be a favorable prognostic finding [83, 124].

## 6.4  Thyroid Hormone and Myelin

Thyroid hormone influences the timing of differentiation and migration of oligodendrocytes in neonatal animals. Along with factors produced by nerve cells themselves, thyroid hormone induces neural stem cells to form oligodendrocytes [180]. Thyroid hormone regulates the expression of several enzymes related to myelination and of the major constituents of the myelin sheath. Binding sites for T3 have been demonstrated in oligodendrocytes both in vivo and in vitro [13]. Thyroid hormone induces differentiation and functional maturation, and the events are independent of each other [13].

Baas and colleagues purified O-2A progenitor cells of neonate rat brain and cultured them with and without T3. Compared to cultures without T3, progenitor cell proliferation was inhibited about twofold, and oligodendrocytes represented 57% of the cells after 6 days of culture compared to 6.8% in the cultures without T3; oligoprogenitor cells decreased from 75% to 24%. In another experiment, 70% of the T3-treated oligodendrocytes had a well-developed network of branched processes, compared to only 18% of untreated oligodendrocytes. T3-treated oligodendrocyte cultures had increased expression of myelin oligodendrocytes glycoprotein (MOG) and glutamine synthetase activity. Schoonover CM et al. showed that thyroid hormone indirectly regulates myelin basic protein mRNA by controlling the number of MBP-expressing oligodendrogyes [135]. Younes-Rapozo et al. showed that T3 deficiency affects neonatal rat oligodendroglial maturation in vitro, which is characterized by less extensive processes and membrane vellum and relative restricted myelin basic protein distribution to the perinuclear region [234]. Thyroid hormone also promotes oligodendrocyte survival from TNF-$\alpha$ and IL-1$\beta$ signal for apoptosis [112].

Remyelination appears similar to virgin myelination in the neonatal brain and spinal cord. In the early active lesions of MS, oligodendrocytes often increase in number, reflecting generation of new oligodendrocytes [33]. Their failure to remyelinate denuded axons is likely multifactorial, but it is reasonable to believe that thyroid hormone plays a significant role. There is growing evidence in the EAE model that this is the case.

## 6.5   Clinical Relevance

Three questions of immediate importance arise when considering the clinical implications of our current level of knowledge about thyroid hormone and MS, but none have clear answers at this time. The first question is whether subclinical hypothyroidism affects disease course and disease symptoms. The second question is whether the development of autoimmune thyroid disease while on immunomodulatory therapy is a good or bad event. The third question is how best to screen for thyroid disease, particularly in the setting of new drug development.

There is currently no agreement on whether everyone with subclinical hypothyroidism should be treated [203, 224]. The more aggressive approach needs to be studied in MS patients, particularly in patients experiencing symptoms that overlap with those of clinical hypothyroidism. Current treatments for MS that have been associated with thyroid antibodies require close monitoring of thyroid status with emphasis on disease course and subsequent hypothyroidism. Finally, new treatments for MS need to be evaluated with respect to their impact on thyroid status, and the meaning of any change in thyroid status should be studied further with respect to its impact on disease.

## 7   Leptin and Ghrelin

## 7.1   Background

Leptin, the obese gene product, was discovered in 1994. It is a peptide hormone produced by adipose tissue; it is structurally and functionally a cytokine that acts on the hypothalamus [44]. Leptin's chief role appears to be maintenance of a minimum level of energy stores during calorie restriction. Low levels are a signal for feeding as well as energy conservation. In that role, it changes activities in the adrenal, gonadal, and thyroid hormone axes. Like other hormones, it also has immunological influences [75, 197]. Leptin receptors (ObRb) are found on mature CD4+ lymphocytes [139].

In 1999, another novel hormone, ghrelin, was identified. This hormone is an amino acid peptide secreted from the stomach, small intestine, and colon. It may also be expressed in the hypothalamus, pituitary, and other tissues. It is an endogenous ligand for the growth hormone secretague receptor. Like leptin, it plays a role in energy homeostasis, but the specifics are not yet elucidated [210]. It may enhance immune cell proliferation but inhibit secretion of proinflammatory cytokines [58, 59, 123].

## 7.2  EAE and Leptin

Matarese et al. showed that EAE could not be induced in the absence of leptin and that leptin supplementation caused a more severe and chronic disease in wild type mice [145]. Leptin administration to increase the proliferative response of T cells was 11-fold over leptin-deficient mice. The IFN-$\gamma$ response was increased 21-fold and inhibited the IL-4 response, shifting the response to a pronounced Th-1 type response.

Sanna et al. showed a relationship between starvation, leptin, and EAE. The serum expression of leptin increased before the onset of EAE in susceptible mice, and starvation delayed onset and attenuated clinical symptoms. Low levels of leptin induced a Th 2 cytokine profile switch. Leptin was expressed in T cells and macrophages in the brain infiltrates and lymph nodes during the acute phase. In vitro, CD4+ T cells produced low but significant levels of leptin [186].

De Rosa et al. showed that anti-leptin treatment caused failure to downregulate the cyclin-dependent kinase inhibitor p27 ( p27 [kip-1]) in autoreactive CD4+ cells, associated with increased tyrosine phosphorylation of ERK 1/2 and hyporesponsiveness of the CD4+ cells to proteolipid protein, and STAT6, known to be involved in Th 2 cytokine secretion. Leptin neutralization reduced expression of ICAM-1 and OX-40 but increased the expression of the very late antigen −4, $\alpha 4\beta 1$ integrin, on CD4+ cells [51]. They hypothesized that this increase $\beta 4\beta 1$ integrin expression was associated with increased migration of cells producing regulatory cytokines into the CNS.

## 7.3  MS and Leptin

In a study of 18 patients with secondary progressive MS, serum leptin production by peripheral blood mononuclear cells showed no significant change overall, but in 12 patients who did not progress on retreatment with IFN-$\beta$, leptin and IL-6 production decreased at 6 and 12 months [8].

Matarese et al. found increased leptin in serum and CSF of 126 RRMS patients compared to 117 age-, gender- and body mass index-matched controls [144]. Leptin levels in the CSF were 1.8-fold higher than serum levels, and leptin levels in CSF correlated with IFN-γ levels. They found an inverse correlation between serum leptin levels and the percentage of T reg (CD4⁺ CD25⁺) cells in the patients, who were all within 4 weeks of the onset of relapse and were naïve to treatment.

## 7.4 MS and Ghrelin

Berilgen et al. studied 40 MS patients with RRMS and SPMS [22]. Fasting levels of ghrelin were determined by radioimmunoassay. MS patients had significantly higher levels than controls, but there was no difference between the two types of MS.

## 7.5 Clinical Relevance

Studies of these novel peptide hormones suggest that they influence MS. They make us reflect on the role of diet in MS and the relationship between the gut and the immune system. The evidence is too slim, however, to make any conclusions or recommendations of clinical usefulness at this time.

## 8 Conclusions

Hormones by their nature have widespread effects on the vital functions of cells, including metabolism, growth, differentiation, survival, and death. They provide communication between different organs and different systems in much the same way as the immune and nervous systems do. When perturbations occur, hormones help to move an organism toward a more healthy equilibrium.

There is mounting evidence that multiple hormones influence MS. The understanding has emerged that each hormone may influence the immune system and influence nervous system alone and in combination. The effects of a given hormone frequently interact with the effects of other hormones to produce parallel effects, synergistic effects, or complementary effects. In contrast, hormones may counterbalance the effects of other hormones helping to establish equilibrium. In the last several decades, the discovery of new hormone receptors or receptor subtypes and the presence of hormone receptors in cells not traditional to their endocrinologic role have resulted in a virtual explosion of new interest. The tools for studying the multiplicity of receptor–hormone interactions and subsequent downstream effects, both genomic and nongenomic, have been developed. This has led to a hope that exploiting hormones for a specific set of actions in a specific disease such as MS will lead to more natural treatments with less, or at least known and manageable, side effect profiles. Sex hormones may eventually bring gender specificity to the treatment of MS and other autoimmune diseases.

The multifunctionality of hormones elegantly enhances their appeal as therapeutic agents. This is especially true in the case of chronic diseases such as MS. Understanding their widespread effects is also the challenge of the research community. Clinicians using hormones should think beyond the previous mindset that hormones have only a specific and narrowly defined role.

There is much to learn. Side effects have been, and will continue to be, an issue with the therapeutic use of hormones. We have experienced the protean problems associated with glucocorticoids. The risks of cancer in the uterus or breast and thrombogenesis dampen enthusiasm for estrogen. Vitamin D appears to be a very attractive hormone for clinical use, since modest doses are well tolerated, it has oral forms, and it is not costly. The possibility of vitamin D enhancing the effect of interferon in humans should be explored quickly given the exciting report in EAE.

Using hormones optimally, perhaps in pulsatile or sequential fashion, may minimize the risks. The development of designer hormones to minimize side effects will, hopefully, further improve the benefit-to-risk ratio.

While not the primary subject of this chapter, study of how MS and its treatment affect hormones is also worthwhile. For example, the link of autoimmune thyroiditis to MS treatments may provide unique insights about the immune dysregulation of both disorders.

# References

1. Abramsky O, Lubetzki-Korn I, Evron S, Brenner T (1984) Suppressive effect of pregnancy on MS and EAE. Prog Clin Biol Res 146:399–406
2. Achiron A, Barak Y, Miron S, Izhak Y, Faibel M, Edelstein S (2003) Alfacalcidol treatment in multiple sclerosis. Clin Neuropharmacol 26:53
3. Achiron A, Kishner I, Dolev M, Stern Y, Dulitzky M, Schiff E, Achiron R (2004) Effect of intravenous immunoglobulin treatment on pregnancy and postpartum-related relapses in multiple sclerosis. J Neurol 251:1133–1137
4. Achiron A, Rotstein Z, Noy S, Mashiach S, Dulitzky M, Achiron R (1996) Intravenous immunoglobulin treatment in the prevention of childbirth-associated acute exacerbations in multiple sclerosis: A pilot study. J Neurol 243:25–28
5. Al-Shammri S, Rawoot P, Azizieh F, AbuQoora A, Hanna M, Saminathan TR, Raghupathy R (2004) Th1/th2 cytokine patterns and clinical profiles during and after pregnancy in women with multiple sclerosis. J Neurol Sci 222:21–27
6. Allan CA, McLachlan RI (2006) Androgen deficiency disorders. In: DeGroot LJ, Jameson JL (eds) Endocrinology. Elsevier Saunders, Philadelphia, pp 3159–3192
7. Anderson GL, Limacher M, Assaf AR, Bassford T, Beresford SA, Black H, Bonds D, Brunner R, Brzyski R, Caan B, Chlebowski R, Curb D, Gass M, Hays J, Heiss G, Hendrix S, Howard BV, Hsia J, Hubbell A, Jackson R, Johnson KC, Judd H, Kotchen JM, Kuller L, LaCroix AZ, Lane D, Langer RD, Lasser N, Lewis CE, Manson J, Margolis K, Ockene J, O'Sullivan MJ, Phillips L, Prentice RL, Ritenbaugh C, Robbins J, Rossouw JE, Sarto G, Stefanick ML, Van Horn L, Wactawski-Wende J, Wallace R, Wassertheil-Smoller S (2004) Effects of conjugated

equine estrogen in postmenopausal women with hysterectomy: The Women's Health Initiative randomized controlled trial. JAMA 291:1701–1712

8. Angelucci F, Mirabella M, Caggiula M, Frisullo G, Patanella K, Sancricca C, Nociti V, Tonali PA, Batocchi AP (2005) Evidence of involvement of leptin and IL-6 peptides in the action of interferon-beta in secondary progressive multiple sclerosis. Peptides 26:2289–2293

9. Annunziata P, Lore F, Venturini E, Morana P, Guarino E, Borghi S, Guazzi GC (1999) Early synthesis and correlation of serum anti-thyroid antibodies with clinical parameters in multiple sclerosis. J Neurol Sci 168:32–36

10. Aoki N (1999) Klinefelter's syndrome, autoimmunity, and associated endocrinopathies. Intern Med 38:838–839

11. Arnason BG, Richman DP (1969) Effect of oral contraceptives on experimental demyelinating disease. Arch Neurol 21:103–108

12. Azar ST, Yamout B (1999) Prolactin secretion is increased in patients with multiple sclerosis. Endocr Res 25:207–214

13. Baas D, Bourbeau D, Sarlieve LL, Ittel ME, Dussault JH, Puymirat J (1997) Oligodendrocyte maturation and progenitor cell proliferation are independently regulated by thyroid hormone. Glia 19:324–332

14. Bansil S, Lee HJ, Jindal S, Holtz CR, Cook SD (1999) Correlation between sex hormones and magnetic resonance imaging lesions in multiple sclerosis. Acta Neurol Scand 99:91–94

15. Barrat FJ, Cua DJ, Boonstra A, Richards DF, Crain C, Savelkoul HF, de Waal-Malefyt R, Coffman RL, Hawrylowicz CM, O'Garra A (2002) In vitro generation of interleukin 10-producing regulatory CD4(+) t cells is induced by immunosuppressive drugs and inhibited by t helper type 1 (th1)- and th2-inducing cytokines. J Exp Med 195:603–616

16. Batuman OA, Ferrero A, Cupp C, Jimenez SA, Khalili K (1995) Differential regulation of transforming growth factor beta-1 gene expression by glucocorticoids in human T and glial cells. J Immunol 155:4397–4405

17. Bebo BF Jr, Dveksler GS (2005) Evidence that pregnancy specific glycoproteins regulate T-cell function and inflammatory autoimmune disease during pregnancy. Curr Drug Targets Inflamm Allergy 4:231–237

18. Bebo BF Jr, Fyfe-Johnson A, Adlard K, Beam AG, Vandenbark AA, Offner H (2001) Low-dose estrogen therapy ameliorates experimental autoimmune encephalomyelitis in two different inbred mouse strains. J Immunol 166:2080–2089

19. Beck RW, Cleary PA, Anderson MM Jr, Keltner JL, Shults WT, Kaufman DI, Buckley EG, Corbett JJ, Kupersmith MJ, Miller NR et al (1992) A randomized, controlled trial of corticosteroids in the treatment of acute optic neuritis. The Optic Neuritis Study Group. N Engl J Med 326:581–588

20. Beck RW, Cleary PA, Trobe JD, Kaufman DI, Kupersmith MJ, Paty DW, Brown CH (1993) The effect of corticosteroids for acute optic neuritis on the subsequent development of multiple sclerosis. The Optic Neuritis Study Group. N Engl J Med 329:1764–1769

21. Behl C, Skutella T, Lezoualc'h F, Post A, Widmann M, Newton CJ, Holsboer F (1997) Neuroprotection against oxidative stress by estrogens: Structure–activity relationship. Mol Pharmacol 51:535–541

22. Berilgen MS, Bulut S, Ustundag B, Tekatas A, Ayar A (2005) Patients with multiple sclerosis have higher levels of serum ghrelin. Neuro Endocrinol Lett 26:819–822

23. Bernton EW, Meltzer MS, Holaday JW (1988) Suppression of macrophage activation and t-lymphocyte function in hypoprolactinemic mice. Science 239:401–404

24. Besedovsky H, del Rey A, Sorkin E, Dinarello CA (1986) Immunoregulatory feedback between interleukin-1 and glucocorticoid hormones. Science 233:652–654

25. Bissay V, De Klippel N, Herroelen L, Schmedding E, Buisseret T, Ebinger G, De Keyser J (1994) Bromocriptine therapy in multiple sclerosis: An open label pilot study. Clin Neuropharmacol 17:473–476

26. Bolton C, O'Neill JK, Allen SJ, Baker D (1997) Regulation of chronic relapsing experimental allergic encephalomyelitis by endogenous and exogenous glucocorticoids. Int Arch Allergy Immunol 114:74–80

27. Bouillon R (2006) Vitamin D: from photosynthesis, metabolism, and action to clinical applications. In: DeGroot LJ, Jameson JL (eds) Endocrinology. Elsevier Saunders, Philadelphia, pp 1435–1463
28. Bouman A, Heineman MJ, Faas MM (2005) Sex hormones and the immune response in humans. Hum Reprod Update 11:411–423
29. Brinar VV, Petelin Z, Brinar M, Djakovic V, Zadro I, Vranjes D (2006) CNS demyelination in autoimmune diseases. Clin Neurol Neurosurg 108:318–826
30. Brunner R, Schaefer D, Hess K, Parzer P, Resch F, Schwab S (2005) Effect of corticosteroids on short-term and long-term memory. Neurology 64:335–337
31. Cantorna MT, Hayes CE, DeLuca HF (1996) 1,25-dihydroxyvitamin d3 reversibly blocks the progression of relapsing encephalomyelitis, a model of multiple sclerosis. Proc Natl Acad Sci U S A 93:7861–7864
32. Carella C, Mazziotti G, Morisco F, Manganella G, Rotondi M, Tuccillo C, Sorvillo F, Caporaso N, Amato G (2001) Long-term outcome of interferon-alpha-induced thyroid autoimmunity and prognostic influence of thyroid autoantibody pattern at the end of treatment. J Clin Endocrinol Metab 86:1925–1929
33. Carroll WM, Jennings AR (1994) Early recruitment of oligodendrocyte precursors in CNS demyelination. Brain 117:563–578
34. Caruso A, Di Giorgi Gerevini V, Castiglione M, Marinelli F, Tomassini V, Pozzilli C, Caricasole A, Bruno V, Caciagli F, Moretti A, Nicoletti F, Melchiorri D (2004) Testosterone amplifies excitotoxic damage of cultured oligodendrocytes. J Neurochem 88:1179–1185
35. Chrousos GP (1995) The hypothalamic–pituitary–adrenal axis and immune-mediated inflammation. N Engl J Med 332:1351–162
36. Chrousos GP, Elenkov IJ (2006) Interactions of the endocrine and immune systems In: DeGroot LJ, Jameson JL (eds) Endocrinology. Elsevier Saunders, Philadelphia, pp 779–818
37. Chrousos GP, Torpy DJ, Gold PW (1998) Interactions between the hypothalamic–pituitary–adrenal axis and the female reproductive system: clinical implications. Ann Intern Med 129:229–240
38. Coles AJ, Cox A, Le Page E, Jones J, Trip SA, Deans J, Seaman S, Miller DH, Hale G, Waldmann H, Compston DA (2006) The window of therapeutic opportunity in multiple sclerosis: evidence from monoclonal antibody therapy. J Neurol 253:98–108
39. Coles AJ, Wing M, Smith S, Coraddu F, Greer S, Taylor C, Weetman A, Hale G, Chatterjee VK, Waldmann H, Compston A (1999) Pulsed monoclonal antibody treatment and autoimmune thyroid disease in multiple sclerosis. Lancet 354:1691–1695
40. Compston DAS, Margolin DH, Haas J, Magner J, Gonzales G, Valente W, Coles A (2006) Two year interim analysis of thyroid abnormalities in a trial of alemtuzumab vs high-dose interferon-beta-1a, for treatment of relapsing-remitting multiple sclerosis. 22nd Congress of the European Committee for the Treatment and Research
41. Confavreux C, Compston A (1998) The natural history of MS. In: McAlpinee D, Compston A, Ebers G, Lassmann H, McDonald I, Matthews B, Wekerle H (eds)Mcalpine's multiple sclerosis. Churchill Livingstone, Edinburgh, pp 183–272
42. Confavreux C, Hutchinson M, Hours MM, Cortinovis-Tourniaire P, Moreau T (1998) Rate of pregnancy-related relapse in multiple sclerosis. Pregnancy in Multiple Sclerosis Group. N Engl J Med 339:285–291
43. Confavreux C, Vukusic S, Adeleine P (2003) Early clinical predictors and progression of irreversible disability in multiple sclerosis: An amnesic process. Brain 126:770–782
44. Coppack SW (2001) Pro-inflammatory cytokines and adipose tissue. Proc Nutr Soc 60:349–356
45. Czock D, Keller F, Rasche FM, Haussler U (2005) Pharmacokinetics and pharmacodynamics of systemically administered glucocorticoids. Clin Pharmacokinet 44:61–98
46. D'Ambrosio D, Cippitelli M, Cocciolo MG, Mazzeo D, Di Lucia P, Lang R, Sinigaglia F, Panina-Bordignon P (1998) Inhibition of il-12 production by 1,25-dihydroxyvitamin D3.

Involvement of NF-kappaB downregulation in transcriptional repression of the p40 gene. J Clin Invest 101:252–262

47. Dalal M, Kim S, Voskuhl RR (1997) Testosterone therapy ameliorates experimental autoimmune encephalomyelitis and induces a T helper 2 bias in the autoantigen-specific T lymphocyte response. J Immunol 159:3–6
48. Damek DM, Shuster EA (1997) Pregnancy and multiple sclerosis. Mayo Clin Proc 72:977–989
49. David PS, Boatwright EA, Tozer BS, Verma DP, Blair JE, Mayer AP, Files JA (2006) Hormonal contraception update. Mayo Clin Proc 81:949–954; quiz 955
50. De Bellis A, Bizzarro A, Pivonello R, Lombardi G, Bellastella A (2005) Prolactin and autoimmunity. Pituitary 8:25–30
51. De Rosa V, Procaccini C, La Cava A, Chieffi P, Nicoletti GF, Fontana S, Zappacosta S, Matarese G (2006) Leptin neutralization interferes with pathogenic t cell autoreactivity in autoimmune encephalomyelitis. J Clin Invest 116:447–455
52. de Seze J, Chapelotte M, Delalande S, Ferriby D, Stojkovic T, Vermersch P (2004) Intravenous corticosteroids in the postpartum period for reduction of acute exacerbations in multiple sclerosis. Mult Scler 10:596–597
53. del Rey A, Klusman I, Besedovsky HO (1998) Cytokines mediate protective stimulation of glucocorticoid output during autoimmunity: Involvement of IL-1. Am J Physiol 275: R1146–R1151
54. Demerens C, Stankoff B, Zalc B, Lubetzki C (1999) Eliprodil stimulates cns myelination: New prospects for multiple sclerosis? Neurology 52:346–350
55. DeRijk RH, Eskandari F, Sternberg EM (2004) Corticosteroid resistance in a subpopulation of multiple sclerosis patients as measured by ex vivo dexamethasone inhibition of LPS induced IL-6 production. J Neuroimmunol 151:180–188
56. Diem R, Hobom M, Maier K, Weissert R, Storch MK, Meyer R, Bahr M (2003) Methylprednisolone increases neuronal apoptosis during autoimmune CNS inflammation by inhibition of an endogenous neuroprotective pathway. J Neurosci 23:6993–7000
57. Dijkstra CD, van der Voort ER, De Groot CJ, Huitinga I, Uitdehaag BM, Polman CH, Berkenbosch F (1994) Therapeutic effect of the d2-dopamine agonist bromocriptine on acute and relapsing experimental allergic encephalomyelitis. Psychoneuroendocrinology 19:135–142
58. Dixit VD, Schaffer EM, Pyle RS, Collins GD, Sakthivel SK, Palaniappan R, Lillard JW Jr, Taub DD (2004) Ghrelin inhibits leptin- and activation-induced proinflammatory cytokine expression by human monocytes and T cells. J Clin Invest 114:57–66
59. Dixit VD, Taub DD (2005) Ghrelin and immunity: A young player in an old field. Exp Gerontol 40:900–910
60. Draca S, Levic Z (1996) The possible role of prolactin in the immunopathogenesis of multiple sclerosis. Med Hypotheses 47:89–92
61. Drew PD, Storer PD, Xu J, Chavis JA (2005) Hormone regulation of microglial cell activation: relevance to multiple sclerosis. Brain Res Brain Res Rev 48:322–327
62. Du C, Khalil MW, Sriram S (2001) Administration of dehydroepiandrosterone suppresses experimental allergic encephalomyelitis in SJL/J mice. J Immunol 167:7094–7101
63. Durelli L, Ferrero B, Oggero A, Verdun E, Bongioanni MR, Gentile E, Isoardo GL, Ricci A, Rota E, Bergamasco B, Durazzo M, Saracco G, Biava MA, Brossa PC, Giorda L, Pagni R, Aimo G (1999) Autoimmune events during interferon beta-1b treatment for multiple sclerosis. J Neurol Sci 162:74–83
64. Durelli L, Ferrero B, Oggero A, Verdun E, Ghezzi A, Montanari E, Zaffaroni M (2001) Thyroid function and autoimmunity during interferon beta-1b treatment: a multicenter prospective study. J Clin Endocrinol Metab 86:3525–3532
65. Durelli L, Oggero A, Verdun E, Isoardo GL, Barbero P, Bergamasco B, Brossa PC, Ghigo E, Maccario M, Faggiano F (2001) Thyroid function and anti-thyroid antibodies in MS patients screened for interferon treatment. A multicenter study. J Neurol Sci 193:17–22

66. El-Etr M, Vukusic S, Gignoux L, Durand-Dubief F, Achiti I, Baulieu EE, Confavreux C (2005) Steroid hormones in multiple sclerosis. J Neurol Sci 233:49–54
67. Elenkov IJ, Wilder RL, Bakalov VK, Link AA, Dimitrov MA, Fisher S, Crane M, Kanik KS, Chrousos GP (2001) Il-12, TNF-alpha, and hormonal changes during late pregnancy and early postpartum: implications for autoimmune disease activity during these times. J Clin Endocrinol Metab 86:4933–4938
68. Elliott GA, Gibbons AJ, Greig ME (1973) A comparison of the effects of melengestrol acetate with a combination of hydrocortisone acetate and medroxyprogesterone acetate and with other steroids in the treatment of experimental alleric encephalomyelitis in Wistar rats. Acta Neuropathol (Berl) 23:95–104
69. Embry AF, Snowdon LR, Vieth R (2000) Vitamin D and seasonal fluctuations of gadolinium-enhancing magnetic resonance imaging lesions in multiple sclerosis. Ann Neurol 48:271–272
70. Erkut ZA, Hofman MA, Ravid R, Swaab DF (1995) Increased activity of hypothalamic corticotropin-releasing hormone neurons in multiple sclerosis. J Neuroimmunol 62:27–33
71. Fassbender K, Schmidt R, Mossner R, Kischka U, Kuhnen J, Schwartz A, Hennerici M (1998) Mood disorders and dysfunction of the hypothalamic-pituitary-adrenal axis in multiple sclerosis: association with cerebral inflammation. Arch Neurol 55:66–72
72. Fernandez M, Giuliani A, Pirondi S, D'Intino G, Giardino L, Aloe L, Levi-Montalcini R, Calza L (2004) Thyroid hormone administration enhances remyelination in chronic demyelinating inflammatory disease. Proc Natl Acad Sci U S A 101:16363–16368
73. Ferrero S, Esposito F, Pretta S, Ragni N (2006) Fetal risks related to the treatment of multiple sclerosis during pregnancy and breastfeeding. Expert Rev Neurother 6:1823–1831
74. Fleming JO, Hummel AL, Beinlich BR, Borowski BJ, Peebles T, Colburn M, Cook TD, Wendt GJ, DeLuca HF (2000) Vitamin d treatment of relapsing-remitting multiple sclerosis (RRMS): A MRI-based pilot study (abstract p05.011). Neurology 54:A338
75. Friedman JM, Halaas JL (1998) Leptin and the regulation of body weight in mammals. Nature 395:763–770
76. Garcia-Ovejero D, Azcoitia I, Doncarlos LL, Melcangi RC, Garcia-Segura LM (2005) Glia-neuron crosstalk in the neuroprotective mechanisms of sex steroid hormones. Brain Res Brain Res Rev 48:273–286
77. Garcia-Segura LM, Cardona-Gomez P, Naftolin F, Chowen JA (1998) Estradiol upregulates Bcl-2 expression in adult brain neurons. Neuroreport 9:593–597
78. Garcion E, Sindji L, Nataf S, Brachet P, Darcy F, Montero-Menei CN (2003) Treatment of experimental autoimmune encephalomyelitis in rat by 1,25-dihydroxyvitamin D3 leads to early effects within the central nervous system. Acta Neuropathol (Berl) 105:438–448
79. Garcion E, Wion-Barbot N, Montero-Menei CN, Berger F, Wion D (2002) New clues about vitamin D functions in the nervous system. Trends Endocrinol Metab 13:100–105
80. Gayo A, Mozo L, Suarez A, Tunon A, Lahoz C, Gutierrez C (1998) Glucocorticoids increase il-10 expression in multiple sclerosis patients with acute relapse. J Neuroimmunol 85:122–130
81. Ghisletti S, Meda C, Maggi A, Vegeto E (2005) 17beta-estradiol inhibits inflammatory gene expression by controlling Nf-kappaB intracellular localization. Mol Cell Biol 25:2957–2968
82. Gilmore W, Arias M, Stroud N, Stek A, McCarthy KA, Correale J (2004) Preliminary studies of cytokine secretion patterns associated with pregnancy in MS patients. J Neurol Sci 224:69–76
83. Gogas H, Ioannovich J, Dafni U, Stavropoulou-Giokas C, Frangia K, Tsoutsos D, Panagiotou P, Polyzos A, Papadopoulos O, Stratigos A, Markopoulos C, Bafaloukos D, Pectasides D, Fountzilas G, Kirkwood JM (2006) Prognostic significance of autoimmunity during treatment of melanoma with interferon. N Engl J Med 354:709–718
84. Gold SM (2006) Neurotrophic factor production by immune cells during testosterone treatment in MS (poster). ACTRIMS

85. Gold SM, Raji A, Huitinga I, Wiedemann K, Schulz KH, Heesen C (2005) Hypothalamo–pituitary–adrenal axis activity predicts disease progression in multiple sclerosis. J Neuroimmunol 165:186–191

86. Goldberg P, Fleming MC, Picard EH (1986) Multiple sclerosis: decreased relapse rate through dietary supplementation with calcium, magnesium and vitamin D. Med Hypotheses 21:193–200

87. Gonzalez Deniselle MC, Lopez-Costa JJ, Saavedra JP, Pietranera L, Gonzalez SL, Garay L, Guennoun R, Schumacher M, De Nicola AF (2002) Progesterone neuroprotection in the wobbler mouse, a genetic model of spinal cord motor neuron disease. Neurobiol Dis 11:457–468

88. Goodman Y, Bruce AJ, Cheng B, Mattson MP (1996) Estrogens attenuate and corticosterone exacerbates excitotoxicity, oxidative injury, and amyloid beta-peptide toxicity in hippocampal neurons. J Neurochem 66:1836–1844

89. Grasser A, Moller A, Backmund H, Yassouridis A, Holsboer F (1996) Heterogeneity of hypothalamic-pituitary-adrenal system response to a combined dexamethasone-CRH test in multiple sclerosis. Exp Clin Endocrinol Diabetes 104:31–37

90. Gregg C, Shikar V, Larsen P, Mak G, Chojnacki A, Yong VW, Weiss S (2007) White matter plasticity and enhanced remyelination in the maternal cns. J Neurosci 27:1812–1823

91. Greig ME, Gibbons AJ, Elliott GA (1970) A comparison of the effects of melengestrol acetate and hydrocortisone acetate on experimental allergic encephalomyelitis in rats. J Pharmacol Exp Ther 173:85–93

92. Haas J (2000) High dose IVIG in the postpartum period for prevention of exacerbations in MS. Mult Scler 6 [Suppl 2]:S18–S20; discussion S33

93. Hammond J, Le Q, Goodyer C, Gelfand M, Trifiro M, LeBlanc A (2001) Testosterone-mediated neuroprotection through the androgen receptor in human primary neurons. J Neurochem 77:1319–1326

94. Harirchian MH, Sahraian MA, Shirani A (2006) Serum prolactin level in patients with multiple sclerosis: a case–control study. Med Sci Monit 12:CR177–CR180

95. Hawkins SA, McDonnell GV (1999) Benign multiple sclerosis? Clinical course, long-term follow up, and assessment of prognostic factors. J Neurol Neurosurg Psychiatry 67:148–152

96. Heesen C, Gbadamosi J, Schoser BG, Pohlau D (2001) Autoimmune hyperthyroidism in multiple sclerosis under treatment with glatiramer acetate – a case report. Eur J Neurol 8:199

97. Heesen C, Gold SM, Bruhn M, Monch A, Schulz KH (2002) Prolactin stimulation in multiple sclerosis – an indicator of disease subtypes and activity? Endocr Res 28:9–18

98. Heesen C, Schulz H, Schmidt M, Gold S, Tessmer W, Schulz KH (2002) Endocrine and cytokine responses to acute psychological stress in multiple sclerosis. Brain Behav Immun 16:282–287

99. Hench PS, Kendall EC, Slocumb CH, et al (1949) The effect of a hormones of the adrenal cortex (17 hydroxy-11-dehydroxcorticosterone: compound e) and of pituitary adrenocorticotropic hormone on rheumatoid arthritis. Mayo Clin Proc 24:181–197

100. Hernan MA, Hohol MJ, Olek MJ, Spiegelman D, Ascherio A (2000) Oral contraceptives and the incidence of multiple sclerosis. Neurology 55:848–854

101. Holmqvist P, Wallberg M, Hammar M, Landtblom AM, Brynhildsen J (2006) Symptoms of multiple sclerosis in women in relation to sex steroid exposure. Maturitas 54:149–153

102. Horai R, Asano M, Sudo K, Kanuka H, Suzuki M, Nishihara M, Takahashi M, Iwakura Y (1998) Production of mice deficient in genes for interleukin (il)-1alpha, il-1beta, il-1alpha/beta, and il-1 receptor antagonist shows that il-1beta is crucial in turpentine-induced fever development and glucocorticoid secretion. J Exp Med 187:1463–1475

103. Huitinga I, De Groot CJ, Van der Valk P, Kamphorst W, Tilders FJ, Swaab DF (2001) Hypothalamic lesions in multiple sclerosis. J Neuropathol Exp Neurol 60:1208–1218

104. Huitinga I, Erkut ZA, van Beurden D, Swaab DF (2003) The hypothalamo-pituitary-adrenal axis in multiple sclerosis. Ann N Y Acad Sci 992:118–128

105. Huitinga I, Erkut ZA, van Beurden D, Swaab DF (2004) Impaired hypothalamus–pituitary–adrenal axis activity and more severe multiple sclerosis with hypothalamic lesions. Ann Neurol 55:37–45
106. Ibanez C, Shields SA, El-Etr M, Leonelli E, Magnaghi V, Li WW, Sim FJ, Baulieu EE, Melcangi RC, Schumacher M, Franklin RJ (2003) Steroids and the reversal of age-associated changes in myelination and remyelination. Prog Neurobiol 71:49–56
107. Institute of Medicine (U.S.). Standing Committee on the Scientific Evaluation of Dietary Reference Intakes (1997) Dietary reference intakes for calcium, phosphorus, magnesium, vitamin D, and fluoride. National Academies Press, Washington DC, p xv
108. Ioppoli C, Meucci G, Mariotti S, Martino E, Lippi A, Gironelli L, Pinchera A, Muratorio A (1990) Circulating thyroid and gastric parietal cell autoantibodies in patients with multiple sclerosis. Ital J Neurol Sci 11:31–36
109. Ito A, Bebo BF Jr, Matejuk A, Zamora A, Silverman M, Fyfe-Johnson A, Offner H (2001) Estrogen treatment down-regulates TNF-alpha production and reduces the severity of experimental autoimmune encephalomyelitis in cytokine knockout mice. J Immunol 167:542–552
110. Jansson L, Olsson T, Holmdahl R (1994) Estrogen induces a potent suppression of experimental autoimmune encephalomyelitis and collagen-induced arthritis in mice. J Neuroimmunol 53:203–207
111. Jiang N, Chopp M, Stein D, Feit H (1996) Progesterone is neuroprotective after transient middle cerebral artery occlusion in male rats. Brain Res 735:101–107
112. Jones SA, Jolson DM, Cuta KK, Mariash CN, Anderson GW (2003) Triiodothyronine is a survival factor for developing oligodendrocytes. Mol Cell Endocrinol 199:49–60
113. Kalman B, Olsson O, Link H, Kam-Hansen S (1989) Estradiol potentiates poke-weed mitogen-induced b cell stimulation in multiple sclerosis and healthy subjects. Acta Neurol Scand 79:340–346
114. Kalueff AV, Tuohimaa P (2007) Neurosteroid hormone vitamin D and its utility in clinical nutrition. Curr Opin Clin Nutr Metab Care 10:12–19
115. Kantarci OH, Barcellos LF, Atkinson EJ, Ramsay PP, Lincoln R, Achenbach SJ, De Andrade M, Hauser SL, Weinshenker BG (2006) Men transmit MS more often to their children vs women: the Carter effect. Neurology 67:305–310
116. Kappas A, Jones HE, Roitt IM (1963) Effects of steroid sex hormones on immunological phenomena. Nature 198:902
117. Kappas A, Palmer RH (1963) Selected aspects of steroid pharmacology. Pharmacol Rev 15:123–167
118. Karssen AM, Meijer OC, van der Sandt IC, De Boer AG, De Lange EC, De Kloet ER (2002) The role of the efflux transporter p-glycoprotein in brain penetration of prednisolone. J Endocrinol 175:251–260
119. Keith AB (1978) Effect of pregnancy on experimental allergic encephalomyelitis in guinea pigs and rats. J Neurol Sci 38:317–326
120. Kim S, Voskuhl RR (1999) Decreased IL-12 production underlies the decreased ability of male lymph node cells to induce experimental autoimmune encephalomyelitis. J Immunol 162:5561–5568
121. Kira J, Harada M, Yamaguchi Y, Shida N, Goto I (1991) Hyperprolactinemia in multiple sclerosis. J Neurol Sci 102:61–66
122. Kirk AD, Hale DA, Swanson SJ, Mannon RB (2006) Autoimmune thyroid disease after renal transplantation using depletional induction with alemtuzumab. Am J Transplant 6:1084–1085
123. Koo GC, Huang C, Camacho R, Trainor C, Blake JT, Sirotina-Meisher A, Schleim KD, Wu TJ, Cheng K, Nargund R, McKissick G (2001) Immune enhancing effect of a growth hormone secretagogue. J Immunol 166:4195–41201
124. Koon H, Atkins M (2006) Autoimmunity and immunotherapy for cancer. N Engl J Med 354:758–760
125. Korn-Lubetzki I, Kahana E, Cooper G, Abramsky O (1984) Activity of multiple sclerosis during pregnancy and puerperium. Ann Neurol 16:229–231

126. Kuiper GG, Carlsson B, Grandien K, Enmark E, Haggblad J, Nilsson S, Gustafsson JA (1997) Comparison of the ligand binding specificity and transcript tissue distribution of estrogen receptors alpha and beta. Endocrinology 138:863–870

127. Kumpfel T, Then Bergh F, Friess E, Uhr M, Yassouridis A, Trenkwalder C, Holsboer F (1999) Dehydroepiandrosterone response to the adrenocorticotropin test and the combined dexamethasone and corticotropin-releasing hormone test in patients with multiple sclerosis. Neuroendocrinology 70:431–438

128. Lassmann H, Wekerle H (1998) The pathology of multiple sclerosis In: McAlpine D, Compston A, Ebers G, Lassmann H, McDonald I, Matthews B, Wekerle H (eds) Mcalpine's multiple sclerosis. Churchill Livingstone, Edinburgh, pp 557–599

129. Lemire JM, Archer DC, Beck L, Spiegelberg HL (1995) Immunosuppressive actions of 1,25-dihydroxyvitamin D3: preferential inhibition of th1 functions. J Nutr 125: 1704S–1708S

130. Leussink VI, Jung S, Merschdorf U, Toyka KV, Gold R (2001) High-dose methylprednisolone therapy in multiple sclerosis induces apoptosis in peripheral blood leukocytes. Arch Neurol 58:91–97

131. Levine S, Sowinski R, Steinetz B (1980) Effects of experimental allergic encephalomyelitis on thymus and adrenal: relation to remission and relapse. Proc Soc Exp Biol Med 165:218–224

132. Li DK, Zhao GJ, Paty DW (2001) Randomized controlled trial of interferon-beta-1a in secondary progressive MS: MRI results. Neurology 56:1505–1513

133. Limberg CC (1948) Demographic distribution of multiple sclerosis and its estimated prevalence in the United States In: Association for Research in Nervous and Mental Disease (ed) Multiple sclerosis and the demyelinating diseases. Conference of the Association for Research in Nervous and Mental Disease, December 10 and 11, 1948, New York. Williams & Wilkins, Baltimore, pp 15–24

134. Limone P, Ferrero B, Calvelli P, Del Rizzo P, Rota E, Berardi C, Barberis AM, Isaia GC, Durelli L (2002) Hypothalamic-pituitary-adrenal axis function and cytokine production in multiple sclerosis with or without interferon-beta treatment. Acta Neurol Scand 105:372–377

135. Lindzey J, Korach KS (2006) Environmental agents and the reproductive system In: DeGroot LJ, Jameson JL (eds) Endocrinology. Elsevier Saunders, Philadelphia, pp 2759–2778

136. Linssen WH, Notermans NC, Hommes OR, Rolland R (1987) Amenorrhea after immunosuppressive treatment of multiple sclerosis. Acta Neurol Scand 76:204–209

137. Liva SM, Voskuhl RR (2001) Testosterone acts directly on CD4+ T lymphocytes to increase IL-10 production. J Immunol 167:2060–2067

138. Lopez C, Comabella M, Tintore M, Sastre-Garriga J, Montalban X (2006) Variations in chemokine receptor and cytokine expression during pregnancy in multiple sclerosis patients. Mult Scler 12:421–427

139. Lord GM, Matarese G, Howard JK, Baker RJ, Bloom SR, Lechler RI (1998) Leptin modulates the T-cell immune response and reverses starvation-induced immunosuppression. Nature 394:897–901

140. Lowe SA (2001) Drugs in pregnancy. Anticonvulsants and drugs for neurological disease. Best Pract Res Clin Obstet Gynaecol 15:863–876

141. Mahon BD, Gordon SA, Cruz J, Cosman F, Cantorna MT (2003) Cytokine profile in patients with multiple sclerosis following vitamin D supplementation. J Neuroimmunol 134:128–132

142. Martinelli V, Gironi M, Rodegher M, Martino G, Comi G (1998) Occurrence of thyroid autoimmunity in relapsing remitting multiple sclerosis patients undergoing interferon-beta treatment. Ital J Neurol Sci 19:65–67

143. Mason D, MacPhee I, Antoni F (1990) The role of the neuroendocrine system in determining genetic susceptibility to experimental allergic encephalomyelitis in the rat. Immunology 70:1–5

144. Matarese G, Carrieri PB, La Cava A, Perna F, Sanna V, De Rosa V, Aufiero D, Fontana S, Zappacosta S (2005) Leptin increase in multiple sclerosis associates with reduced number of CD4(+)CD25+ regulatory t cells. Proc Natl Acad Sci U S A 102:5150–1515

145. Matarese G, Di Giacomo A, Sanna V, Lord GM, Howard JK, Di Tuoro A, Bloom SR, Lechler RI, Zappacosta S, Fontana S (2001) Requirement for leptin in the induction and progression of autoimmune encephalomyelitis. J Immunol 166:5909–5916

146. Mattner F, Smiroldo S, Galbiati F, Muller M, Di Lucia P, Poliani PL, Martino G, Panina-Bordignon P, Adorini L (2000) Inhibition of Th1 development and treatment of chronic-relapsing experimental allergic encephalomyelitis by a non-hypercalcemic analogue of 1,25-dihydroxyvitamin D(3). Eur J Immunol 30:498–508

147. Mattson D, Petrie M, Srivastava DK, McDermott M (1995) Multiple sclerosis. Sexual dysfunction and its response to medications. Arch Neurol 52:862–868

148. Michelson D, Stone L, Galliven E, Magiakou MA, Chrousos GP, Sternberg EM, Gold PW (1994) Multiple sclerosis is associated with alterations in hypothalamic–pituitary–adrenal axis function. J Clin Endocrinol Metab 79:848–853

149. Monzani F, Caraccio N, Casolaro A, Lombardo F, Moscato G, Murri L, Ferrannini E, Meucci G (2000) Long-term interferon beta-1b therapy for MS: is routine thyroid assessment always useful? Neurology 55:549–552

150. Morales LB, Loo KK, Liu HB, Peterson C, Tiwari-Woodruff S, Voskuhl RR (2006) Treatment with an estrogen receptor alpha ligand is neuroprotective in experimental autoimmune encephalomyelitis. J Neurosci 26:6823–6833

151. Munck A, Naray-Fejes-Toth A (2006) Glucocorticoid physiology In: DeGroot LJ, Jameson JL (eds) Endocrinology. Elsevier Saunders, Philadelphia, pp 2287–2307

152. Munger KL, Zhang SM, O'Reilly E, Hernan MA, Olek MJ, Willett WC, Ascherio A (2004) Vitamin d intake and incidence of multiple sclerosis. Neurology 62:60–65

153. Muthian G, Raikwar HP, Rajasingh J, Bright JJ (2006) 1,25 dihydroxyvitamin-d3 modulates JAK-stat pathway in il-12/ifngamma axis leading to Th1 response in experimental allergic encephalomyelitis. J Neurosci Res 83:1299–1309

154. Nagy E, Berczi I, Wren GE, Asa SL, Kovacs K (1983) Immunomodulation by bromocriptine. Immunopharmacology 6:231–243

155. Nataf S, Garcion E, Darcy F, Chabannes D, Muller JY, Brachet P (1996) 1,25 dihydroxyvitamin d3 exerts regional effects in the central nervous system during experimental allergic encephalomyelitis. J Neuropathol Exp Neurol 55:904–914

156. Niederwieser G, Buchinger W, Bonelli RM, Berghold A, Reisecker F, Koltringer P, Archelos JJ (2003) Prevalence of autoimmune thyroiditis and non-immune thyroid disease in multiple sclerosis. J Neurol 250:672–675

157. NMMS Society (2006) A phase 2 study of estriol therapy combined with glatiramer. Research/Clinical Update, Nov 10

158. Noseworthy J, Confavreaux C, Compston A (1998) Treatment of the acute relapse. In: McAlpine D, compston A, Ebers G, Lassmann H, McDonald I, Matthews B, Wekerle H (eds) Mcalpine's multiple sclerosis.Churchill Livingstone, Edinburgh , pp 683–699

159. Obendorf M, Patchev VK (2004) Interactions of sex steroids with mechanisms of inflammation. Curr Drug Targets Inflamm Allergy 3:425–433

160. Obradovic D, Gronemeyer H, Lutz B, Rein T (2006) Cross-talk of vitamin D and glucocorticoids in hippocampal cells. J Neurochem 96:500–509

161. Orton SM, Herrera BM, Yee IM, Valdar W, Ramagopalan SV, Sadovnick AD, Ebers GC (2006) Sex ratio of multiple sclerosis in Canada: a longitudinal study. Lancet Neurol 5:932–936

162. Ostensen M, Villiger PM (2002) Immunology of pregnancy: pregnancy as a remission inducing agent in rheumatoid arthritis. Transpl Immunol 9:155–160

163. Palaszynski KM, Loo KK, Ashouri JF, Liu HB, Voskuhl RR (2004) Androgens are protective in experimental autoimmune encephalomyelitis: implications for multiple sclerosis. J Neuroimmunol 146:144–152

164. Palaszynski KM, Smith DL, Kamrava S, Burgoyne PS, Arnold AP, Voskuhl RR (2005) A yin-yang effect between sex chromosome complement and sex hormones on the immune response. Endocrinology 146:3280–3285

165. Parry S, Strauss JF. Placental hormones. In: DeGroot LJ, Jameson JL (eds) Endocrinology. Elsevier Saunders, Philadelphia, pp 3353–3368

166. Patwardhan AJ, Eliez S, Bender B, Linden MG, Reiss AL (2000) Brain morphology in Klinefelter syndrome: Extra X chromosome and testosterone supplementation. Neurology 54:2218–2223

167. Penhale WJ, Farmer A, Irvine WJ (1975) Thyroiditis in t cell-depleted rats. Influence of strain, radiation dose, adjuvants and antilymphocyte serum. Clin Exp Immunol 21:362–375

168. Perretti M, Ahluwalia A (2000) The microcirculation and inflammation: site of action for glucocorticoids. Microcirculation 7:147–161

169. Petanceska SS, Nagy V, Frail D, Gandy S (2000) Ovariectomy and 17beta-estradiol modulate the levels of Alzheimer's amyloid beta peptides in brain. Neurology 54:2212–2217

170. Petek-Balci B, Yayla V, Ozer F (2005) Multiple sclerosis and hashimoto thyroiditis: Two cases. Neurologist 11:301–4

171. Pittock SJ, Weinshenker BG, Lucchinetti CF, Wingerchuk DM, Corboy JR, Lennon VA (2006) Neuromyelitis optica brain lesions localized at sites of high aquaporin 4 expression. Arch Neurol 63:964–968

172. Poser S, Raun NE, Wikstrom J, Poser W (1979) Pregnancy, oral contraceptives and multiple sclerosis. Acta Neurol Scand 59:108–118

173. Pozzi S, Benedusi V, Maggi A, Vegeto E (2006) Estrogen action in neuroprotection and brain inflammation. Ann N Y Acad Sci 1089:302–323

174. Pozzilli C, Falaschi P, Mainero C, Martocchia A, D'Urso R, Proietti A, Frontoni M, Bastianello S, Filippi M (1999) MRI in multiple sclerosis during the menstrual cycle: relationship with sex hormone patterns. Neurology 53:622–624

175. Pozzilli C, Tomassini V, Marinelli F, Paolillo A, Gasperini C, Bastianello S (2003) 'gender gap' in multiple sclerosis: magnetic resonance imaging evidence. Eur J Neurol 10:95–97

176. Reder AT, Lowy MT (1993) Serum prolactin levels in active multiple sclerosis and during cyclosporin treatment. J Neurol Sci 117:192–196

177. Reder AT, Lowy MT, Meltzer HY, Antel JP (1987) Dexamethasone suppression test abnormalities in multiple sclerosis: Relation to ACTH therapy. Neurology 37:849–853

178. Reder AT, Thapar M, Jensen MA (1994) A reduction in serum glucocorticoids provokes experimental allergic encephalomyelitis: implications for treatment of inflammatory brain disease. Neurology 44:2289–2294

179. Riskind PN, Massacesi L, Doolittle TH, Hauser SL (1991) The role of prolactin in autoimmune demyelination: suppression of experimental allergic encephalomyelitis by bromocriptine. Ann Neurol 29:542–547

180. Rogister B, Ben-Hur T, Dubois-Dalcq M (1999) From neural stem cells to myelinating oligodendrocytes. Mol Cell Neurosci 14:287–300

181. Roitt IM (2006) Control mechanisms. In: Delves PJ, Martin SJ, Buron DR, Roitt IM (eds) Roitt's essential immunology. Blackwell Science, Oxford, pp 223–228

182. Roof RL, Duvdevani R, Heyburn JW, Stein DG (1996) Progesterone rapidly decreases brain edema: treatment delayed up to 24 hours is still effective. Exp Neurol 138:246–251

183. Rossouw JE, Anderson GL, Prentice RL, LaCroix AZ, Kooperberg C, Stefanick ML, Jackson RD, Beresford SA, Howard BV, Johnson KC, Kotchen JM, Ockene J (2002) Risks and benefits of estrogen plus progestin in healthy postmenopausal women: principal results from the women's health initiative randomized controlled trial. JAMA 288:321–333

184. Rotondi M, Oliviero A, Profice P, Mone CM, Biondi B, Del Buono A, Mazziotti G, Sinisi AM, Bellastella A, Carella C (1998) Occurrence of thyroid autoimmunity and dysfunction throughout a nine-month follow-up in patients undergoing interferon-beta therapy for multiple sclerosis. J Endocrinol Invest 21:748–752

185. Sanchez-Ramon S, Navarro AJ, Aristimuno C, Rodriguez-Mahou M, Bellon JM, Fernandez-Cruz E, de Andres C (2005) Pregnancy-induced expansion of regulatory T-

lymphocytes may mediate protection to multiple sclerosis activity. Immunol Lett 96:195–201

186. Sanna V, Di Giacomo A, La Cava A, Lechler RI, Fontana S, Zappacosta S, Matarese G (2003) Leptin surge precedes onset of autoimmune encephalomyelitis and correlates with development of pathogenic T cell responses. J Clin Invest 111:241–250

187. Santizo RA, Anderson S, Ye S, Koenig HM, Pelligrino DA (2000) Effects of estrogen on leukocyte adhesion after transient forebrain ischemia. Stroke 31:2231–2235

188. Schumacher M, Guennoun R, Robert F, Carelli C, Gago N, Ghoumari A, Gonzalez Deniselle MC, Gonzalez SL, Ibanez C, Labombarda F, Coirini H, Baulieu EE, De Nicola AF (2004) Local synthesis and dual actions of progesterone in the nervous system: neuroprotection and myelination. Growth Horm IGF Res 14 [Suppl A]:S18–S33

189. Schumann EM, Kumpfel T, Then Bergh F, Trenkwalder C, Holsboer F, Auer DP (2002) Activity of the hypothalamic-pituitary-adrenal axis in multiple sclerosis: correlations with gadolinium-enhancing lesions and ventricular volume. Ann Neurol 51:763–767

190. Schwid SR, Goodman AD, Mattson DH (1997) Autoimmune hyperthyroidism in patients with multiple sclerosis treated with interferon beta-1b. Arch Neurol 54:1169–1190

191. Sena AH, Pedrosa RG, Cascais MJ, Andrade ML, Ferret-Sena VM, Morais MG (2006) Oral contraceptive use in patients with multiple sclerosis (abstract p04.120). Neurology 66:A229

192. Shah AK, Tselis A, Mason B (2000) Acute disseminated encephalomyelitis in a pregnant woman successfully treated with plasmapheresis. J Neurol Sci 174:147–151

193. Sicotte L, Giesser BS, Tandon V, Steiner B, Klutch R, Drain A, Shattuck DW, Hull L, Swerdloff R, Voskuhl RR (2006) A pilot study of testosterone treatment for men with relapsing remitting multiple sclerosis (abstract p01.070). Neurology Suppl 2:A30

194. Sicotte NL, Liva SM, Klutch R, Pfeiffer P, Bouvier S, Odesa S, Wu TC, Voskuhl RR (2002) Treatment of multiple sclerosis with the pregnancy hormone estriol. Ann Neurol 52:421–428

195. Smith DL, Du S, Wetmore KM, Arnold AP, Singh RR, Voskuhl RR (2006) The XX sex chromosome complement, as compared to the XY, confers greater susceptibility to experimental autoimmune encephalomyelitis and lupus. ACTRIMS Meeting 2006

196. Smith R, Studd JW (1992) A pilot study of the effect upon multiple sclerosis of the menopause, hormone replacement therapy and the menstrual cycle. J R Soc Med 85:612–613

197. Smith SR, Ravussin E (2006) Role of the adipocyte in metabolism and endocrine function. In: DeGroot LJ, Jameson JL (eds) Endocrinology. Elsevier Saunders, Philadelphia, pp 1045–1062

198. Soilu-Hanninen M, Airas L, Mononen I, Heikkila A, Viljanen M, Hanninen A (2005) 25-hydroxyvitamin D levels in serum at the onset of multiple sclerosis. Mult Scler 11:266–271

199. Soldan SS, Alvarez Retuerto AI, Sicotte NL, Voskuhl RR (2003) Immune modulation in multiple sclerosis patients treated with the pregnancy hormone estriol. J Immunol 171:6267–6274

200. Stefferl A, Linington C, Holsboer F, Reul JM (1999) Susceptibility and resistance to experimental allergic encephalomyelitis: Relationship with hypothalamic-pituitary-adrenocortical axis responsiveness in the rat. Endocrinology 140:4932–4938

201. Stefferl A, Storch MK, Linington C, Stadelmann C, Lassmann H, Pohl T, Holsboer F, Tilders FJ, Reul JM (2001) Disease progression in chronic relapsing experimental allergic encephalomyelitis is associated with reduced inflammation-driven production of corticosterone. Endocrinology 142:3616–3624

202. Subramanian S, Matejuk A, Zamora A, Vandenbark AA, Offner H (2003) Oral feeding with ethinyl estradiol suppresses and treats experimental autoimmune encephalomyelitis in SJL mice and inhibits the recruitment of inflammatory cells into the central nervous system. J Immunol 170:1548–1555

203. Surks MI, Ortiz E, Daniels GH, Sawin CT, Col NF, Cobin RH, Franklyn JA, Hershman JM, Burman KD, Denke MA, Gorman C, Cooper RS, Weissman NJ (2004) Subclinical thyroid disease: scientific review and guidelines for diagnosis and management. JAMA 291:228–238

204. Tellez N, Comabella M, Julia E, Rio J, Tintore M, Brieva L, Nos C, Montalban X (2006) Fatigue in progressive multiple sclerosis is associated with low levels of dehydroepiandrosterone. Mult Scler 12:487–494

205. Then Bergh F, Grasser A, Trenkwalder C, Backmund H, Holsboer F, Rupprecht R (1999) Binding characteristics of the glucocorticoid receptor in peripheral blood lymphocytes in multiple sclerosis. J Neurol 246:292–298

206. Then Bergh F, Kumpfel T, Grasser A, Rupprecht R, Holsboer F, Trenkwalder C (2001) Combined treatment with corticosteroids and moclobemide favors normalization of hypothalamo-pituitary-adrenal axis dysregulation in relapsing-remitting multiple sclerosis: a randomized, double blind trial. J Clin Endocrinol Metab 86:1610–1615

207. Thomas AJ, Nockels RP, Pan HQ, Shaffrey CI, Chopp M (1999) Progesterone is neuroprotective after acute experimental spinal cord trauma in rats. Spine 24:2134–2138

208. Thorogood M, Hannaford PC (1998) The influence of oral contraceptives on the risk of multiple sclerosis. Br J Obstet Gynaecol 105:1296–1299

209. Tomassini V, Onesti E, Mainero C, Giugni E, Paolillo A, Salvetti M, Nicoletti F, Pozzilli C (2005) Sex hormones modulate brain damage in multiple sclerosis: MRI evidence. J Neurol Neurosurg Psychiatry 76:272–275

210. Tritos NA, Kokkotou EG (2006) The physiology and potential clinical applications of ghrelin, a novel peptide hormone. Mayo Clin Proc 81:653–660

211. Trooster WJ, Teelken AW, Gerrits PO, Lijnema TH, Loof JG, Minderhoud JM, Nieuwenhuis P (1996) The effect of gonadectomy on the clinical course of chronic experimental allergic encephalomyelitis. Clin Neurol Neurosurg 98:222–226

212. Trooster WJ, Teelken AW, Kampinga J, Loof JG, Nieuwenhuis P, Minderhoud JM (1993) Suppression of acute experimental allergic encephalomyelitis by the synthetic sex hormone 17-alpha-ethinylestradiol: An immunological study in the Lewis rat. Int Arch Allergy Immunol 102:133–140

213. Van Etten E, Decallonne B, Verlinden L, Verstuyf A, Bouillon R, Mathieu C (2003) Analogs of 1alpha,25-dihydroxyvitamin d3 as pluripotent immunomodulators. J Cell Biochem 88:223–226

214. van Walderveen MA, Tas MW, Barkhof F, Polman CH, Frequin ST, Hommes OR, Valk J (1994) Magnetic resonance evaluation of disease activity during pregnancy in multiple sclerosis. Neurology 44:327–329

215. van Winsen LM, Muris DF, Polman CH, Dijkstra CD, van den Berg TK, Uitdehaag BM (2005) Sensitivity to glucocorticoids is decreased in relapsing remitting multiple sclerosis. J Clin Endocrinol Metab 90:734–740

216. VanAmerongen BM, Dijkstra CD, Lips P, Polman CH (2004) Multiple sclerosis and vitamin D: an update. Eur J Clin Nutr 58:1095–1109

217. vanEtten E, Gysemans C, Branisteaunu DD et al (2007) Novel insights in the immune function of the vitamin d system: synergism with interferon beta. J Steroid Biochem Mol Biol 103:546–551

218. Vegeto E, Belcredito S, Etteri S, Ghisletti S, Brusadelli A, Meda C, Krust A, Dupont S, Ciana P, Chambon P, Maggi A (2003) Estrogen receptor-alpha mediates the brain antiinflammatory activity of estradiol. Proc Natl Acad Sci U S A 100:9614–9619

219. Vegeto E, Bonincontro C, Pollio G, Sala A, Viappiani S, Nardi F, Brusadelli A, Viviani B, Ciana P, Maggi A (2001) Estrogen prevents the lipopolysaccharide-induced inflammatory response in microglia. J Neurosci 21:1809–1818

220. Vieth R, Chan PC, MacFarlane GD (2001) Efficacy and safety of vitamin D3 intake exceeding the lowest observed adverse effect level. Am J Clin Nutr 73:288–294

221. Vieth R, Ladak Y, Walfish PG (2003) Age-related changes in the 25-hydroxyvitamin D versus parathyroid hormone relationship suggest a different reason why older adults require more vitamin D. J Clin Endocrinol Metab 88:185–191

222. Villard-Mackintosh L, Vessey MP (1993) Oral contraceptives and reproductive factors in multiple sclerosis incidence. Contraception 47:161–168

311

223 Vukusic S, Hutchinson M, Hours M, Moreau T, Cortinovis-Tourniaire P, Adeleine P, Confavreux C, The Pregnancy In Multiple Sclerosis G (2004) Pregnancy and multiple sclerosis (the PRIMS study): clinical predictors of post-partum relapse. Brain 127:1353–1360

224. Wartofsky L, Van Nostrand D, Burman KD (2006) Overt and 'subclinical' hypothyroidism in women. Obstet Gynecol Surv 61:535–542

225. Wassertheil-Smoller S, Hendrix SL, Limacher M, Heiss G, Kooperberg C, Baird A, Kotchen T, Curb JD, Black H, Rossouw JE, Aragaki A, Safford M, Stein E, Laowattana S, Mysiw WJ (2003) Effect of estrogen plus progestin on stroke in postmenopausal women: the Women's Health Initiative: a randomized trial. JAMA 289:2673–2684

226. Weatherby SJ, Mann CL, Davies MB, Fryer AA, Haq N, Strange RC, Hawkins CP (2000) A pilot study of the relationship between gadolinium-enhancing lesions, gender effect and polymorphisms of antioxidant enzymes in multiple sclerosis. J Neurol 247:467–470

227. Wei T, Lightman SL (1997) The neuroendocrine axis in patients with multiple sclerosis. Brain 120:1067–1076

228. Weinshenker BG, Bass B, Rice GP, Noseworthy J, Carriere W, Baskerville J, Ebers GC (1989) The natural history of multiple sclerosis: a geographically based study. 2. Predictive value of the early clinical course. Brain 112:1419–1428

229. Weiss RE, Wu SY, Refetoff S (2006) Diagnostic tests of the thyroid IN: Endocrinology. Ed: LJ DeGroot and JL Jameson. Philadelphia: Elsevier Saunders 2006, 1899–1962

230. Wiersinga WM. Hypothyroidism and myxedema coma. In: DeGroot LJ, Jameson JL (eds) Endocrinology. Elsevier Saunders, Philadelphia, pp 2081–2099

231. Windaus A, Linsert O (1928) Vitamin D 1. Ann Chem 465:148

232. Wingerchuk DM, Lesaux J, Rice GP, Kremenchutzky M, Ebers GC (2005) A pilot study of oral calcitriol (1,25-dihydroxyvitamin d3) for relapsing-remitting multiple sclerosis. J Neurol Neurosurg Psychiatry 76:1294–1296

233. Wingerchuk DM, Rodriguez M (2006) Premenstrual multiple sclerosis pseudoexacerbations: role of body temperature and prevention with aspirin. Arch Neurol 63:1005–1008

234. Younes-Rapozo V, Berendonk J, Savignon T, Manhaes AC, Barradas PC (2006) Thyroid hormone deficiency changes the distribution of oligodendrocyte/myelin markers during oligodendroglial differentiation in vitro. Int J Dev Neurosci 24:445–453

235. Zivadinov R, Rudick RA, De Masi R, Nasuelli D, Ukmar M, Pozzi-Mucelli RS, Grop A, Cazzato G, Zorzon M (2001) Effects of iv methylprednisolone on brain atrophy in relapsing-remitting MS. Neurology 57:1239–1247

236. Zorgdrager A, De Keyser J (1997) Menstrually related worsening of symptoms in multiple sclerosis. J Neurol Sci 149:95–97

237. Zorgdrager A, De Keyser J (2002) The premenstrual period and exacerbations in multiple sclerosis. Eur Neurol 48:204–206

# Statins and Demyelination

**M.S. Weber and S.S. Zamvil(✉)**

**Abstract** Statins are inhibitors of the 3-hydroxy-3-methylglutaryl coenzyme A reductase, which are widely prescribed for their cholesterol-lowering properties in order to reduce atherogenesis and cardiovascular morbidity. Moreover, statins have been shown to exert pleiotropic immunomodulatory effects that might be of therapeutic benefit in autoimmune disorders. Statins appear to alter immune function largely independent of lipid lowering and rather through inhibition of posttranslational protein prenylation of small regulatory GTP-binding proteins. In experimental autoimmune encephalomyelitis (EAE), the murine model for multiple sclerosis (MS), statins were shown to reverse established paralysis and to exert synergistic benefit in combination with agents approved for MS therapy. Based upon these encouraging findings in treatment of EAE, statins are now being tested in clinical trials in patients with MS.

S.S. Zamvil
Department of Neurology, University of California, San Francisco, 513 Parnassus Avenue, S-268, San Francisco, CA 94143-0435, USA
e-mail: zamvil@ucsf.neuroimmunol.org

M. Rodriguez (ed.), *Advances in Multiple Sclerosis and Experimental Demyelinating Diseases. Current Topics in Microbiology and Immunology 318.*
© Springer-Verlag Berlin Heidelberg 2008

# 1 Introduction

Currently, FDA-approved disease-modifying drugs for multiple sclerosis (MS) are only partially effective. Thus, the search for novel therapies and new treatment regimes must continue. Statins inhibit the enzyme 3-hydroxy-3-methylglutaryl coenzyme A (HMG-CoA) reductase. The enzyme HMG-CoA reductase catalyzes the conversion of HMG-CoA to L-mevalonate, the key intermediate in the biosynthesis of cholesterol [17]. Over decades, statins have established themselves as generally safe and well-tolerated drugs [1, 2, 22] and are prescribed to more than 25 million people worldwide today. The family of statins includes naturally occurring members (lovastatin, mevastatin, pravastatin, and simvastatin) and synthetic members (fluvastatin, atorvastatin, and rosuvastatin), which differ in their lipophilicity, half-life, and potency.

Statins studied in animal models of autoimmune diseases demonstrate immunomodulatory properties independent of their cholesterol-lowering properties that might be of benefit in treatment of neuroinflammatory disorders. Orally administered statins are particularly attractive candidates for treatment of MS; all currently approved drugs, such as interferon-beta, glatiramer acetate (GA), mitoxantrone, and natalizumab, are administered parenterally and have side effects and potential toxicities.

# 2 Mechanism of Action

In 1995, the potential impact of statins on immune function surfaced with a study demonstrating that cardiac transplant patients treated with pravastatin had a reduced incidence of hemodynamically significant rejection episodes and showed decreased mortality that did not correlate with cholesterol reduction [25]. Numerous subsequent studies further elaborated the anti-inflammatory properties of statins [43].

Rather recent studies have elucidated the molecular mechanisms that may be responsible for statin-mediated immune modulation. One report suggested that statins directly bind the cellular adhesion molecule leukocyte function antigen 1 (LFA-1), primarily resulting in reduced migration of pro-inflammatory leukocytes [50]. The majority of statin-mediated immunomodulatory effects, however, appear related to the competitive displacement of HMG-CoA from the HMG-CoA reductase, as these effects can be reversed by addition of its downstream product mevalonate. Importantly, mevalonate is the key metabolite, not only for the synthesis of cholesterol, but also for the synthesis of isoprenoid intermediates, such as farnesylpyrophosphate (FPP) and geranylgeranylpyrophosphate (GGPP). These molecules are responsible for the prenylation of GTP-binding proteins [56], such as Ras and Rho, which have important roles in multiple signaling pathways regulating cellular differentiation and proliferation [46]. Posttranslational isoprenylation of these proteins is necessary for their attachment to the cytoplasmic surface of the plasma membrane, where they function. Thus, by inhibiting isoprenylation of Ras and Rho, statins modulate cellular functions that are also required for the activation of immune cells (Fig. 1).

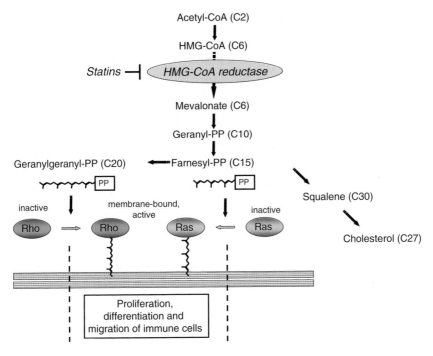

**Fig. 1** Proliferation, differentiation, and migration of immune cells

# 3 Statins in Treatment of Experimental Autoimmune Encephalomyelitis

The potential benefit of statins in central nervous system (CNS) autoimmune diseases primarily relates to studies in murine experimental autoimmune encephalomyelitis (EAE). In EAE, activated myelin-reactive CD4+ T cells cause demyelination of axons resulting in chronic or relapsing paralysis. Oral statin treatment at the EAE onset prevented the development of chronic or relapsing paralysis and could even reverse EAE when statin treatment was initiated after paralysis was established [4, 42, 53]. These studies suggest that statin treatment targets several steps in the pathogenesis of EAE including inhibition of myelin antigen presentation, which is required for T-cell activation, differentiation of T cells into pro-inflammatory T cells and recruitment of leukocytes into the CNS.

## 3.1  Modulation of Cellular Immune Function by Statins

### 3.1.1  Effects on Antigen-Presenting Cells

For the activation of CD4[+] T cells, linear peptide antigen must be presented in the context of the major histocompatibility complex (MHC) class II molecules on the surface of antigen-presenting cells (APCs). The MHC class II transactivator (CIITA) directs inducible MHC class II expression on nonprofessional APCs and constitutive expression on professional APCs [10]. It has been demonstrated that atorvastatin inhibits upregulation of MHC class II on a variety of APCs [27, 53, 55], including microglia, a residential APC population that may have an important role in antigen presentation within the central nervous system (CNS). Inhibition of MHC class II upregulation is reversed by mevalonate, indicating that this statin effect is mediated through inhibition of the mevalonate pathway. Similarly, simvastatin inhibits expression of MHC class II on human endothelial cells, an effect reversed by mevalonate and GGPP, but not by squalene, suggesting the involvement of GTP-binding proteins in MHC class II inhibition [38].

Besides antigen recognition in the context of the MHC class II molecule, a second signal is necessary for T cell activation [13]. Antigen-activated T cells express CD40 ligand, which recognizes the co-stimulatory molecule CD40 on the surface of APCs. This cross-linking of CD40 enhances APC expression of further co-stimulatory molecules on APC, such as B7-1 (CD80) and B7-2 (CD86), which interact with CD28 on the surface of T cells. Simvastatin and atorvastatin prevent cytokine-induced maturation of professional APCs, resulting in a strongly reduced ability to activate T cells [51]. This appears to be mediated through inhibition of the mevalonate pathway as APC maturation and subsequent T cell activation are restored by addition of either mevalonate or GGPP. Similarly, atorvastatin inhibits IFN-γ-inducible expression of CD40, CD80, and CD86 molecules on microglial cells [53]. Decreased expression of these molecules was found to be associated with reduced secretion of APC-derived cytokines involved in the differentiation of T cells into pro-inflammatory T cells [44].

### 3.1.2  Modulation of T Cell Proliferation and Differentiation

Independent of their effects on antigen presentation, statins appear to exert a direct inhibitory effect on T cell activation. In vitro treatment of purified T cells inhibit proliferation when antigen is presented by untreated APCs [53]. Aktas and colleagues demonstrated that inhibition of antigen-induced T cell proliferation by statins is linked to negative regulation of cell-cycle progression, which is consistent with inhibition of GTPase-mediated cell proliferation [4]. In a subsequent publication, the same group identified atorvastatin-mediated phosphorylation of ERK1 to be responsible for T cell anergy [48]. Interestingly, statin-related T cell inhibition apparently depends on the activation status of T cells, suggesting that atorvastatin preferentially targets activated T cells [31].

CD4+ T cells can be categorized into Th1, Th2, and Th17 subsets, primarily on the profile of cytokines secreted [3]. CD4+ Th1 cells, which have a key role in initiating EAE [5, 23], secrete pro-inflammatory cytokines such as IFN-γ, interleukin (IL)-2 and IL-12 and tumor necrosis factor α (TNF-α). Another subset of pathogenic T cells, IL-17-secreting Th17 cells, may participate primarily in perpetuation of EAE [26]. Th2 cytokines, such as IL-4, IL-5, IL-10, and IL-13, have downregulatory properties on the inflammatory cascade in EAE and may have a beneficial effect in MS pathogenesis.

Several independent EAE studies indicate that myelin-specific CD4+ T cells become less reactive to antigen-specific stimulation during statin treatment and secrete lower amounts of the pro-inflammatory Th1 cytokines. Statin-mediated T cell immune deviation is associated with a reduced phosphorylation of STAT4 (signal transducer and activator of transcription 4), which is required for IL-12-dependent Th1-differentiation [53]. Conversely, statin treatment induces secretion of anti-inflammatory Th2 cytokines (IL-4, IL-5, and IL-10) and enhanced phosphorylation of STAT6, which is involved in IL-4-dependent Th2 differentiation [53]. Nath and collegues further demonstrated that in vitro statin treatment of T cells promotes expression of GATA-binding protein 3 (GATA3) [32], a transcription factor associated with Th2 differentiation. These immunomodulatory effects of statins on T cell activation and differentiation appear to be related to inhibition of prenylation of regulatory proteins [12]. Atorvastatin treatment inhibits production of FPP and GGPP in T cells. Reduced levels of these isoprenoid intermediates decreased the membrane association of Ras and Rho and compromised the downstream activation of ERK and DNA binding of the c-fos transcription factor. As c-fos transactivates the IFN-γ promoter and represses the IL-4 promoter [21], these findings may explain how atorvastatin biases T cells to produce higher amounts of IL-4 in the early period of antigen signaling and subsequently trigger GATA-3 expression and the Th2 program of differentiation.

## 3.2  Inhibition of Leukocyte Recruitment into the CNS

Leukocyte migration into the CNS involves multiple steps including chemoattraction, cell adhesion, extravasation, and proteolytic degradation of biological membranes. Lymphocyte function-associated antigen 1 (LFA-1) and its ligand, intracellular adhesion molecule 1 (ICAM-1), have an important role in leukocyte adhesion to brain endothelium. Both molecules have been identified on the surface of inflammatory cells and endothelial cells in perivascular MS lesions [9]. Independent of its effect on HMG CoA reductase, lovastatin binds LFA-1 and directly inhibits LFA-1- and ICAM-1-mediated cell adhesion [50]. Further studies demonstrated that in vitro treatment of brain endothelium cells with lovastatin [19] and simvastatin [20] indeed inhibit transendothelial leukocyte migration. Following their passage across the endothelial barriers, leukocytes still must traverse the basement membrane (basal lamina) of brain venuoles to access CNS parenchyma.

Matrix metalloproteinases (MMPs) are proteolytic enzymes considered to be the physiologic mediators of cell migration through biological membranes and extracellular matrix [52]. Two independent reports demonstrated that statins reduce the secretion of MMP-9 by monocytes [6, 16]. Taken together, statins appear to interfere with multiple steps of leukocyte recruitment and migration into the CNS.

## 3.3   Potential Neuroprotective Effects

In addition to their effect on function and migration of immune cells, statins apparently exert direct effects on neuronal and glial cells, which might be particularly important for recovery in relapsing-remitting CNS autoimmune disease. Statins protect cultured neurons from excitotoxic death, a form of neuronal death caused primarily by brain ischemia [54]. This neuroprotective effect appears to correlate directly to inhibition of neuronal cholesterol biosynthesis abrogated by addition of either mevalonate or cholesterol. In rat primary astrocytes, microglia, and macrophages, lovastatin inhibits induction of damaging free radicals such as nitric oxide [35], which might also be therapeutically relevant for neurodegenerative disorders such as Alzheimer's disease [29]. In a study focusing on the potential effect of statins on remyelination, lovastatin inhibited degeneration of oligodendrocyte progenitors [36], a process that may be responsible for impaired remyelination after inflammatory damage of the myelin sheath. In fact, lovastatin treatment increased expression of myelin proteins and transcription factors associated with differentiating oligodendrocytes, restored remyelination in the spinal cord of mice with EAE [36] and effectively alleviated neurodegeneration in combination with 5-aminoimidazole-4-carboxamide-1-beta-D-ribofuranoside, an immunomodulating agent that activates AMP-activated protein kinase [37]. Interestingly, short-term in vitro treatment of oligodendrocyte progenitors with simvastatin induced robust process extension, whereas prolonged treatment caused process retraction and increased cell death [30]. Another study reported that statins may inhibit neurite outgrowth after axonal damage. In vitro atorvastatin treatment led to neurite loss and, ultimately, to the cell death of a neuronal cell line and rat primary cortical neurons [39]. Addition of GGPP alone completely restored neuronal function and viability, indicating that GGPP, rather than cholesterol or FFP, is critical for neurite outgrowth and survival.

## 4   Statins in Treatment of MS

Based on the encouraging findings in treatment of EAE, one may anticipate the translation of statin-mediated immunomodulation to human CNS autoimmune disease. In vitro, statins inhibit the expression of ICAM-1 and various chemokine receptors on activated peripheral mononuclear cells [34]. Further, when peripheral blood APC is cultured in the presence of statins, expression of HLA-DR decreases, which correlates with decreased antigen presentation and T cell activation.

Regarding the immunomodulatory potential of statins in treatment of autoimmune disease, a clinical trial of atorvastatin in patients with rheumatoid arthritis (RA), another Th1-mediated autoimmune disease, yielded encouraging data [28]. The trial treated 116 patients with active RA with 40 mg atorvastatin or placebo daily, added to their ongoing disease-modifying antirheumatic drug therapy. The group receiving atorvastatin not only showed decreased levels of inflammation but also experienced a significant benefit compared to the active placebo group.

As some patients with MS receive statins for the indication of hypercholesterolemia, epidemiological evidence may already exist supporting their use in MS. This question is difficult to address for several reasons. First, various statins differ in their efficacy for treatment of hypercholesterolemia and thus are likely to differ in their capability to induce immune modulation. Second, the majority of patients treated for hypercholesterolemia receive lower approved doses of statins; however, data from animal studies suggest that statin-mediated immune modulation is evident only at higher dosages. Third, it is possible that statins are beneficial in the earlier, inflammatory phase of MS. The mean age of onset of MS is 32, whereas the mean age of an individual receiving statin treatment for hypercholesterolemia is 62 [8], a time when the majority of MS patients have already entered a more advanced or secondary progressive phase primarily associated with degeneration. Thus, to date, the evidence supporting use of statins in MS is insufficient, and physicians and patients should wait for the results of controlled clinical trials before using these drugs in treatment of MS.

So far, two smaller clinical studies have been published on the treatment effects of statins in MS patients. A 12-month open-label study tested 20 mg lovastatin in seven patients with relapsing-remitting MS with an active disease course [40]. Although no clinical changes were observed in this small cohort, lovastatin treatment had beneficial effects on surrogate MRI markers. Another small open-label trial tested simvastatin in patients with clinically definite relapsing-remitting MS [47]. Over 6 months, 30 patients with at least one gadolinium-enhancing lesion in the 3-month pretreatment period received the highest FDA-approved dose of 80 mg simvastatin per day. Treatment was well tolerated, and again, the mean number and volume of gadolinium-enhancing lesions declined by 44% and 41%, respectively.

Notwithstanding these encouraging findings, these data need to be interpreted cautiously. In open-label trials with a small enrollment, decreased inflammatory activity might reflect the regression to the mean following a comparably active disease course at the time of enrollment. A larger, double-blinded placebo-controlled trial is currently being conducted to address these open questions. In 14 centers throughout North America, a total of 152 patients who have experienced their first demyelinating attack or clinically isolated syndrome are being treated for 12 months with 80 mg atorvastatin or placebo. The primary endpoint of the study is either a further clinical exacerbation, resulting in clinically definite relapsing-remitting MS, or more than three new T2 or gadolinium-enhancing lesions in the 3-monthly brain MRIs. Investigators eagerly await the results of this trial.

## *4.1   Statins in Combination with Existing MS Drugs*

Ongoing trials might determine that statins – similar to approved MS drugs – are only partially effective as monotherapy in treatment of MS. In that case, statins might be useful in combination with existing disease-modifying medications, especially as they are well tolerated and orally administered. Medications chosen for combination therapy should ideally have a different mode of action without overlapping toxicities to provide an additive or synergistic effect. In this regard, an in vitro study revealed that the combination of IFN-$\beta$ and statins has an additive effect on the inhibition of T cell activation [34]. A small clinical trial is currently being conducted to test the combination of high-dose IFN-$\beta$ 1a (Rebif®, 44 µg three times per week) with atorvastatin in patients with relapsing-remitting MS [7]. Combination therapy with intermediate- (40 mg/day) and high-dose atorvastatin (80 mg/day) was well tolerated with no clinical relapses. Serial MRIs, however, revealed increased numbers of T2 and gadolinium-enhancing lesions in two out of four patients receiving combination therapy compared to baseline, raising concern that the combination of atorvastatin and high-dose IFN-$\beta$ may not be beneficial in treatment of relapsing-remitting MS [7].

GA is another particularly well-tolerated therapy for MS that appears to cause a preferential Th2 deviation of T cells, including myelin-reactive T cells [11, 33]. Recent data indicate that GA also exerts immunomodulatory activity on APCs, promoting secretion of Th2-polarizing cytokines and inhibiting the secretion of proinflammatory Th1-polarizing cytokines [24, 49]. One can envisage that an agent that augments the immunomodulatory activity of GA on myelin-reactive lymphocytes or APCs might enhance the efficacy of GA in MS therapy. In this regard, it was recently reported that the combination of GA and atorvastatin synergistically prevents and reverses paralysis in EAE [45], which is associated with a combined effect on anti-inflammatory Th2 differentiation of myelin-reactive T cells. In vitro studies revealed that atorvastatin and GA also alter the cytokine secretion by activated monocytes in an additive manner. Based primarily on these findings, trials testing atorvastatin in combination with GA are anticipated.

## *4.2   Potential Toxicities of Statin Treatment*

Generally, statins are considered safe and well tolerated. Nevertheless, statins do have side effects to consider, particularly when they are administered in combination with other agents. Statins are metabolized by the cytochrome P450 pathway and occasionally cause hepatotoxicity (in most cases with a reversible elevation of transaminases). Myopathy is another rare side effect that occurs in less than 0.2% of statin-treated patients [1, 2, 22]. In severe cases of rhabdomyolysis (<0.05%), myoglobinuria can result in kidney failure [18]. In 2001, cerivastatin (Lipobay®) was removed from the US market after the incidence of fatal rhabdomyolysis in association with cerivastatin therapy was found to be 16–80 times higher than for any other statin [41]. Importantly, the occurrence of rhabdomyolysis was more likely when statins were used in combination with other lipid-lowering drugs including fibrates or compounds generally metabolized through the cytochrome P450 pathway. Polyneuropathy, for which the mechanism remains elusive, might be another occasional side effect of statin therapy. However, a study on the relative risk of polyneuropathy under statin treatment revealed that the incidence was only slightly higher in users of statins (0.73 per 10,000 person-years) than in the hyperlipidemia nontreated cohort and the general population cohort (0.40 vs 0.46 per 10,000 person-years) [14, 15], so that it remains unclear whether a true association exists.

# References

1. Anonymous (1994) Randomised trial of cholesterol lowering in 4444 patients with coronary heart disease: The Scandinavian Simvastatin Survival Study (4 s). Lancet 344: 1383–1389
2. Anonymous (1998) Prevention of cardiovascular events and death with pravastatin in patients with coronary heart disease and a broad range of initial cholesterol levels. The Long-Term Intervention with Pravastatin in Ischaemic Disease (Lipid) Study Group. N Engl J Med 339:1349–1357
3. Abbas AK, Murphy KM, Sher A (1996) Functional diversity of helper T lymphocytes. Nature 383:787–793
4. Aktas O, Waiczies S, Smorodchenko A, Dorr J, Seeger B, Prozorovski T, Sallach S, Endres M, Brocke S, Nitsch R, Zipp F (2003) Treatment of relapsing paralysis in experimental encephalomyelitis by targeting Th1 cells through atorvastatin. J Exp Med 197:725–733
5. Begolka WS, Vanderlugt CL, Rahbe SM, Miller SD (1998) Differential expression of inflammatory cytokines parallels progression of central nervous system pathology in two clinically distinct models of multiple sclerosis. J Immunol 161:4437–4446
6. Bellosta S, Via D, Canavesi M, Pfister P, Fumagalli R, Paoletti R, Bernini F (1998) HMG-COA reductase inhibitors reduce MMP-9 secretion by macrophages. Arterioscler Thromb Vasc Biol 18:1671–1678
7. Birnbaum G, Irfan A (2005) A double blind, placebo controlled combination trial of interferon beta 1a (Rebif) and atorvastatin (Lipitor) in patients with relapsing remitting multiple sclerosis. Paper presented at the AAN, 2005
8. Bonet S, Garcia Villena I, Tomas Santos P, Tapia Mayor I, Gussinye Canabal P, Mundet Tuduri X (1999) When and how do we treat our hypercholesterolemic patients?. Aten Primaria 24:397–403
9. Cannella B, Raine CS (1995) The adhesion molecule and cytokine profile of multiple sclerosis lesions. Ann Neurol 37:424–435
10. Chang CH, Flavell RA (1995) Class ii transactivator regulates the expression of multiple genes involved in antigen presentation. J Exp Med 181:765–767
11. Duda PW, Schmied MC, Cook SL, Krieger JI, Hafler DA (2000) Glatiramer acetate (Copaxone) induces degenerate, th2-polarized immune responses in patients with multiple sclerosis. J Clin Invest 105:967–976
12. Dunn SE, Youssef S, Goldstein MJ, Prod'homme T, Weber MS, Zamvil SS, Steinman L (2006) Isoprenoids determine Th1/Th2 fate in pathogenic T cells, providing a mechanism of modulation of autoimmunity by atorvastatin. J Exp Med 203:401–412
13. Dustin ML, Shaw AS (1999) Costimulation: building an immunological synapse. Science 283:649–650

14. Gaist D, Garcia Rodriguez LA, Huerta C, Hallas J, Sindrup SH (2001) Are users of lipid-lowering drugs at increased risk of peripheral neuropathy? Eur J Clin Pharmacol 56:931–933
15. Gaist D, Jeppesen U, Andersen M, Garcia Rodriguez LA, Hallas J, Sindrup SH (2002) Statins and risk of polyneuropathy: a case-control study. Neurology 58:1333–1337
16. Ganne F, Vasse M, Beaudeux JL, Peynet J, Francois A, Mishal Z, Chartier A, Tobelem G, Vannier JP, Soria J, Soria C (2000) Cerivastatin, an inhibitor of HMG-COA reductase, inhibits urokinase/urokinase-receptor expression and MMP-9 secretion by peripheral blood monocytes – a possible protective mechanism against atherothrombosis. Thromb Haemost 84:680–688
17. Ginsberg HN (1998) Effects of statins on triglyceride metabolism. Am J Cardiol 81:32B–35B
18. Graham DJ, Staffa JA, Shatin D, Andrade SE, Schech SD, La Grenade L, Gurwitz JH, Chan KA, Goodman MJ, Platt R (2004) Incidence of hospitalized rhabdomyolysis in patients treated with lipid-lowering drugs. JAMA 292:2585–2590
19. Greenwood J, Walters CE, Pryce G, Kanuga N, Beraud E, Baker D, Adamson P (2003) Lovastatin inhibits brain endothelial cell Rho-mediated lymphocyte migration and attenuates experimental autoimmune encephalomyelitis. FASEB J 17:905–907
20. Ifergan I, Wosik K, Cayrol R, Kebir H, Auger C, Bernard M, Bouthillier A, Moumdjian R, Duquette P, Prat A (2006) Statins reduce human blood–brain barrier permeability and restrict leukocyte migration: relevance to multiple sclerosis. Ann Neurol 60:45–55
21. Jorritsma PJ, Brogdon JL, Bottomly K (2003) Role of TCR-induced extracellular signal-regulated kinase activation in the regulation of early IL-4 expression in naive CD4+ T cells. J Immunol 170:2427–2434
22. Jukema JW, Bruschke AV, van Boven AJ, Reiber JH, Bal ET, Zwinderman AH, Jansen H, Boerma GJ, van Rappard FM, Lie KI et al (1995) Effects of lipid lowering by pravastatin on progression and regression of coronary artery disease in symptomatic men with normal to moderately elevated serum cholesterol levels. The Regression Growth Evaluation Statin Study (REGRESS). Circulation 91:2528–2540
23. Khoury SJ, Hancock WW, Weiner HL (1992) Oral tolerance to myelin basic protein and natural recovery from experimental autoimmune encephalomyelitis are associated with downregulation of inflammatory cytokines and differential upregulation of transforming growth factor beta, interleukin 4, and prostaglandin E expression in the brain. J Exp Med 176:1355–1364
24. Kim HJ, Ifergan I, Antel JP, Seguin R, Duddy M, Lapierre Y, Jalili F, Bar-Or A (2004) Type 2 monocyte and microglia differentiation mediated by glatiramer acetate therapy in patients with multiple sclerosis. J Immunol 172:7144–7153
25. Kobashigawa JA, Katznelson S, Laks H, Johnson JA, Yeatman L, Wang XM, Chia D, Terasaki PI, Sabad A, Cogert GA et al (1995) Effect of pravastatin on outcomes after cardiac transplantation. N Engl J Med 333:621–627
26. Komiyama Y, Nakae S, Matsuki T, Nambu A, Ishigame H, Kakuta S, Sudo K, Iwakura Y (2006) IL-17 plays an important role in the development of experimental autoimmune encephalomyelitis. J Immunol 177:566–573
27. Kwak B, Mulhaupt F, Myit S, Mach F (2000) Statins as a newly recognized type of immunomodulator. Nat Med 6:1399–1402
28. McCarey DW, McInnes IB, Madhok R, Hampson R, Scherbakov O, Ford I, Capell HA, Sattar N (2004) Trial of Atorvastatin in Rheumatoid Arthritis (TARA): double-blind, randomised placebo-controlled trial. Lancet 363:2015–2021
29. Menge T, Hartung HP, Stuve O (2005) Statins – a cure-all for the brain? Nat Rev Neurosci 6:325–331
30. Miron VE, Rajasekharan S, Jarjour AA, Zamvil SS, Kennedy TE, Antel JP (2007) Simvastatin regulates oligodendroglial process dynamics and survival. Glia 55:130–143
31. Mix E, Ibrahim SM, Pahnke J, Glass A, Mazon-Pelaez I, Lemcke S, Koczan D, Gimsa U, Bansemer S, Scheel T, Karopka T, Bottcher T, Muller J, Dazert E, Antipova V, Hoffrogge R, Wree A, Zschiesche M, Strauss U, Kundt G, Warzok R, Gierl L, Rolfs A (2006) 3-hydroxy-3-methylglutaryl coenzyme a reductase inhibitor atorvastatin mediated effects depend on the activation status of target cells in PLP-EAE. J Autoimmun 27:251–265

32. Nath N, Giri S, Prasad R, Singh AK, Singh I (2004) Potential targets of 3-hydroxy-3-methylglu-taryl coenzyme a reductase inhibitor for multiple sclerosis therapy. J Immunol 172:1273–1286
33. Neuhaus O, Farina C, Wekerle H, Hohlfeld R (2001) Mechanisms of action of glatiramer ace-tate in multiple sclerosis. Neurology 56:702–708
34. Neuhaus O, Strasser-Fuchs S, Fazekas F, Kieseier BC, Niederwieser G, Hartung HP, Archelos JJ (2002) Statins as immunomodulators: comparison with interferon-beta 1b in MS. Neurology 59:990–997
35. Pahan K, Sheikh FG, Namboodiri AM, Singh I (1997) Lovastatin and phenylacetate inhibit the induction of nitric oxide synthase and cytokines in rat primary astrocytes, microglia, and macrophages. J Clin Invest 100:2671–2679
36. Paintlia AS, Paintlia MK, Khan M, Vollmer T, Singh AK, Singh I (2005) HMG-COA reduct-ase inhibitor augments survival and differentiation of oligodendrocyte progenitors in animal model of multiple sclerosis. FASEB J 19:1407–1421
37. Paintlia AS, Paintlia MK, Singh I, Singh AK (2006) Immunomodulatory effect of combination therapy with lovastatin and 5-aminoimidazole-4-carboxamide-1-beta-d-ribofuranoside allevi-ates neurodegeneration in experimental autoimmune encephalomyelitis. Am J Pathol 169:1012–1025
38. Sadeghi MM, Tiglio A, Sadigh K, O'Donnell L, Collinge M, Pardi R, Bender JR (2001) Inhibition of interferon-gamma-mediated microvascular endothelial cell major histocompati-bility complex class II gene activation by HMG-COA reductase inhibitors. Transplantation 71:1262–1268
39. Schulz JG, Bosel J, Stoeckel M, Megow D, Dirnagl U, Endres M (2004) HMG-COA reductase inhibition causes neurite loss by interfering with geranylgeranylpyrophosphate synthesis. J Neurochem 89:24–32
40. Sena A, Pedrosa R, Graca Morais M (2003) Therapeutic potential of lovastatin in multiple sclerosis. J Neurol 250:754–755
41. Staffa JA, Chang J, Green L (2002) Cerivastatin and reports of fatal rhabdomyolysis. N Engl J Med 346:539–540
42. Stanislaus R, Gilg AG, Singh AK, Singh I (2002) Immunomodulation of experimental autoim-mune encephalomyelitis in the Lewis rats by lovastatin. Neurosci Lett 333:167–170
43. Steinman L (2004) Immune therapy for autoimmune diseases. Science 305:212–216
44. Stuve O, Youssef S, Weber MS, Nessler S, von Budingen HC, Hemmer B, Prod'homme T, Sobel RA, Steinman L, Zamvil SS (2006) Immunomodulatory synergy by combination of atorvastatin and glatiramer acetate in treatment of CNS autoimmunity. J Clin Invest 116:1037–1044
45. Stüve O, Youssef S, Weber MS, Prod'homme T, Dunn SE, Steinman L, Zamvil SS (2004) The combination of atorvastatin and glatiramer acetate induces a Th2 phenotype and shows enhanced clinical efficacy in experimental autoimmune encephalomyelitis. J Neuroimmunol 154:77
46. Takai Y, Sasaki T, Matozaki T (2001) Small GTP-binding proteins. Physiol Rev 81:153–208
47. Vollmer T, Key L, Durkalski V, Tyor W, Corboy J, Markovic-Plese S, Preiningerova J, Rizzo M, Singh I (2004) Oral simvastatin treatment in relapsing-remitting multiple sclerosis. Lancet 363:1607–1608
48. Waiczies S, Prozorovski T, Infante-Duarte C, Hahner A, Aktas O, Ullrich O, Zipp F (2005) Atorvastatin induces T cell anergy via phosphorylation of ERK1. J Immunol 174:5630–5635
49. Weber MS, Starck M, Wagenpfeil S, Meinl E, Hohlfeld R, Farina C (2004) Multiple sclerosis: glatiramer acetate inhibits monocyte reactivity in vitro and in vivo. Brain 127:1370–1378
50. Weitz-Schmidt G, Welzenbach K, Brinkmann V, Kamata T, Kallen J, Bruns C, Cottens S, Takada Y, Hommel U (2001) Statins selectively inhibit leukocyte function antigen-1 by bind-ing to a novel regulatory integrin site. Nat Med 7:687–692
51. Yilmaz A, Reiss C, Tantawi O, Weng A, Stumpf C, Raaz D, Ludwig J, Berger T, Steinkasserer A, Daniel WG, Garlichs CD (2004) HMG-COA reductase inhibitors suppress maturation of human dendritic cells: new implications for atherosclerosis. Atherosclerosis 172:85–93
52. Yong VW, Krekoski CA, Forsyth PA, Bell R, Edwards DR (1998) Matrix metalloproteinases and diseases of the CNS. Trends Neurosci 21:75–80

53. Youssef S, Stuve O, Patarroyo JC, Ruiz PJ, Radosevich JL, Hur EM, Bravo M, Mitchell DJ, Sobel RA, Steinman L, Zamvil SS (2002) The HMG-COA reductase inhibitor, atorvastatin, promotes a Th2 bias and reverses paralysis in central nervous system autoimmune disease. Nature 420:78–84

54. Zacco A, Togo J, Spence K, Ellis A, Lloyd D, Furlong S, Piser T (2003) 3-hydroxy-3-methyl-glutaryl coenzyme a reductase inhibitors protect cortical neurons from excitotoxicity. J Neurosci 23:11104–11111

55. Zeinstra E, Wilczak N, Chesik D, Glazenburg L, Kroese FG, De Keyser J (2006) Simvastatin inhibits interferon-gamma-induced MHC class II up-regulation in cultured astrocytes. J Neuroinflammation 3:16

56. Zhang FL, Casey PJ (1996) Protein prenylation: molecular mechanisms and functional consequences. Annu Rev Biochem 65:241–269

# Role of Uric Acid in Multiple Sclerosis

**S. Spitsin and H. Koprowski(✉)**

**Abstract**  In the past decade, a growing number of evidence has implicated free radicals in a variety of pathophysiological conditions including aging, cancer, and coronary heart disease. Analyses of different aspects of multiple sclerosis (MS) pathology with respect to oxidative damage have also revealed evidence of free radical injury to the central nervous system (CNS), although attempts to protect the CNS using various antioxidants have met with only moderate success. Several recent studies have reported lower levels of uric acid (UA), a major scavenger of reactive nitrogen species, in MS patients, while other studies found no such correlation. Here, we discuss these studies as well as current efforts to manipulate serum UA levels in MS patients.

## 1   Uric Acid in Evolution

The fate of uric acid (UA) in vertebrate evolution is a remarkable story in itself. The appearance of UA as an end product of purine metabolism dates back to the period when the first vertebrates emerged from an aquatic to an oxygen-rich environment [27]. In an atmosphere containing 30%–35% oxygen, early amphibians and reptiles underwent much higher oxidative stresses than did aquatic animals [9]. Loss of several enzymes responsible for sequential degradation of UA led to an

H. Koprowski
Thomas Jefferson University, 1020 Locust St, JAH Room M85, Philadelphia, PA 19107, USA
e-mail: hilary.koprowski@jefferson.edu

M. Rodriguez (ed.), *Advances in Multiple Sclerosis and Experimental*                    325
*Demyelinating Diseases. Current Topics in Microbiology and Immunology 318.*
© Springer-Verlag Berlin Heidelberg 2008

accumulation of this powerful radical scavenger in the first terrestrial vertebrates. For about 200 million years, UA persisted as the end product of purine metabolism in reptiles. Mammals, however, returned to an earlier pathway and began converting UA into allantoin [27], a more soluble substance but without radical scavenging properties. For small, relatively short-lived early mammals, the advantages of easily excretable allantoin outweighed the benefits of accruing the poorly soluble antioxidant UA; however, with increased lifespan and the development of a more complex CNS, the need for better protection against free radicals became apparent. Between 25 and 15 million years ago, serum levels of UA increased tenfold in hominoids due to a nonsense mutation in codon 33 of the uricase (urate oxidase) gene [84, 85]. The enzyme uricase degrades UA to allantoin and is active in most mammals. The codon 33 mutation is shared among humans, chimpanzees, gorillas, and orangutans. Interestingly, independent evolutionary events led to the inactivation of the same gene in some other primates. A 13-base pair deletion in exon 2 accounts for inactivated uricase in the gibbon lineage, while other not fully characterized events, most likely mutations in a promoter region, result in reduced uricase activity in New World monkeys and, to a lesser extent, in Old World monkeys [58]. These findings suggest the presence of a common evolutionary pressure that impairs uricase activity, thereby selecting for retention of UA in most primates.

Evolutionary selection for UA occurred, even though it predisposed the organism to gout and kidney stones and probably also required some adjustments in the secretory pathways of early primates. Homozygous uricase-knockout mice, but not their heterozygous counterparts, die several weeks after birth since their kidneys cannot handle large loads of UA [83]. Perhaps the original mutation of uricase in early primates was also lethal when homozygous. Nevertheless, mutation was selected in evolution along with some adjustments to purine metabolism. Resulting serum UA levels, between 210 and 450 μM (3.5–8.0 mgdl$^{-1}$), are higher than any other natural antioxidants. However, they are dangerously close to saturation, which can be as low as 8–10 mgdl$^{-1}$ depending on minor variations in physiological conditions.

Another unsolved puzzle is the gain of UA in hominids during a similar time frame when the ability to synthesize another important radical scavenger, ascorbic acid, was lost [9]. Although hominids still depend on a dietary supply of vitamin C, normal serum levels of UA are four- to sixfold greater than those of ascorbic acid, raising the possibility that UA is partially replaced vitamin C as an antioxidant in higher primates.

Of note, there are alternative views on the role of UA in primate evolution; for example, UA may have helped to maintain blood pressure in low-salt dietary conditions encountered by early hominids during the Miocene epoch [79]. According to this hypothesis, UA merely contributes to the epidemic of cardiovascular disease and hypertension that plagues modern humans on high-salt diets. However, this does not address the question of why primates, rather than grazing animals, would be the target of pressure to adapt to low-salt conditions. Although this hypothesis is not currently in the mainstream, certain negative actions of UA cannot be disregarded. Indeed, some evidence indicates a pathogenic role for high UA levels in the development of hypertension, vascular disease, and renal disease in humans [38].

Animals other than primates demonstrate the importance of UA as a radical scavenger. Birds generally have a longer lifespan than mammals of comparable body size, body temperature, and metabolic rate [31]; they inherited UA as purine metabolic end product from reptiles and have high serum UA levels. Insects also have high levels of UA, and a potential role for UA in insect free-radical defense has been suggested based on the observation that urate-null mutants of *Drosophila melanogaster* are more susceptible to various aspects of oxidative stress than are the wild type [33]. Another study linked aging in *Drosophila* with the ability to produce UA [55].

# 2  Uric Acid and Free Radicals

UA, or urate at physiological conditions, is a powerful and selective antioxidant [1, 4, 80]. It is highly reactive with hydroxyl radicals and hypochlorous acid. Urate interferes minimally with nitric oxide (NO·), a free radical with low toxicity but with important physiological functions. Urate is an efficient scavenger of several reactive nitrogen species that form in vitro and in vivo after reaction of NO with other radicals and biological molecules [8, 81]. Free radical interactions in living organisms are extremely complex. Originally UA was described as a singlet oxygen and hydroxyl radical scavenger [1, 4]. Later, when the importance of the chemistry of NO and reactive nitrogen species became clear, UA was shown to protect live cells from the damaging actions of peroxynitrite ($ONOO^-$), the product of the reaction between NO and superoxide ($O^{2-}$) [8, 47]. Then it was shown that the chemistry of $ONOO^-$ may be even more complex. In a biological milieu, highly reactive peroxynitrite rapidly interacts with bicarbonate/carbon dioxide to form a nitrosoperoxycarbonate anion ($ONOOCO^{2-}$) with enhanced capacity to nitrate aromatics [18, 53] and generate intermediate radicals, such as ·NO2 and CO3$^-$ with damaging properties [71, 72]. Despite the incomplete understanding of various proposed reactions of nitrogen species in vivo, it is clear that UA can protect living cells, including CNS cells, from the damaging actions of free radicals [13, 62, 71, 77].

A high concentration of UA in human sera is another critical factor for efficient radical scavenging. The average human body contains 1–2 g of UA, which represents a higher concentration than other nonenzymatic scavengers such as ascorbate, tocopherols, methionine, and glutathione. UA likely provides 30%–65% of the peroxyl-radical scavenging capacity in human blood plasma [4].

Biosynthesis of UA from xanthine may lead to superoxide radical production through the action of xanthine oxidase, especially under hypoxic conditions. The drug allopurinol routinely inhibits xanthine oxidase and prevents hypoxia reperfusion injury. However, under normal physiological conditions, xanthine dehydrogenase, another form of the same enzyme, oxidizes purines at the expense of NADH without significant production of free radicals [17]. Although small amounts of xanthine dehydrogenase are expressed in many organs, most of the enzyme is produced in the small intestine and the liver followed by lung and heart, making those organs particularly sensitive to hypoxia reperfusion injury [49]. In contrast, the UA produced by xanthine dehydrogenase spreads throughout the body via the bloodstream, providing protection from oxidative damage to various tissues, including the CNS.

## 3    Role of Free Radicals in Multiple Sclerosis: Lessons from Experimental Allergic Encephalomyelitis and Other Models

There are multiple sources of oxidative stress in MS brain. Glutamate excitoxicity is linked to activation of metabolic pathways that lead to free radical production (reviewed in Gilgun-Sherki et al. [24]). Free radicals are generated in mitochondria of all CNS cells and in particularly high quantities by resident microglia and infiltrating macrophages (Fig. 1) (reviewed in Gilgun-Sherki et al. [25] ). Activated microglia, macrophages, astrocytes, and endothelial cells can also produce $NO^{\cdot}$ and generate $ONOO^{-}$ [8]. Iron, which is present in some regions of the brain, is catalytic for the free radical reactions (reviewed in Levine and Chakrabarty 2004 [51]).

Several lines of evidence have implicated oxidative stress in the pathogenesis of MS and other neurogenerative diseases [24, 25]. In vitro studies have demonstrated that neurons, postmitotic cells, are more sensitive to oxidative stress than other CNS cells [6, 10]. Various antioxidants, including UA, protect neurons from free radical damage in tissue culture [62, 86].

The first evidence of $ONOO^{-}$ formation in brain of MS patients was reported by Bagasra et al. [3]. Since then, several independent studies have confirmed the formation of peroxynitrite in brain, cerebrospinal fluid (CSF), and blood of patients with MS and animals with experimental allergic encephalomyelitis (EAE) [15, 16, 34, 52, 63, 78]. $ONOO^{-}$ can induce a variety of effects, including oxidation of DNA and proteins, lipid peroxidation, inhibition of mitochondrial respiration, and tyrosine nitration [7, 8, 23, 29]. In addition, $ONOO^{-}$ may mediate cell death via DNA single-strand breakage and activation of the nuclear enzyme poly(ADP-ribose) polymerase (PARP) [74]. While the precise $ONOO^{-}$-dependent chemical reactivity remains unknown, there is a little doubt that $ONOO^{-}$ is a key contributor to MS and EAE.

Evidence of free radical involvement in EAE-related damage came from attempts to treat EAE symptoms with radical scavengers. Studies in various models showed a wide spectrum of natural and synthetic antioxidants to delay or suppress EAE symptoms [11, 19, 26, 28, 54, 61]. UA administration also inhibited the development of clinical EAE and ameliorated preexisting signs of the disease [34, 36, 37, 70].

Besides EAE, other CNS conditions associated with $ONOO^{-}$-related damage have been treated successfully with UA. Increased UA levels are effective against viral and bacterial infections of the CNS. In rats infected with Borna virus, UA treatment substantially delays development of symptoms and inhibited formation of nitrotyrosine and production of proinflammatory cytokines [35]. In a rat model of pneumococcal meningitis, UA exerts dose-dependent anti-inflammatory effect at blood levels in the human physiological range [42, 43]. UA administration at the

# Circulation

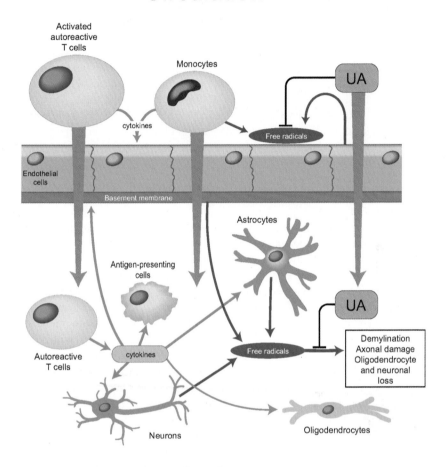

# CNS

**Fig. 1** Role of free radicals in demyelination. During the early stages of inflammatory response, free radicals are produced by circulating and endothelial cells and may contribute to the loss of BBB integrity through direct damage to endothelial cells or promotion of lymphocyte adhesion and infiltration. UA does not readily cross the intact BBB. During the early stages of inflammation, inactivation of certain radicals, including peroxynitrite by UA, may protect the integrity of BBB. During the late stages of CNS inflammation, free radicals are produced by a variety of resident and infiltrating cells and may cause either direct damage or participate in regulation of a variety of cytokines, chemokines, matrix metalloproteinases, and adhesion molecules. During this stage, BBB becomes compromised. UA penetrates areas of active lesions and contributes to containment of CNS pathology attributed to free radical damage such as mitochondrial dysfunction, DNA and protein damage, lipid peroxidation, myelin injury, etc

onset of spinal cord injury in a mouse model inhibits several pathological changes in the spinal cord including general tissue damage, nitrotyrosine formation, lipid peroxidation, activation of poly(ADP-ribose) polymerase, and neutrophil invasion; more importantly, UA treatment improved functional recovery from the injury [62].

Based on the encouraging results in animal studies, investigators are looking into the potential benefit of dietary antioxidants for MS patients (reviewed in Carlson and Rose [12]). Thus far, no human studies have proven this hypothesis. However, it is well known that many MS patients take multiple vitamins and other purportedly antioxidant food supplements. Currently, the field of MS research lacks well-designed clinical trials to address issues of antioxidant composition, intake, and effectiveness.

# 4   Serum Uric Acid Levels in Patients with Multiple Sclerosis

In vitro and in vivo findings have rendered UA the most studied antioxidant in MS. In a seminal study by Hooper et al. [37], analysis of the records of 20,212,505 patients enrolled in Medicare and Medicaid for diagnosis of MS and gout revealed only four patients with both conditions instead of the 62 expected, making MS and gout almost mutually exclusive (Table 1). The same authors also observed that serum UA levels among a group of 46 MS patients were significantly lower ($p<0.001$) than in the control population comprised of patients with spinal cord injuries, cerebral palsy, Parkinson's disease, and other conditions with similar degrees of disability. Patients receiving drugs known to modulate serum UA levels were excluded from the study. To control for the significant influence of diet on serum UA levels, the institutionalized subjects all received the same diet for 5 days before collection of serum, and all subjects donated blood samples before breakfast. However, this pioneering study did not take disease activity into account. Magnetic resonance imaging (MRI) performed after the study on a selected group of 20 patients revealed gadolinium-enhancing lesions in only two patients (10%). Another study by these authors [68] analyzed sets of twins in which only one sibling had MS; the MS-affected siblings consistently revealed lower UA levels than the healthy siblings in both homo- and heterozygous twin pairs.

Since those initial reports, at least ten other independent studies on UA and MS have been conducted with somewhat conflicting results; i.e., half of the studies confirmed the low UA levels in the MS population, but the other half found no differences from controls. Drulovic et al. [21], for example, observed that average serum UA levels were about 8% lower in MS patients than in patients with other neurological diseases (OND). The difference increased to about 15% and was statistically significant for patients with active MS. Those investigators also demonstrated UA fluctuation in serum of relapsing-remitting patients with MS (RRMS), significantly higher UA levels detected during remission than during relapse ($p=0.006$), and differences reaching 20%.

In an analysis of sera of 124 MS patients vs 124 sex- and age-matched OND patients, Sotgiu et al. [67] observed a 13% reduction in serum UA levels of MS patients.

**Table 1** Studies on serum UA levels in MS patients

| Study | Population | Serum UA levels | Remarks |
|---|---|---|---|
| Hooper et al. 1998 | 46 MS patients vs 46 non-MS patients with other OND and similar degree of disabilities, sex- and age- matched. Strict dietary control. No information on disease activity | Lower in MS patients by about 10% ($p < 0.01$) | Selective MRI on 20 patients several months after the study revealed that only 10% had active lesions (unpublished) |
| Hooper et al. 1998 | Statistical analysis of 20,212,505 Medicare and Medicaid records, including 36,733 gout and 34,607 MS. No information on disease activity | 15-Fold decrease of incidence of MS in patients with gout. No direct information on serum UA levels | Strongly suggestive that high serum UA levels may protect against MS |
| Karg et al. 1999 | 25 MS patients vs nine controls. 72% Males in MS population versus 50% among controls | No difference | Small study with other primary objectives. Male predominance in MS group likely influences the outcome |
| Drulovic et al. 2001 | 240 MS patients vs 104 patients with OND, sex- and age- matched | Lower in MS patients by 8% (not significant) and by 15% in patients with active MS ($p < 0.05$) | Suggested that UA may be a marker of MS activity |
| Spitsin et al. 2001 | 132 Sets of twins with one sibling affected by MS, including 88 sets of the same sex and 52 monozygotic pairs. No information on disease activity | Lower in twin with MS for all 132 sets by 11%. Lower in 88 sets of the same sex by 10% and for 52 monozygotic pairs by 12%. ($p$ Multiple Sclerosis $< 0.05$ for all sets) | Similar decrease in UA levels in mono- and di-zygotic twins. Data from Monozygotic twins strongly support hypothesis that UA level can be driven down by MS |
| Sotgiu et al. 2002 | 124 MS patients versus 124 OND sex- and age- matched patients | Lower in MS patients by 13% ($p = 0.001$) | UA levels did not significantly correlate with disease activity, duration, disability or course |
| Toncev et al. 2002 | 63 MS patients vs 20 OIND and 20 healthy controls, sex- and age-matched | Lower in MS patients by 28% ($p < 0.001$) | Strong correlation between UA and MS activity. UA levels were lower in patients with disrupted blood–brain barrier ($p < 0.001$) |

(continued)

**Table 1** (continued)

| Study | Population | Serum UA levels | Remarks |
|---|---|---|---|
| Knapp et al. 2004 | 21 Patients with optic neuritis. Separate statistics for males and females. 17 Females with ON vs 22 healthy controls and four males with ON versus 16 controls | Lower in patients with optic neuritis; 22% decrease in females ($p = 0.006$); 7% decrease in males (not significant) | Five of 21 patients with optic neuritis were also diagnosed with MS |
| Becker et al. 2004 | 18 MS patients vs 26 healthy controls, 11 facial palsy, 18 Guillain-Barré syndrome and 15 bacterial meningitis | No difference | Insufficient data on MS activity |
| Kastenbauer et al. 2005 | 70 MS patients vs 24 OND. At least 18 MS patients had active lesions at the time of blood collection | No difference | No evidence of increased degradation of urate to allantoin found in MS patients |
| Mostert et al. 2005 | 60 MS patients vs 29 healthy controls, sex- and age-matched. No MRI data | No difference | All MS patients were nonrelapsing |
| Ramsaransing et al. 2005 | 82 MS patients vs 29 healthy controls sex- and age-matched. No MRI data | No difference between MS patients and controls. No difference between benign and progressive MS | All MS patients were nonrelapsing |
| Rentzos et al. 2006 | 190 MS patients including 35 with MRI activity and 29 CIS vs 58 OND, including 28 with OIND, sex- and age-matched. Dietary controls | Lower in MS patients by about 20% ($p > < 0.03$). No difference between active and nonactive MS ($p > < 0.003$) | Although sex and age matching was done for the entire MS and non-MS groups, data on sex distribution in the active MRI group were not provided |

*OND*, other neurological diseases; *OIND*, other inflammatory neurological diseases; CIS, clinically isolated syndrome, represented by patients with high risk of developing MS, with two or more silent lesions and clinical features such as optic neuritis, diplopia, hemiparesis, or cerebral ataxia

However, UA levels analyzed in MS patients selected according to disease activity showed only a 2.5%–5% reduction in active MS, and the difference was not significant. MRI data were available only for 21 patients in that study (13 with active lesions and eight with inactive), and gender distribution information was not given. Thus, the accuracy of conclusions about UA and MS activity in that study remains unclear.

Toncev et al. [76] analyzed 63 MS patients, 20 patients with other inflammatory neurological diseases (OIND), and 20 healthy controls. They reported up to a 28% reduction in UA levels in MS vs non-MS patients and a 20% reduction in MS vs patients with OIND. Both relapsing patients and those with active lesions had significantly lower UA levels than did patients in remission and without active lesions.

Recently Rentzos et al. [60] confirmed the presence of lower UA levels in MS patients in analysis of 190 MS versus 58 OND patients. However, they found no correlation between UA levels and MS activity. In fact, they reported UA levels in 35 patients with active lesions to be actually about 6% higher than in patients without lesions. They suggested that lower UA levels in MS represent a primary, constitutive loss of protection against nitric oxide and CNS inflammation.

Knapp et al. [45] reported lower serum UA levels in patients with optic neuritis (an inflammatory demyelinating condition affecting the optic nerve and closely related to MS) than in control individuals.

Two somewhat overlapping studies [57, 59] found no significant difference between MS patients and healthy controls in UA levels; they may reflect patient populations without relapse in the 3 months before the studies. Indeed, MS patients in both studies had normal serum UA levels (340 μM for males and 250 μM for females), consistent with levels reported in all previous studies for controls. About 20% of the MS patients took β-interferon, which is known to increase serum UA levels. However, β-interferon users and nonusers in these studies had similar UA levels. Patient descriptions did not allow speculation about dietary contributions to serum UA levels. No differences in UA levels were seen between patients with benign and patients with progressive MS [59]. While MS patients' NO production by peripheral blood leukocytes increased about twofold, this increase did not affect serum UA levels [57].

Three other studies also found no reduction in serum UA levels in MS patients [5, 40, 41]. In the first two studies, the MS patient population was small (25 and 18 patients, respectively), and comparison of UA levels was not a primary objective so that critical factors such as disease activity and sex distribution were not fully considered. Kastenbauer et al. [41] compared serum UA levels of 70 MS patients (at least 18 with active lesions and 36 with acute exacerbation) with those in 24 OND patients. Although the OND control group was small and heterogeneous, average serum UA levels for the MS group (238 μM) were closer to those of the OND control than to MS populations reported in other studies.

Recently, Koch and Keyser [46] suggested that MS patients are not primarily deficient in UA but that serum UA decreases with inflammatory disease activity. Thus, UA levels might be a marker of MS activity rather than a protective factor. In fact, a substantial amount of data supports this hypothesis. In most reported cases, serum UA levels of MS patients are only 10%–15% lower than those in normal controls or patients with OND. It seems unlikely that such a small difference in antioxidant defense could be so critical in the development of MS. Data from monozygotic twins also support an environmental rather than a genetic basis for the differences in UA levels [69]. Benign and progressive MS populations reported no differences between serum UA levels, although higher levels might be expected in the benign MS group. Oxidative stress may act to decrease UA levels in MS patients. Allantoin is one of the possible products of UA oxidation by free radicals. Increased allantoin levels were detected in human sera and CSF of patients with other inflammatory conditions; however, limited studies did not reveal an increase in samples from MS patients [5, 41]. On the other hand, Kanabrocki et al. [39] demonstrated an altered relationship between serum NO and UA in MS patients. Temporal reduction in serum UA level apparently correlates with increased ONOO⁻ production in MS patients.

Methodological issues may account for the lack of correlation between MS activity and serum UA levels reported in some studies. For example, human serum UA levels are dependent on gender, age, diet, medication, and other factors, and not all studies could address these factors equally. Moreover, disease activity can be monitored by the presence of gadolinium-enhancing lesions and/or clinical relapses, but both criteria have their own limitations. MS patients also often have evidence of activation in different lymphocyte populations; however, most studies could not take account for conditions of the peripheral immune system. Small patient sample size may be another critical factor. A study demonstrating lower serum UA levels in MS patients enrolled a total of 795 MS patients and 21 patients with optic neuritis but looked at a total of 195 patients when no difference was found and included an apparently overlapping patient population [5, 41, 57, 59]. Definite conclusions about the primary or secondary role of UA levels in the development of MS await further research. In our experience, about 10% of MS patients have very low UA levels ($\leq 3$ mgdL⁻¹). Possibly, slightly lower UA levels reflect disease activity in some patients, and very low UA levels predispose them to MS. We need appropriately designed studies to answer this question.

Generally, 50 patients should be sufficient to apply logistic regression analysis and/or $t$-tests to demonstrate a 10%–15% reduction in serum UA levels. However, due to differences in UA levels between male and female populations, a total of 200 people (four groups: MS/non-MS, male/female) are needed for such a study. Further attempts to break the MS cohort into groups (e.g., relapsing-remitting, primary progressive, secondary progressive, benign) require bringing the number of patients in each group to 50 for proper statistical analyses.

Although logical attempts have been made to correlate serum UA levels and disease severity, these studies may not fully address whether UA deficiency is a primary or secondary function in MS. This is because UA level is only one of several factors contributing to the development of MS symptoms including genetic background and environmental factors. Conceivably, a person with a weak predisposition for MS may develop symptoms because of a lower UA level. On the other hand, higher UA levels may partially diminish a stronger predisposition for MS. As a result, disease severity will be similar in both cases. Consequently, studying existing cases of MS may not address the question about a primary or secondary role of UA. Another approach involves monitoring serum UA levels in individuals before the development of MS. This type of study requires a very large population. Even by performing the study in individuals with a genetic predisposition (risk for the development of MS, 1%–2%), 5,000 to 10,000 individuals highly predisposed to MS would need to submit to monitoring of serum UA levels from childhood through adulthood.

One finding clearly stands out among all others: the significant inverse correlation between incidence of MS and gout suggests that gout protects against development of MS [37]. However, patients with gout have a substantially larger increase in serum UA levels when compared with the difference between MS and non-MS populations in these levels. Most patients with gout have UA levels greater than 8.0 mgdl$^{-1}$; i.e., about twofold higher than the average level in men. Another feature of gout is formation of urate crystals, mainly in the joints but also throughout the body. These crystals may trigger a local inflammatory response that activates macrophages and produces various cytokines. Whether those events might suppress the development of MS remains to be addressed.

# 5 Possible Mechanisms of Uric Acid Action in Multiple Sclerosis, Protection of Blood–Brain Barrier Integrity

There are at least two components underlying MS pathogenesis: inflammation and neurodegeneration (reviewed in Hauser and Oksenberg [30]). Both components may be associated with free radical-related damage.

In vitro experiments have shown UA to block multiple actions of ONOO$^{-}$ and some other free radicals [1, 4, 80]. Findings in both MS and EAE demonstrate that UA treatment suppresses the permeability changes in the blood–brain barrier (BBB). In turn, immune cell invasion into the CNS is inhibited, and TNF-$\alpha$ production and ICAM-1 upregulation in CNS tissue are blocked [36, 44, 65]. On the other hand, the presence of UA does not alter immune function parameters such as antigen presentation, T cell proliferation, antibody production, and monocyte activation [44, 70]. Similar effects of UA have been described in other models such as neurotropic virus-induced encephalitis [35], bacterial meningitis [42, 43], and spinal cord injury in mice [62]. Thus, certain ONOO$^{-}$-dependent reactions may play a key role in the functional changes occurring at the BBB in EAE and other CNS inflammatory diseases [64]. They may directly modify structural elements of the BBB or modulate neurovascular endothelial cell function through an effect on signal transduction by ONOO$^{-}$-mediated, UA-sensitive reactions. UA treatment restores the integrity of the BBB and blocks 3-nitrotyrosine formation, but not inducible nitric oxide synthase (iNOS) expression, in focal areas of inflammation [36].

Only limited data exists on possible mechanisms of CNS protection by UA. However, in a pilot human clinical trial aimed at increasing serum UA levels in MS patients, disappearance or reduction of gadolinium-enhanced lesions and decreased nitrotyrosine blood levels were observed ([48, 68] and unpublished observations). This suggests that the mechanisms of UA action in humans are similar to those observed in animal models and are directed at maintaining BBB integrity. Of note, UA does not penetrate the intact BBB in either animals or humans; thus, normal CNS concentrations of urate are approximately tenfold lower than in the blood stream. However, UA has constant access to CNS microvasculature and can penetrate the compromised BBB in both human MS and mouse EAE conditions [66, 69]. As a result, UA levels are higher in areas of active lesions [50].

Recently, it has become evident that axonal degeneration is an important factor in MS pathogenesis (reviewed in Hendriks [32] and Andrews et al. [2]). While the mechanisms underlying this phenomenon are not fully understood, free radicals generated by activated resident and infiltrating cells as well as by mitochondria of demyelinated axons are likely to contribute to axonal loss. Increased UA levels in these areas may be protective against such damage. For example, recently it was reported that UA protects spinal cord neurons in vitro against glutamate toxicity by a mechanism other than purely binding peroxynitrite [22].

# 6   Treatment of MS Patients by Raising UA Levels

Although more research is needed to pinpoint the exact mechanisms of CNS protection by UA, initial attempts to manipulate UA levels in MS patients have been made. From the data discussed in Sect. 4 of this review, it is unlikely that raising UA levels in MS patients by 10%–20% (the difference between MS and non-MS populations) will produce any therapeutic effect. More likely, serum UA levels of 8 mgdl$^{-1}$ or higher, such as those observed in gout patients, are needed for protection [37]. On the other hand, levels much higher than 8 mgdl$^{-1}$ might precipitate a gout attack and/or kidney stone formation. In the original attempt to raise serum UA levels in MS patients and maintain these levels at around 8 mgdl$^{-1}$, UA was administered orally [69]. However, oral UA proved ineffective in raising serum UA levels due to poor absorption and sensitivity to bacterial uricase in the gut. Thus, investigators chose the UA precursor to raise the typically low serum UA levels of MS patients. Inosine is approved for human consumption as a food supplement and a muscle performance enhancer. Although the capacity of inosine to act as a muscle stimulant remains controversial [20, 56, 73, 82], professional athletes use it routinely and extensively at dosages of 1–6 g per day for periods ranging from several days [73, 82] to weeks [20] and years [14] with no reported side effects. The EAE animal model of MS confirmed inosine's efficacy as a therapeutic agent [66]. A phase I clinical trial proved that inosine administration effectively raised UA levels of MS patients into the high/normal range [69]. Only two of the 11 enrolled patients had gadolinium-enhancing lesions, and all 11 were free of active lesions after 1 year of inosine therapy. At least two more trials followed. Toncev [75] reported that 32 MS patients receiving 1–2 g of inosine per day for approximately

3 years had significantly lower relapse rates and smaller increases in EDSS score than 32 patients in a nontreated control group matched for age, gender, disability, and disease duration. Daily doses of 1–2 g of inosine have boosted serum UA levels in treated patients from an average of 200 μM (3.4 mgdl⁻¹) to 250–300 μM (4.2–5.0 mgdl⁻¹). Thus, even modest increases in serum UA levels might provide a therapeutic value for MS patients.

A current, more comprehensive phase I/II clinical trial is assessing the therapeutic efficacy of raising UA levels by inosine administration in a larger group of MS patients with active disease. Of particular importance is the effect of treatment on quantifiable BBB permeability and on lesion activity evaluated by gadolinium-enhancing MRI. This study is still in progress, but preliminary results for the first group of 11 patients who have completed 1 year of study are available for discussion. The patient with the highest number of active lesions prior to treatment showed the most dramatic improvement (Fig. 2). During 6 months of inosine treatment, the average serum UA level in this individual increased from 4.2 to 8.7 mgdl⁻¹ ($p<0.001$), the number of active lesions decreased from an average of ten to one by the end of the trial ($p<0.001$), and the Kurtzke expanded disability status scale (EDSS) score dropped from 2.0 to 1.0.

The remaining patients had fewer active lesions than the patient presented above. Nevertheless, analysis of the combined data for these patients revealed a significant correlation ($p<0.007$ by two-sided Fisher's exact test) between raising serum UA level and reduction in disease activity (Table 2). This suggests that UA may naturally protect against the loss of BBB integrity and inhibit lesion formation. Experiments to assess possible measures of disease activity in sera have revealed nitrotyrosine levels to be the most active predictor of treatment outcome.

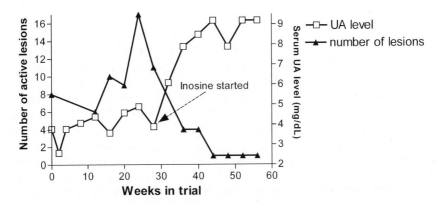

**Fig. 2** Reduction of disease activity during inosine treatment in an MS patient with high lesion burden. Patient was treated with placebo for the first 6 months and with inosine for the second 6 months. Blood drawings and gadolinium-enhanced MRI were performed monthly

**Table 2** Comparison of serum UA levels and disease activity in MS patients during placebo/inosine treatment

| Serum UA level | Number of visits | Visits with active lesions | Visits with exacerbations |
| --- | --- | --- | --- |
| >6.5 mg/dl | 49 | 3 | 0 |
| <6.5 mg/dl | 29 | 11 | 4 |
| Total | 78 | 14 | 4 |

The association between UA level and lesion activity is significant by Fisher's exact test (two-sided) $p<0.007$. The association between UA level and exacerbation is significant by Fisher's exact test (two-sided) $p<0.03$

# Conclusions

UA acts as a part of a sophisticated, but not infallible, antioxidant defense system consisting of multiple components [9]. To be fully effective, UA must interact with numerous enzymes, scavengers, and quenchers. A better understanding of these mechanisms may aid the development of optimal therapeutic approaches to target free radicals in MS. Low UA levels apparently reflect disease activity in the majority of MS patients and can be used as a diagnostic tool. A high UA level, approaching those in patients with gout, may be a therapeutic tool in itself or in combination with other treatments. The question of whether the very low serum UA levels found in some MS patients might predispose to the development of MS remains to be answered.

**Acknowledgements** We are thankful to Dr. Clyde Markowitz and medical staff of the Department of Neurology, University of Pennsylvania, for collaborating in clinical trial of inosine in the treatment of multiple sclerosis, and to Dr. Brian Jones for assistance with statistics.

# References

1. Ames BN, Cathcart R, Schwiers E, Hochstein P (1981) Uric acid provides an antioxidant defense in humans against oxidant- and radical-caused aging and cancer: a hypothesis. Proc Natl Acad Sci U S A 78:6858–6862
2. Andrews HE, Nichols PP, Bates D, Turnbull DM (2005) Mitochondrial dysfunction plays a key role in progressive axonal loss in Multiple Sclerosis. Med Hypotheses 64:669–677
3. Bagasra O, Michaels FH, Zheng YM, Bobroski LE, Spitsin SV, Fu ZF, Tawadros R, Koprowski H (1995) Activation of the inducible form of nitric oxide synthase in the brains of patients with multiple sclerosis. Proc Natl Acad Sci U S A 92:12041–1205
4. Becker BF (1993) Towards the physiological function of uric acid. Free Radic Biol Med 14:615–631
5. Becker BF, Kastenbauer S, Kodel U, Kiesl D, Pfister HW (2004) Urate oxidation in CSF and blood of patients with inflammatory disorders of the nervous system. Nucleosides Nucleotides Nucleic Acids 23:1201–1204
6. Beckman JS (1991) The double-edged role of nitric oxide in brain function and superoxide-mediated injury. J Dev Physiol 15:53–59

7. Beckman JS (1996) Oxidative damage and tyrosine nitration from peroxynitrite. Chem Res Toxicol 9:836–844
8. Beckman JS, Koppenol WH (1996) Nitric oxide, superoxide, and peroxynitrite: the good, the bad, and ugly. Am J Physiol 271:C1424–C1437
9. Benzie IF (2000) Evolution of antioxidant defence mechanisms. Eur J Nutr 39:53–61
10. Bolanos JP, Heales SJ, Land JM, Clark JB (1995) Effect of peroxynitrite on the mitochondrial respiratory chain: differential susceptibility of neurones and astrocytes in primary culture. J Neurochem 64:1965–1972
11. Brenner T, Brocke S, Szafer F, Sobel RA, Parkinson JF, Perez DH, Steinman L (1997) Inhibition of nitric oxide synthase for treatment of experimental autoimmune encephalomyelitis. J Immunol 158:2940–2946
12. Carlson NG, Rose JW (2006) Antioxidants in multiple sclerosis: do they have a role in therapy? CNS Drugs 20:433–441
13. Chamorro A, Planas AM, Muner DS, Deulofeu R (2004) Uric acid administration for neuroprotection in patients with acute brain ischemia. Med Hypotheses 62:173–176
14. Cheng Y, Jiang DH (1990) Therapeutic effect of inosine in Tourette syndrome and its possible mechanism of action. Chin J Neurol Psychiatry 23:90–93, 126–127
15. Cross AH, Manning PT, Keeling RM, Schmidt RE, Misko TP (1998) Peroxynitrite formation within the central nervous system in active multiple sclerosis. J Neuroimmunol 88:45–56
16. Cross AH, Manning PT, Stern MK, Misko TP (1997) Evidence for the production of peroxynitrite in inflammatory CNS demyelination. J Neuroimmunol 80:121–130
17. Cross AR, Jones OT (1991) Enzymic mechanisms of superoxide production. Biochim Biophys Acta 1057:281–298
18. Denicola A, Freeman BA, Trujillo M, Radi R (1996) Peroxynitrite reaction with carbon dioxide/bicarbonate: kinetics and influence on peroxynitrite-mediated oxidations. Arch Biochem Biophys 333:49–58
19. Ding M, Zhang M, Wong JL, Rogers NE, Ignarro LJ, Voskuhl RR (1998) Antisense knockdown of inducible nitric oxide synthase inhibits induction of experimental autoimmune encephalomyelitis in SJL/J mice. J Immunol 160:2560–2564
20. Dragan I, Baroga M, Eremia N, Georgescu E (1993) Studies regarding some effects of inosine in elite weightlifters. Rom J Physiol 30:47–50
21. Drulovic J, Dujmovic I, Stojsavljevic N, Mesaros S, Andjelkovic S, Miljkovic D, Peric V, Dragutinovic G, Marinkovic J, Levic Z, Mostarica Stojkovic M (2001) Uric acid levels in sera from patients with multiple sclerosis. J Neurol 248:121–126
22. Du Y, Chen CP, Tseng CY, Eisenberg Y, Firestein BL (2007) Astroglia-mediated effects of uric acid to protect spinal cord neurons from glutamate toxicity. Glia 55:463–472
23. Ducrocq C, Blanchard B, Pignatelli B, Ohshima H (1999) Peroxynitrite: an endogenous oxidizing and nitrating agent. Cell Mol Life Sci 55:1068–1077
24. Gilgun-Sherki Y, Melamed E, Offen D (2001) Oxidative stress induced-neurodegenerative diseases: the need for antioxidants that penetrate the blood–brain barrier. Neuropharmacology 40:959–975
25. Gilgun-Sherki Y, Melamed E, Offen D (2004) The role of oxidative stress in the pathogenesis of multiple sclerosis: the need for effective antioxidant therapy. J Neurol 251:261–268
26. Gilgun-Sherki Y, Offen D, Panet H, Melamed E, Atlas D (2003) A novel brain-targeted low molecular weight hydrophobic antioxidant compound demonstrates neuroprotective effect in mice with chronic EAE. Multiple Sclerosis 9:S16
27. Gutman AB (1965) Significance of uric acid as a nitrogenous waste in vertebrate evolution. Arthritis Rheum 8:614–626
28. Hall ED (1992) Novel inhibitors of iron-dependent lipid peroxidation for neurodegenerative disorders. Ann Neurol [32 Suppl]:S137–S142
29. Halliwell B, Zhao K, Whiteman M (1999) Nitric oxide and peroxynitrite. The ugly, the uglier and the not so good: a personal view of recent controversies. Free Radic Res 31:651–669
30. Hauser SL, Oksenberg JR (2006) The neurobiology of multiple sclerosis: genes, inflammation, and neurodegeneration. Neuron 52:61–76

31. Hediger MA, Johnson RJ, Miyazaki H, Endou H (2005) Molecular physiology of urate transport. Physiology (Bethesda) 20:125–133
32. Hendriks JJ, Teunissen CE, de Vries HE, Dijkstra CD (2005) Macrophages and neurodegeneration. Brain Res Brain Res Rev 48:185–195
33. Hilliker AJ, Duyf B, Evans D, Phillips JP (1992) Urate-null rosy mutants of Drosophila melanogaster are hypersensitive to oxygen stress. Proc Natl Acad Sci U S A 89:4343–4347
34. Hooper DC, Bagasra O, Marini JC, Zborek A, Ohnishi ST, Kean R, Champion JM, Sarker AB, Bobroski L, Farber JL, Akaike T, Maeda H, Koprowski H (1997) Prevention of experimental allergic encephalomyelitis by targeting nitric oxide and peroxynitrite: implications for the treatment of multiple sclerosis. Proc Natl Acad Sci U S A 94:2528–2533
35. Hooper DC, Kean RB, Scott GS, Spitsin SV, Mikheeva T, Morimoto K, Bette M, Rohrenbeck AM, Dietzschold B, Weihe E (2001) The central nervous system inflammatory response to neurotropic virus infection is peroxynitrite dependent. J Immunol 167:3470–3477
36. Hooper DC, Scott GS, Zborek A, Mikheeva T, Kean RB, Koprowski H, Spitsin SV (2000) Uric acid, a peroxynitrite scavenger, inhibits CNS inflammation, blood–CNS barrier permeability changes, and tissue damage in a mouse model of multiple sclerosis. FASEB J 14:691–698
37. Hooper DC, Spitsin S, Kean RB, Champion JM, Dickson GM, Chaudhry I, Koprowski H (1998) Uric acid, a natural scavenger of peroxynitrite, in experimental allergic encephalomyelitis and multiple sclerosis. Proc Natl Acad Sci U S A 95:675–680
38. Johnson RJ, Kang DH, Feig D, Kivlighn S, Kanellis J, Watanabe S, Tuttle KR, Rodriguez-Iturbe B, Herrera-Acosta J, Mazzali M (2003) Is there a pathogenetic role for uric acid in hypertension and cardiovascular and renal disease? Hypertension 41:1183–1190
39. Kanabrocki EL, Ryan MD, Hermida RC, Ayala DE, Scott GS, Murray D, Bremner WF, Third JL, Johnson MC, Foley S, Van Cauteren J, Shah F, Shirazi P, Nemchausky BA, Hooper DC (2004) Altered circadian relationship between serum nitric oxide, carbon dioxide, and uric acid in multiple sclerosis. Chronobiol Int 21:739–758
40. Karg E, Klivenyi P, Nemeth I, Bencsik K, Pinter S, Vecsei L (1999) Nonenzymatic antioxidants of blood in multiple sclerosis. J Neurol 246:533–539
41. Kastenbauer S, Kieseier BC, Becker BF (2005) No evidence of increased oxidative degradation of urate to allantoin in the CSF and serum of patients with multiple sclerosis. J Neurol 252:611–612
42. Kastenbauer S, Koedel U, Becker BF, Pfister HW (2001) Experimental meningitis in the rat: protection by uric acid at human physiological blood concentrations. Eur J Pharmacol 425:149–152
43. Kastenbauer S, Koedel U, Pfister HW (1999) Role of peroxynitrite as a mediator of pathophysiological alterations in experimental pneumococcal meningitis. J Infect Dis 180:1164–1170
44. Kean RB, Spitsin SV, Mikheeva T, Scott GS, Hooper DC (2000) The peroxynitrite scavenger uric acid prevents inflammatory cell invasion into the central nervous system in experimental allergic encephalomyelitis through maintenance of blood-central nervous system barrier integrity. J Immunol 165:6511–6518
45. Knapp CM, Constantinescu CS, Tan JH, McLean R, Cherryman GR, Gottlob I (2004) Serum uric acid levels in optic neuritis. Mult Scler 10:278–280
46. Koch M, De Keyser J (2006) Uric acid in multiple sclerosis. Neurol Res 28:316–319
47. Kooy NW, Royall JA, Ischiropoulos H, Beckman JS (1994) Peroxynitrite-mediated oxidation of dihydrorhodamine 123. Free Radic Biol Med 16:149–156
48. Koprowski H, Spitsin SV, Hooper DC (2000) Prospects for the treatment of multiple sclerosis by raising serum levels of uric acid, a scavenger of peroxynitrite. Ann Neurol 49:139
49. Kurosaki M, Li Calzi M, Scanziani E, Garattini E, Terao M (1995) Tissue- and cell-specific expression of mouse xanthine oxidoreductase gene in vivo: regulation by bacterial lipopolysaccharide. Biochem J 306:225–234
50. Langemann H, Kabiersch A, Newcombe J (1992) Measurement of low-molecular-weight antioxidants, uric acid, tyrosine and tryptophan in plaques and white matter from patients with multiple sclerosis. Eur Neurol 32:248–252
51. Levine SM, Chakrabarty A (2004) The role of iron in the pathogenesis of experimental allergic encephalomyelitis and multiple sclerosis. Ann N Y Acad Sci 1012:252–266

52. Liu JS, Zhao ML, Brosnan CF, Lee SC (2001) Expression of inducible nitric oxide synthase and nitrotyrosine in multiple sclerosis lesions. Am J Pathol 158:2057–2066
53. Lymar S, Hurst J (1995) Rapid reaction between peroxynitrite ion and carbon dioxide: implications for biological activity. J Am Chem Soc 117:8867–8868
54. Malfroy B, Doctrow SR, Orr PL, Tocco G, Fedoseyeva EV, Benichou G (1997) Prevention and suppression of autoimmune encephalomyelitis by EUK-8, a synthetic catalytic scavenger of oxygen-reactive metabolites. Cell Immunol 177:62–68
55. Massie HR, Shumway ME, Whitney SJ (1991) Uric acid content of Drosophila decreases with aging. Exp Gerontol 26:609–614
56. McNaughton L, Dalton B, Tarr J (1999) Inosine supplementation has no effect on aerobic or anaerobic cycling performance. Int J Sport Nutr 9:333–344
57. Mostert JP, Ramsaransing GS, Heersema DJ, Heerings M, Wilczak N, De Keyser J (2005) Serum uric acid levels and leukocyte nitric oxide production in multiple sclerosis patients outside relapses. J Neurol Sci 231:41–44
58. Oda M, Satta Y, Takenaka O, Takahata N (2002) Loss of urate oxidase activity in hominoids and its evolutionary implications. Mol Biol Evol 19:640–653
59. Ramsaransing GS, Heersema DJ, De Keyser J (2005) Serum uric acid, dehydroepiandrosterone sulphate, and apolipoprotein E genotype in benign vs. progressive multiple sclerosis. Eur J Neurol 12:514–518
60. Rentzos M, Nikolaou C, Anagnostouli M, Rombos A, Tsakanikas K, Economou M, Dimitrakopoulos A, Karouli M, Vassilopoulos D (2006) Serum uric acid and multiple sclerosis. Clin Neurol Neurosurg 108:527–531
61. Schreibelt G, Musters RJ, Reijerkerk A, de Groot LR, van der Pol SM, Hendrikx EM, Dopp ED, Dijkstra CD, Drukarch B, de Vries HE (2006) Lipoic acid affects cellular migration into the central nervous system and stabilizes blood–brain barrier integrity. J Immunol 177:2630–2637
62. Scott GS, Cuzzocrea S, Genovese T, Koprowski H, Hooper DC (2005) Uric acid protects against secondary damage after spinal cord injury. Proc Natl Acad Sci U S A 102:3483–8
63. Scott GS, Hake P, Kean RB, Virag L, Szabo C, Hooper DC (2001) Role of poly(ADP-ribose) synthetase activation in the development of experimental allergic encephalomyelitis. J Neuroimmunol 117:78–86
64. Scott GS, Hooper DC (2001) The role of uric acid in protection against peroxynitrite-mediated pathology. Med Hypotheses 56:95–100
65. Scott GS, Kean RB, Fabis MJ, Mikheeva T, Brimer CM, Phares TW, Spitsin SV, Hooper DC (2004) ICAM-1 upregulation in the spinal cords of PLSJL mice with experimental allergic encephalomyelitis is dependent upon TNF-alpha production triggered by the loss of blood–brain barrier integrity. J Neuroimmunol 155:32–42
66. Scott GS, Spitsin SV, Kean RB, Mikheeva T, Koprowski H, Hooper DC (2002) Therapeutic intervention in experimental allergic encephalomyelitis by administration of uric acid precursors. Proc Natl Acad Sci U S A 99:16303–16308
67. Sotgiu S, Pugliatti M, Sanna A, Sotgiu A, Fois ML, Arru G, Rosati G (2002) Serum uric acid and multiple sclerosis. Neurol Sci 23:183–188
68. Spitsin S, Hooper DC, Leist T, Streletz LJ, Mikheeva T, Koprowskil H (2001) Inactivation of peroxynitrite in multiple sclerosis patients after oral administration of inosine may suggest possible approaches to therapy of the disease. Mult Scler 7:313–319
69. Spitsin S, Hooper DC, Mikheeva T, Koprowski H (2001) Uric acid levels in patients with multiple sclerosis: analysis in mono- and dizygotic twins. Mult Scler 7:165–166
70. Spitsin SV, Scott GS, Kean RB, Mikheeva T, Hooper DC (2000) Protection of myelin basic protein immunized mice from free-radical mediated inflammatory cell invasion of the central nervous system by the natural peroxynitrite scavenger uric acid. Neurosci Lett 292:137–141
71. Squadrito GL, Cueto R, Splenser AE, Valavanidis A, Zhang H, Uppu RM, Pryor WA (2000) Reaction of uric acid with peroxynitrite and implications for the mechanism of neuroprotection by uric acid. Arch Biochem Biophys 376:333–337

72. Squadrito GL, Pryor WA (1998) Oxidative chemistry of nitric oxide: the roles of superoxide, peroxynitrite, and carbon dioxide. Free Radic Biol Med 25:392–403

73. Starling RD, Trappe TA, Short KR, Sheffield-Moore M, Jozsi AC, Fink WJ, Costill DL (1996) Effect of inosine supplementation on aerobic and anaerobic cycling performance. Med Sci Sports Exerc 28:1193–1198

74. Szabo C (1996) DNA strand breakage and activation of poly-ADP ribosyltransferase: a cytotoxic pathway triggered by peroxynitrite. Free Radic Biol Med 21:855–869

75. Toncev G (2006) Therapeutic value of serum uric acid levels increasing in the treatment of multiple sclerosis. Vojnosanit Pregl 63:879–882

76. Toncev G, Milicic B, Toncev S, Samardzic G (2002) High-dose methylprednisolone therapy in multiple sclerosis increases serum uric acid levels. Clin Chem Lab Med 40:505–508

77. Touil T, Deloire-Grassin MS, Vital C, Petry KG, Brochet B (2001) In vivo damage of CNS myelin and axons induced by peroxynitrite. Neuroreport 12:3637–3644

78. van der Veen RC, Hinton DR, Incardonna F, Hofman FM (1997) Extensive peroxynitrite activity during progressive stages of central nervous system inflammation. J Neuroimmunol 77:1–7

79. Watanabe S, Kang DH, Feng L, Nakagawa T, Kanellis J, Lan H, Mazzali M, Johnson RJ (2002) Uric acid, hominoid evolution, and the pathogenesis of salt-sensitivity. Hypertension 40:355–3560

80. Whiteman M, Halliwell B (1996) Protection against peroxynitrite-dependent tyrosine nitration and alpha 1-antiproteinase inactivation by ascorbic acid. A comparison with other biological antioxidants. Free Radic Res 25:275–283

81. Whiteman M, Ketsawatsakul U, Halliwell B (2002) A reassessment of the peroxynitrite scavenging activity of uric acid. Ann N Y Acad Sci 962:242–259

82. Williams MH, Kreider RB, Hunter DW, Somma CT, Shall LM, Woodhouse ML, Rokitski L (1990) Effect of inosine supplementation on 3-mile treadmill run performance and VO2 peak. Med Sci Sports Exerc 22:517–522

83. Wu X, Wakamiya M, Vaishnav S, Geske R, Montgomery C Jr, Jones P, Bradley A, Caskey CT (1994) Hyperuricemia and urate nephropathy in urate oxidase-deficient mice. Proc Natl Acad Sci U S A 91:742–746

84. Wu XW, Lee CC, Muzny DM, Caskey CT (1989) Urate oxidase: primary structure and evolutionary implications. Proc Natl Acad Sci U S A 86:9412–9416

85. Wu XW, Muzny DM, Lee CC, Caskey CT (1992) Two independent mutational events in the loss of urate oxidase during hominoid evolution. J Mol Evol 34:78–84

86. Yu ZF, Bruce-Keller AJ, Goodman Y, Mattson MP (1998) Uric acid protects neurons against excitotoxic and metabolic insults in cell culture, and against focal ischemic brain injury in vivo. J Neurosci Res 53:613–625

# Neuromyelitis Optica: Clinical Syndrome and the NMO-IgG Autoantibody Marker

B.G. Weinshenker(☒) and D.M. Wingerchuk

**Abstract** Neuromyelitis optica (NMO) is a severe demyelinating disease of the CNS that preferentially affects the optic nerves and spinal cord, tends to relapse, and results in early permanent disability for most affected patients. A new autoantibody marker called neuromyelitis optica immunoglobulin G (NMO-IgG), which targets the water channel protein aquaporin-4, is highly specific for NMO. The marker has demonstrated that the NMO spectrum of disorders is wider than previously known and includes some patients with single-episode or recurrent longitudinally extensive myelitis, recurrent isolated optic neuritis, Asian optic–spinal multiple sclerosis, and patients with co-existing systemic autoimmune diseases such as lupus erythematosus or Sjögren's syndrome. We review the place of NMO within the nosology of CNS demyelinating diseases, the discovery of NMO-IgG and its impact on the definition of NMO and its spectrum, implications for understanding NMO pathogenesis, and informing treatment decisions.

B.G. Weinshenker
Mayo Clinic College of Medicine, 200 First Street SW, Rochester, MN 55901, USA
e-mail: weinb@mayo.edu

M. Rodriguez (ed.), *Advances in Multiple Sclerosis and Experimental*
*Demyelinating Diseases. Current Topics in Microbiology and Immunology 318.*
© Springer-Verlag Berlin Heidelberg 2008

# 1  All that Relapses is not MS

What's in a name? That which we call a rose by any other name would smell as sweet.

William Shakespeare, *Romeo and Juliet*, act 2 scene 2

For neurological diagnosis, a name is the essential starting point for diagnosis, prognosis, and treatment. Names and classifications evolve, and new classifications either embrace entities previously regarded as distinct or more specific as the molecular pathogenesis of a disease is elucidated. For example, Duchenne's and Becker's muscular dystrophy are both dystrophinopathy; Miller Fisher syndrome is a GQ1b-associated variant of acute inflammatory demyelinating polyneuropathy. However, for many idiopathic diseases, neurologists still rely upon the temporal evolution, clinical manifestations, and pathology to characterize the illness, e.g. chronic inflammatory demyelinating polyneuropathy, Lennox-Gastaut syndrome, and frontotemporal dementia. The name applied for the last century to characterize relapsing CNS demyelinating disease is multiple sclerosis (MS). Just as epilepsy has been defined by the tendency of seizures to recur in an unprovoked fashion, MS has been defined by "lesions disseminated in time and space"; in other words, recurrent attacks of clinically defined CNS inflammatory disease with biopsy documentation of inflammation rarely obtained. The faulty logic—if MS relapses, then all conditions that relapse are MS—has dominated clinical practice. Only limited qualifications were applied to the principle of dissemination in time and space; lesions were required to affect the central nervous system white matter pathways and must not be better explained by an alternative diagnosis. It had been long recognized that the differential diagnosis of MS is extensive and that many other diseases that are neither inflammatory nor demyelinating may fulfill that criterion, including stroke, cancer, and other inflammatory disorders such as sarcoidosis and vasculitis, among others. However, despite continuing concerns about their homogeneity, inflammatory demyelinating diseases that relapse have been treated as a single entity with protean manifestations and variable, but generally unpredictable outcome. Lassmann et al. have recently characterized immunopathological differences among inflammatory demyelinating diseases [14]. Those differences may even account for differential response to certain acute interventions, such as the differential response of patients with MS to plasma exchange [10]; however, the clinical, radiological, and treatment differences between the immunopathological subtypes are not yet well understood, and the distinction between them is only possible with biopsy of an active lesion or at autopsy. Although MS had been initially regarded as a relapsing remitting disease, increasingly it has been appreciated that some MS patients do not have (clinically) definable relapses and present with progressive course. Typically, patients with primary progressive MS have similar multifocal lesions that might have been expected, had they been symptomatic, to cause a relapsing illness.

The converse is also true: patients with a single clinical event (monophasic course) have by definition been excluded from the rubric of MS and been defined as having acute disseminated encephalomyelitis (ADEM) by analogy to the postvaccinial syndrome recognized in humans who developed a monophasic inflammatory demyelinating disorder after rabies vaccine and by analogy with the animal model induced by immunization with a variety of myelin preparations with appropriate adjuvant. The same faulty logic has been applied to the definition of ADEM—since ADEM is monophasic, any monophasic inflammatory demyelinating disease may be a form of ADEM.

The diagnostic approach of relapsing and monophasic demyelinating diseases of the central nervous system is being rewritten by recent studies of neuromyelitis optica (NMO). NMO is a form of demyelinating disease long considered unique by virtue of its apparently selective and severe involvement of the optic nerves and spinal cord and the rapidity of its evolution, often to death, reflecting the severity of manifestations and the short interval that typically occurs between index attacks. Albutt was the first to recognize the association between optic neuritis and myelitis in 1870 [2], but Devic gets credit for the recognition of this syndrome. His description of a case and review of a total of 16 cases in the contemporary medical literature in a thesis by his student Gault in 1894 led to Devic's eponymous association with the disease [7]. Initially regarded as a monophasic illness, the interval allowed between the index attacks was variably defined and extended from months to years in reports over the latter half of the twentieth century. However, optic neuritis and myelitis occur both in NMO and MS, and this led to obvious confusion in the differential diagnosis between these two entities and an understandable inclination to downplay the significance of differences between these entities when no definitive way of separating them existed. Despite reports that relapsing forms of NMO exist, the dogma that inflammatory demyelinating diseases should be classified exclusively based on their temporal profile limited the acceptance of relapsing forms of NMO; relapsing cases of NMO are now recognized to vastly outnumber monophasic cases. Relapsing NMO was generally classified until the past decade as MS. However, advances over the past decade changed the concept of NMO and may challenge the singular importance of temporal course in arriving at a diagnosis of MS. First, clinical differences, not only in the individual episodes of optic neuritis and myelitis but in the frequency, distribution, and sequelae of attacks, were recognized between NMO and MS [6, 23, 24, 36]. Secondly, MRI revealed distinctive differences between NMO and MS, especially the tendency for long, central spinal cord lesions to be present at the time of attacks of myelitis, which correlate with the presence of complete, symmetric transverse myelitis [36]. Finally, a recently discovered biomarker, NMO-IgG, is approximately 70% sensitive and 90% specific for NMO [16]. This antibody biomarker has not only proved to be a valuable diagnostic and prognostic marker, but the recent discovery of its target antigen, the water channel protein aquaporin-4 (AQP4) [15], promises to unravel the pathogenesis of this disorder and identify mechanisms underlying demyelination and the basis of lesion localization within the central nervous system in inflammatory demyelinating disease.

## 2 NMO is Distinct: The Clinical Clues

Until recently, the diagnosis of NMO was applied almost exclusively to cases conforming to the traditional definition of a severe disorder in which bilateral optic neuritis and myelitis occurred simultaneously and resulted in substantial permanent disability but without future clinical relapses. This restricted perspective naturally led to the conclusion that NMO was extremely rare because milder cases, those that relapsed, and those with symptoms or signs suggesting CNS disease outside of the optic nerve and spinal cord were diagnosed as severe MS or atypical MS. The advent of several technologies, especially magnetic resonance imaging (MRI), facilitated the still-evolving recognition of the clinical spectrum of NMO. It was noted that brain MRI scans from NMO patients were usually normal or revealed only nonspecific white matter lesions that did not meet MS radiological criteria. Over time, most patients accrue more such lesions, but their clinical course is dominated by recurrent optic neuritis and myelitis attacks. Patients studied with spinal cord MRI scans during acute myelitis attacks were usually found to have longitudinally extensive lesions, defined as extending continuously over the length of three or more vertebral segments [36]. Cerebrospinal fluid (CSF) analysis performed in the first days or weeks after the clinical onset of myelitis often demonstrated findings that were unusual for MS, including a prominent pleocytosis of 50–1,000 leukocytes per microliter (or/$\mu$L) and containing polymorphonuclear cells, which are virtually never seen in MS. These MRI and CSF characteristics were gradually recognized as features that could aid the neurologist in distinguishing NMO from MS even early in the disease course. Moreover, many reported NMO cases and series exhibited clusters of optic neuritis and myelitis relapses over many years yet maintained normal brain MRI scans. Some patients had experienced bouts of unilateral, rather than bilateral, optic neuritis. In the 1990s, several case series recognized the core features of NMO as relapsing, severe optic neuritis and myelitis with normal (or nearly so) brain MRI scans at disease onset and distinctive spinal cord MRI scans and CSF profiles. A Mayo Clinic study of 73 NMO patients established that the disease course was the same for individuals who experienced unilateral optic neuritis as for those with bilateral disease and that the index events of optic neuritis and myelitis were usually not simultaneous; rather, they were typically weeks or even years apart, heralding a future relapsing course [36]. These observations culminated in the development of liberalized NMO diagnostic criteria published in 1999 and later validated in many world regions [5, 8, 24].

The cumulative NMO case series literature provided additional insights into characteristics such as demographics and disease associations. Most NMO patients are female, with the sex ratio approaching 9:1 in some series. Although most reports from North America and Europe include a high proportion of Caucasian patients, non-Caucasians such as African-Americans, Hispanics, and Asians are clearly overrepresented in NMO compared to MS. The age of disease onset of NMO is later (median 39 years) than that of MS (median 29 years). Finally, up to half of NMO patients demonstrate the presence of multiple autoantibodies such as antinuclear antibody, anti-double-stranded DNA, and extractable nuclear antigen or have evidence of clinically manifest systemic autoimmunity. (Thyroid disorders are most common, but myasthenia gravis occurs at much higher frequency than expected [13], and multiple autoimmune diseases may occur in patients with NMO.)

Although not everyone had accepted NMO as a distinct disease, it became incontrovertible that patients meeting the demographic profile and diagnostic criteria described above usually have a poor prognosis. We now recognize that milder attacks and favorable recovery can occur in NMO. However, most patients experience severe attacks leading to a stepwise accrual of disability. In a 1999 study, more than half of patients were blind (visual acuity less than 20/200) in at least one eye or required at least unilateral gait assistance 5 years after disease onset [36]. In addition, one-third of patients died of myelitis that extended to the upper cervical spinal cord and not infrequently into the brain stem, resulting in neurogenic respiratory failure. Although more recent advances in understanding the spectrum of NMO have shown that milder cases do occur, these morbidity and mortality data stand in stark contrast to multiple sclerosis disability data [26].

The clinical, CSF, and neuroimaging variables that defined NMO also led to advances toward demonstrating that NMO is pathologically distinct from MS. Biopsy and autopsy specimens studied with advanced immunohistochemical techniques showed that NMO lesions are associated with markers of antibody-mediated immunopathology [17]. Acute lesions are characterized by demyelination but also by severe inflammatory infiltrates containing polymorphonuclear cells, eosinophils, macrophages, and necrosis. Penetrating spinal arteries have a thickened and hyalinized appearance. Whereas pattern 2 MS lesions reveal deposition of complement components and immunoglobulin in areas of active demyelination, these features in NMO lesions are located around penetrating microvessels. They stain with characteristic ring and rosette patterns, now suspected to reflect the distribution of the molecular target on the astrocytes targeted by these antibodies (see Sect. 3). Overall, the findings suggest that the perivascular region is targeted by an antibody-dependent, complement-mediated immune attack possibly amplified by eosinophil recruitment with local degranulation. The severity of the inflammatory process, the unusual cell differential profile, and the distribution of the complement and immunoglobulin deposition all suggest that the pathophysiological mechanisms underlying NMO are primarily driven by humoral mechanisms.

# 3 A Tool: Discovery of a Biomarker and Its Target

Believing that NMO and MS were clinically, radiologically, pathologically, and prognostically distinct, investigators searched for a marker antibody to add further weight to the argument. Sera from several patients was sent to the Clinical Neuroimmunology Laboratory at Mayo Clinic, a lab that tests patient sera for CNS-specific reactive antibodies using indirect immunofluorescence, largely to confirm a suspected diagnosis of a paraneoplastic disorders. A pattern, previously detected in other patients but of unknown clinical significance, was observed in the first two patients tested [16]. This pattern of immunofluorescence suggested that the target antigen was localized at the abluminal surface of mouse brain microvessels in the midbrain and cerebellum as well as the pia, subpial glia, and the linings of the Virchow-Robin spaces; it did not stain microvessels in other organs, although it did stain the distal renal tubules and the gastric mucosal crypts. Clinical follow-up of previously identified patients with this immunofluorescence pattern of unknown significance determined that the pattern correctly identified patients with typical symptoms of NMO in 12 of 14 patients on whom adequate clinical information could be obtained. These patients were derived from tens of thousands of samples that had been processed, of which a small minority, by the nature of the paraneo-plastic syndromes for which these samples were most commonly submitted, were expected to have NMO or symptoms thereof. Hence, the identification of clinical symptoms of NMO in almost all these patients was a clear indicator of an important association of this new biomarker with NMO.

Subsequent testing at Mayo Clinic in prospective studies confirmed the associa-tion of NMO-IgG with both NMO and other syndromes that were immediately recognized as limited forms of NMO, such as recurrent optic neuritis without mye-litis and recurrent longitudinally extensive transverse myelitis without optic neuritis [16]. These results have been confirmed by independent laboratories, which also find that this or related assays for aquaporin-4 are highly specific for NMO and the aforementioned limited forms of NMO [9, 39].

While initial studies were conducted using clinical classification and laboratory assay in blinded fashion, we utilized the established specificity of NMO-IgG in second-phase studies to address whether the existence of NMO is broader than pre-viously recognized. This issue is considered in Sect. 4.

The staining characteristics of NMO-IgG have informed the identification of its target antigen. The staining of both abluminal surfaces of microvessels and the staining of the subpia implicated a lesion in astrocyte foot processes in the glia limitans, which represents the conglomeration of such foot processes at these sites; this is a site critically important to the blood–brain barrier. The identification of the target antigen was further informed by staining of the distal renal collecting tubules and the depths of the gastric mucosal crypts, suggesting a shared antigen between these two sites. Aquaporin-4 became a logical and highly plausible candidate.

A series of experiments definitively established aquaporin-4 as the molecular target of NMO-IgG [15]. First, staining of mouse CNS tissues with NMO patient sera provided an identical pattern and co-localized by confocal microscopy with that yielded by staining with aquaporin-4-specific antiserum. Staining was abolished in aquaporin-4 knockout mice. Staining by NMO patient serum resulted in HEK-293 cell lines that did not exhibit any endogenous immunostaining for aquaporin-4 after transfection with constructs expressing aquaporin-4. Finally, in this cell line, Lennon et al. were able to immunoprecipitate aquaporin-4 but no other component of the cell cytoskeletal complex known to anchor aquaporin-4 to the cell membrane.

Although these experiments established the specificity of this biomarker, they did not prove that the antibody is pathogenic. Certain clues, including the co-localization of immunopathological findings in NMO to the abluminal surface of microvessels, provided strong clues that the antigen at this site was the target of the characteristic immunopathology of the disease [17] but did not prove that it was. Data that has since emerged in support of the pathogenic nature of this autoantibody are discussed in Sect. 5.

# 4 Uncertainties (Boundaries, Forme Frustes, OSMS vs NMO, etc.)

NMO has broken barriers of "what is MS" and "what is ADEM." NMO may be either monophasic or relapsing, suggesting that sole reliance on temporal course is an unsatisfactory way of defining idiopathic inflammatory demyelinating disease. Furthermore, it suggests that a molecular marker defines this syndrome as well as, and in some instances, better than clinical criteria; patients with early symptoms not yet sufficient to lead to a definite clinical diagnosis had positive serological tests [34]. Our group had to wrestle with the imperfect sensitivity of the assay, and legitimate arguments were raised that an immune response may be an epiphenomenon rather than pathogenic in its own right. What were the limits defining NMO? Having established the specificity of the marker, we began to explore the spectrum of NMO-related disorders, using the antibody as a tool. This naturally put us at risk of circular reasoning and using the data from antibody testing to define a disease for which there was no gold standard, and we were careful to use these exploratory analyses only after a first-level analysis using the existing clinical diagnostic criteria as the gold standard established the specificity of NMO-IgG beyond any question. Clinical criteria are imperfect, in part because the necessary information (e.g., whether there was a longitudinally extensive spinal cord lesion) is often unavailable and because there are alternative causes for optic neuritis and myelitis syndromes. In fact, a specific diagnosis has never been possible for a large proportion of myelitis and optic neuritis cases. Many cases are diagnosed as idiopathic optic neuritis or myelitis. Through a combination of analysis of clinical factors adding specificity and longitudinal follow-up to document that the clinical course did not converge with that of prototypic MS, we have tentatively suggested, in part but not exclusively based on NMO-IgG testing, that the spectrum of NMO is broader than previously recognized.

Disorders that exist on the fringe of NMO include the following.

## 4.1 Limited Versions of NMO

Most cases of NMO, particularly relapsing cases, begin with optic neuritis or myelitis, and the inevitable conclusion is that patients with early symptoms cannot be diagnosed based on clinical criteria requiring both optic neuritis and myelitis. Furthermore, we recognized that a large proportion of patients seropositive for

NMO-IgG had either recurrent or single events of longitudinally extensive transverse myelitis or recurrent optic neuritis, but not both. These would have been unclassifiable as NMO. A prospective follow-up study of patients with a first longitudinally extensive transverse myelitis event indicated a greater than 50% risk of relapse with transverse myelitis or optic neuritis over 1 year in those seropositive for NMO-IgG, whereas those seronegative were free of recurrent neurological events [34]. Practically, this indicated NMO-IgG as a useful predictive test to guide the decision of whether to institute preventative therapy in patients with longitudinally extensive transverse myelitis.

## 4.2   Asian Forms of Optic–Spinal MS

The strong similarities between Asian forms of optic–spinal MS and NMO have long been appreciated [12]. However, the presence of a longitudinally extensive lesion was not considered essential for the diagnosis of Asian optic–spinal MS, and brain lesions were permitted when confined to the brainstem. As optic neuritis and myelitis could be symptoms of either prototypic MS or NMO, additional criteria were necessary for a specific diagnosis, and the presence of a long cord lesion and the absence of brain involvement were both useful in that regard. However, we also began to recognize the relatively common occurrence in patients with NMO of brainstem lesions as well as other brain lesions, including occasional cerebral hemisphere lesions, even ones involving the corpus callosum that might closely simulate MS [27]. Typically, such lesions did not occur at the onset of disease, although few absolute rules could be established. Similarly, the presence of longitudinally extensive cord lesions of the spinal cord on MRI scans obtained at the time of an acute attack provided good discrimination between patients who later pursued a course typical of MS and those who pursued a course more typical of NMO [37]. The incongruities in the diagnostic criteria for Asian optic–spinal MS and NMO likely explain much of the differences in specificity of the antibody between Asian and Western studies. However, the same distinctive pathology seen in Western NMO patients has been identified in Japanese cases [19, 20]. Seropositivity in Japanese optic–spinal MS cases is associated with severe visual loss and other features typical of NMO. Western-type MS occurs in Japan and these cases are NMO-IgG-seronegative.[21] Further agreement on diagnostic criteria is expected to resolve differences in clinical and MRI features between those diagnosed with NMO and those with optic–spinal MS.

## 4.3   NMO Symptoms in the Setting of Systemic
##        Autoimmune Disease

We and others have recognized the association of NMO with autoimmune disease [23, 36]; some patients have multiple systemic autoimmune diseases, including relatively uncommon diseases such as myasthenia gravis, which have been recognized to coexist with NMO much more frequently than expected by its prevalence [13]. Patients with preexisting systemic autoimmune diseases, such as systemic lupus erythematosus or Sjögren's syndrome, are assumed to be experiencing neurological complications of their systemic autoimmune disease when they develop optic neuritis or myelitis. However, we have recently shown that patients with these systemic autoimmune diseases who do not have optic neuritis or myelitis are never seropositive for NMO-IgG, whereas those who develop these neurological syndromes are seropositive for NMO-IgG at the same frequency as those who do not have systemic autoimmune disease [32]. These findings point to a coexistence of NMO with other autoimmune diseases, rather than a direct causation by systemic lupus erythematosus or Sjögren's. Had these autoimmune conditions been directly causative, we would have expected patients with underlying systemic autoimmune diseases to be seronegative for NMO-IgG, as are virtually all patients with these conditions who do not experience these specific neurological complications.

Although the evidence for the existence of a wider spectrum of NMO-related disorders is compelling, these observations are preliminary and are not yet embraced by the general neurological community. Others have also reported that a high proportion of recurrent myelitis cases in adults are seropositive for NMO-IgG, but further studies, especially in children, will be necessary before this can be generalized. We have proposed revised diagnostic criteria for fully developed NMO [37] (Table 1).

# 5 Toward an Understanding of NMO Pathogenesis

The discovery by Lennon and colleagues of NMO-IgG and identification of its target, aquaporin-4, may represent a major milestone on the path to understanding NMO pathogenesis and proving its distinction from MS [15]. Aquaporins are membrane water channel proteins fundamental to maintenance of fluid homeostasis, especially when cells are challenged by physiological stressors such as ischemia, osmotic disturbances, or metabolic imbalances [1]. The CNS contains aquaporin types 1, 4, and 9 from the roster of more than a dozen members of the

**Table 1** Revised neuromyelitis optica diagnostic criteria (2006)

Diagnosis requires fulfillment of absolute criteria *and* at least two of three supportive criteria:
Absolute criteria:
1. Optic neuritis
2. Acute myelitis
Supportive criteria:
1. Negative brain MRI at disease onset
2. Spinal cord MRI with contiguous T2-weighted signal abnormality extending over three or more vertebral segments
3. NMO-IgG seropositivity

aquaporin family. Aquaporin-4 is the most abundant. It plays an important role in CNS diseases, and alterations in its regulation or expression have been implicated in disorders such as stroke, epilepsy, pre-eclampsia, and cerebral trauma, among others.

In the rat CNS, aquaporin-4 is found along endothelial tight junctions on astrocytic foot processes (to which it is anchored by the dystroglycan complex), on the abluminal aspect of microvessels, cerebellar Purkinje cells, and the hypothalamus [3, 22]. There are intriguing parallels between the CNS distribution of aquaporin-4 and a distinct brain MRI lesional pattern seen in a minority of NMO-IgG-seropositive patients in which T2-weighted signal changes involve the third ventricle, hypothalamus, periaqueductal and peri-fourth ventricular regions, periependymal regions surrounding the lateral ventricles, superior cerebellar peduncle, and subpial regions of the cerebellar hemispheres [27–29]. Recent evaluation of human optic nerve and spinal cord revealed that aquaporin-4 expresses in a vasculocentric pattern reminiscent of the pattern of immune complex deposition observed in NMO lesions [30].

The specificity and diagnostic utility of NMO-IgG for NMO and related disorders is now well established, but its relevance to the pathophysiology of the disorder is not yet known. It is tempting to consider NMO as an autoimmune channelopathy. The sites of spinal cord aquaporin-4 immunoreactivity (abluminal surface of blood vessels and astrocytic foot processes) coincide with areas of immunoglobulin and complement deposition in NMO pathological specimens. To cause disease, peripheral NMO-IgG would need to access CNS aquaporin-4, either at sites where the blood–brain barrier is absent (e.g., circumventricular organs), susceptible (possibly the spinal cord), or damaged. Lennon et al. [15] hypothesized that NMO-IgG activates complement, either directly by binding with aquaporin-4 or indirectly by interfering with aquaporin-regulated fluid homeostatic mechanisms resulting in endothelial leakage and secondary complement activation. It is notable that demyelination is present in NMO yet the antibody targets an astrocytic protein. This observation suggests that reassessment of the role of the astrocyte as a potential primary target may also be worthwhile for multiple sclerosis.

Early pathological studies of spinal cord from NMO patients detected loss of aquaporin-4 in central grey matter, especially in perivascular regions near deposits of complement and immunoglobulin. This loss, however, corresponded in some regions to areas of necrosis and cavitation where glial fibrillary acidic protein (GFAP) staining was also reduced or lost [19, 20]. In contrast, MS lesions showed preservation or upregulation of AQP4 in demyelinated lesions. These early reports did not include information about the stage of demyelinating activity of NMO and MS lesions. A recent study evaluating patterns of CNS aquaporin-4 immunoreactivity in tissues from patients with NMO, MS, stroke, or no CNS disease showed that all NMO lesions exhibited severe aquaporin-4 loss regardless of the stage of demyelination [30]. In contrast, MS lesions showed stage-dependent loss. A novel NMO lesion type involving the spinal cord, medullary tegmentum, and area postrema was also recognized; it was characterized by inflammation, edema, and aquaporin-4 loss but neither demyelination nor necrosis. In NMO patients, foci of aquaporin-4 loss coincided with sites of intense vasculocentric immune complex deposition.

The cumulative clinical, immunohistochemical, and pathological findings from NMO patients and controls support the hypothesis that NMO lesions are initiated by a complement-activating aquaporin-4-specific autoantibody. However, definitive proof that NMO-IgG is the primary effector and that NMO is a distinct disease will require passive transfer of disease with anti-aquaporin-4 antibody or by active immunization with aquaporin-4.

## 6   How Has Current Knowledge Affected the Therapeutic Approach to NMO?

Anecdotal reports and case series suggest immunosuppressive therapies as beneficial to NMO by preventing future relapses [38]. Many of these observations were made well in advance of most of the advances in understanding NMO pathophysiology outlined earlier in this chapter. The case for treatments aimed at reducing activity of the humoral arm of the immune system continues to strengthen.

The wide-ranging, albeit nonspecific, anti-inflammatory treatment effects of corticosteroids seem to limit the severity of NMO attacks. Despite the use of high-dose corticosteroids over several days, some patients experience progression of neurological symptoms. In this circumstance, evidence from a randomized, blinded, crossover trial supports the use of plasmapheresis as second-line therapy. Weinshenker and colleagues compared plasmapheresis vs sham exchange in patients with very severe, corticosteroid-refractory CNS inflammatory/demyelinating events in settings such as MS, NMO, and recurrent or single-event transverse myelitis [33]. Eight of 19 patients (42.1%) had moderate or greater improvement in their targeted neurological deficit (coma, aphasia, hemiplegia, paraplegia, or quadriplegia) during that treatment phase compared with one of 19 (5.9%) demonstrating improvement during sham exchange. Included among responders were patients with NMO or acute transverse myelitis. A separate retrospective study noted that six of ten NMO patients with myelitis attacks that failed to respond to corticosteroids experienced moderate or marked improvement within 2 weeks of treatment initiation [11].

These data are consistent with the hypothesis that plasmapheresis benefits NMO by removing one or more humoral factors such as pathogenic antibodies, circulating immune complexes, complement or activated complement components, or cytokines [33]. Plasmapheresis responders in the controlled trial sustained their clinical improvement up to at least the final examination visit (208 days after treatment). One interpretation of this observation is that plasmapheresis contributed to disease stabilization by interrupting a humorally mediated inflammatory cascade.

Two therapeutic observations in NMO are consistent with the hypothesis that humoral autoimmunity is clinically relevant: (1) standard MS immunomodulatory therapies fail to significantly impact the disease and (2) general or B cell directed immunosuppression is associated with induction of remissions lasting at least 12–18 months in patients with previously active and treatment-resistant disease [38]. Both observations remain anecdotal but are becoming generally accepted.

Standard MS treatments such as beta-interferons and glatiramer acetate act primarily through T cell-mediated immunological pathways and, therefore, might be expected to exert little or no effect on NMO pathophysiology. There are no randomized controlled trials that have formally evaluated the efficacy of these agents for NMO. A Japanese MS study included optic–spinal MS patients but was not powered to determine a treatment effect for this specific subgroup. Some case series suggest that beta-interferons are detrimental to the course of NMO [25, 31].

Several small observational series support the likely benefit of immunosuppression. In a case series of seven patients, the combination of prednisone and azathioprine was associated with up to 18 months of attack freedom [18]. Mitoxantrone favorably impacted the course of five NMO patients with active disease [35]. Other immunosuppressive therapies, such as mycophenolate mofetil, cyclophosphamide, and methotrexate, appear to induce short-term remissions. The mechanism of these nonspecific immunosuppressive drugs includes effects on B cells and antibody production in addition to alteration of T cell responses.

More specific B cell-directed immunotherapy data come from a case series of active NMO patients treated with the monoclonal antibody rituximab [4]. Rituximab is a chimeric murine/human anti-CD20 monoclonal antibody that produces specific and long-lasting depletion of pre-B and mature B cells but not memory B cells or plasma cells. Eight patients with active, relapsing NMO that failed to respond to other immunotherapies (including beta-interferon, glatiramer acetate, azathioprine, intravenous immunoglobulin, and mitoxantrone) improved for an average of 12 months (range 6–18 months) after therapy with four weekly 375 mg/m$^2$ intravenous infusions of rituximab. When flow cytometry detected re-emergence of CD19-positive cells, retreatment was offered with two consecutive infusions of 1,000 mg administered 2 weeks apart. The median annualized attack rate fell from 2.6 attacks/patient/year in the pretreatment period to 0 attacks/patient/year after rituximab therapy ($p=0.0078$). Seven of eight patients had significant recovery of neurological function with reduction in the median Expanded Disability Status Scale score from 7.5 before treatment to 5.5 at final posttreatment examination ($p=0.013$). These pilot data represent a potential important advance in development of treatments derived from the growing understanding of NMO pathophysiology. The target specificity of rituximab seems advantageous, but the emergence of cases of progressive multifocal leukoencephalopathy in treated patients requires careful long-term study to determine whether the risk–benefit calculation truly favors rituximab over other approaches to immunosuppression.

# Conclusion

Neuromyelitis optica, long considered a peculiar and severe MS variant, has characteristic clinical, immunohistochemical and neuroimaging features that move it ever closer to distinct disease status. The discovery of NMO-IgG, and pursuit of its clinicopathological correlations, has resulted in expansion of the clinical spectrum of

NMO. Future investigation into the possibility that NMO represents the first of a newly identified class of autoimmune aquaporin channelopathies has just begun.

# References

1. Agre P, Kozono D (2003) Aquaporin water channels: molecular mechanisms for human diseases. FEBS Lett 555:72–78
2. Albutt TC (1870) On the ophthalmoscopic signs of spinal disease. Lancet 1:76–78
3. Amiry-Moghaddam M, Ottersen OP (2003) The molecular basis of water transport in the brain. Nat Rev Neurosci 4:991–1001
4. Cree BA, Lamb S, Morgan K, Chen A, Waubant E, Genain C (2005) An open label study of the effects of rituximab in neuromyelitis optica. Neurology 64:1270–1272
5. de Seze J, Lebrun C, Stojkovic T, Ferriby D, Chatel M, Vermersch P (2003) Is Devic's neuromyelitis optica a separate disease? A comparative study with multiple sclerosis. Mult Scler 9:521–525
6. de Seze J, Stojkovic T, Ferriby D, Gauvrit JY, Montagne C, Mounier-Vehier F, Verier A, Pruvo JP, Hache JC, Vermersch P (2002) Devic's neuromyelitis optica: clinical, laboratory, MRI and outcome profile. J Neurol Sci 197:57–61
7. Devic E (1894) Myélite aigue compliquée de névrite optique. Bull Med (Paris) 8:1033–1034
8. Ghezzi A, Bergamaschi R, Martinelli V, Trojano M, Tola MR, Merelli E, Mancardi L, Gallo P, Filippi M, Zaffaroni M, Comi G (2004) Clinical characteristics, course and prognosis of relapsing Devic's neuromyelitis optica. J Neurol 251:47–52
9. Jarius S, Franciotta D, Bergamaschi R, Wright H, Littleton E, Palace J, Hohlfeld R, Vincent A (2007) NMO-IgG in the diagnosis of neuromyelitis optica. Neurology 68:1076–1077
10. Keegan M, Konig F, McClelland R, Bruck W, Morales Y, Bitsch A, Panitch H, Lassmann H, Weinshenker B, Rodriguez M, Parisi J, Lucchinetti CF (2005) Relation between humoral pathological changes in multiple sclerosis and response to therapeutic plasma exchange. Lancet 366:579–582
11. Keegan M, Pineda AA, McClelland RL, Darby CH, Rodriguez M, Weinshenker BG (2002) Plasma exchange for severe attacks of CNS demyelination: predictors of response. Neurology 58:143–146
12. Kira J (2003) Multiple sclerosis in the Japanese population. Lancet Neurol 2:117–127
13. Kister I, Gulati S, Boz C, Bergamaschi R, Piccolo G, Oger J, Swerdlow ML (2006) Neuromyelitis optica in patients with myasthenia gravis who underwent thymectomy. Arch Neurol 63:851–856
14. Lassmann H, Bruck W, Lucchinetti C (2001) Heterogeneity of multiple sclerosis pathogenesis: implications for diagnosis and therapy. Trends Mol Med 7:115–121
15. Lennon VA, Kryzer TJ, Pittock SJ, Verkman AS, Hinson SR (2005) IgG marker of optic-spinal multiple sclerosis binds to the aquaporin-4 water channel. J Exp Med 202:473–477
16. Lennon VA, Wingerchuk DM, Kryzer TJ, Pittock SJ, Lucchinetti CF, Fujihara K, Nakashima I, Weinshenker BG (2004) A serum autoantibody marker of neuromyelitis optica: distinction from multiple sclerosis. Lancet 364:2106–2112
17. Lucchinetti CF, Mandler RN, McGavern D, Bruck W, Gleich G, Ransohoff RM, Trebst C, Weinshenker B, Wingerchuk D, Parisi JE, Lassmann H (2002) A role for humoral mechanisms in the pathogenesis of Devic's neuromyelitis optica. Brain 125:1450–1461
18. Mandler RN, Ahmed W, Dencoff JE (1998) Devic's neuromyelitis optica: a prospective study of seven patients treated with prednisone and azathioprine. Neurology 51:1219–1220
19. Misu T, Fujihara K, Nakamura M, Murakami K, Endo M, Konno H, Itoyama Y (2006) Loss of aquaporin-4 in active perivascular lesions in neuromyelitis optica: a case report. Tohoku J Exp Med 209:269–275

20. Misu T, Kakita A, Fujihara K et al (2005) A comparative neuropathological analysis of Japanese cases of neuromyelitis optica and multiple sclerosis. Neurology 64:A39
21. Nakashima I, Fujihara K, Miyazawa I, Misu T, Narikawa K, Nakamura M, Watanabe S, Takahashi T, Nishiyama S, Shiga Y, Sato S, Weinshenker BG, Itoyama Y (2006) Clinical and MRI features of Japanese patients with multiple sclerosis positive for NMO-IgG. J Neurol Neurosurg Psychiatry 77:1073–1075
22. Nielsen S, Nagelhus EA, Amiry-Moghaddam M, Bourque C, Agre P, Ottersen OP (1997) Specialized membrane domains for water transport in glial cells: high-resolution immunogold cytochemistry of aquaporin-4 in rat brain. J Neurosci 17:171–180
23. O'Riordan JI, Gallagher HL, Thompson AJ, Howard RS, Kingsley DP, Thompson EJ, McDonald WI, Miller DH (1996) Clinical, CSF, and MRI findings in Devic's neuromyelitis optica. J Neurol Neurosurg Psychiatry 60:382–387
24. Papais-Alvarenga RM, Miranda-Santos CM, Puccioni-Sohler M, de Almeida AM, Oliveira S, Basilio De Oliveira CA, Alvarenga H, Poser CM (2002) Optic neuromyelitis syndrome in Brazilian patients. J Neurol Neurosurg Psychiatry 73:429–435
25. Papeix C, de Seze J (2005) French therapeutic experience of Devic's disease: a retrospective study of 33 cases. Neurology 64 [Suppl1]:A328–A329
26. Pittock SJ, Mayr WT, McClelland RL, Jorgensen NW, Weigand SD, Noseworthy JH, Rodriguez M (2004) Disability profile of MS did not change over 10 years in a population-based prevalence cohort. Neurology 62:601–606
27. Pittock SJ, Lennon VA, Krecke K, Wingerchuk DM, Lucchinetti CF, Weinshenker BG (2006) Brain abnormalities in neuromyelitis optica. Arch Neurol 63:390–396
28. Pittock SJ, Weinshenker BG, Lucchinetti CF, Wingerchuk DM, Corboy JR, Lennon VA (2006) Neuromyelitis optica brain lesions localized at sites of high aquaporin 4 expression. Arch Neurol 63:964–968
29. Poppe AY, Lapierre Y, Melancon D, Lowden D, Wardell L, Fullerton LM, Bar-Or A (2005) Neuromyelitis optica with hypothalamic involvement. Mult Scler 11:617–621
30. Roemer SF, Parisi JE, Lennon VA, Benarroch EE, Lassmann H, Bruck W, Mandler RN, Weinshenker BG, Pittock SJ, Wingerchuk DM, Lucchinetti CF (2007) Pattern-specific loss of aquaporin-4 immunoreactivity distinguishes neuromyelitis optica from multiple sclerosis. Brain 130:1194–1205
31. Warabi Y, Matsumoto Y, Hayashi H (2006) Interferon beta-1b exacerbates multiple sclerosis with severe optic nerve and spinal cord demyelination. J Neurol Sci 252:57–61
32. Weinshenker B, Pittock S, de Seze J, Vermersch P, Wingerchuk D, Zephir H, Homberger H, Lucchinetti C, Lennon V (2006) The relationship between neuromyelitis optica and systemic autoimmune disease. Mult Scler 12:S16
33. Weinshenker BG, O'Brien PC, Petterson TM, Noseworthy JH, Lucchinetti CF, Dodick DW, Pineda AA, Stevens LN, Rodriguez M (1999) A randomized trial of plasma exchange in acute central nervous system inflammatory demyelinating disease. Ann Neurol 46:878–886
34. Weinshenker BG, Wingerchuk DM, Vukusic S, Linbo L, Pittock SJ, Lucchinetti CF, Lennon VA (2006) Neuromyelitis optica IgG predicts relapse after longitudinally extensive transverse myelitis. Ann Neurol 59:566–569
35. Weinstock-Guttman B, Ramanathan M, Lincoff N, Napoli SQ, Sharma J, Feichter J, Bakshi R (2006) Study of mitoxantrone for the treatment of recurrent neuromyelitis optica (Devic disease). Arch Neurol 63:957–963
36. Wingerchuk DM, Hogancamp WF, O'Brien PC, Weinshenker BG (1999) The clinical course of neuromyelitis optica (Devic's syndrome). Neurology 53:1107–1114
37. Wingerchuk DM, Lennon VA, Pittock SJ, Lucchinetti CF, Weinshenker BG (2006) Revised diagnostic criteria for neuromyelitis optica. Neurology 66:1485–1489
38. Wingerchuk DM, Weinshenker BG (2005) Neuromyelitis optica. Curr Treat Options Neurol 7:173–182
39. Zuliani L, Lopez de Munain A, Ruiz Martinez J, Olascoaga J, Graus F, Saiz A (2006) Anticuerpos IgG-NMO en la neuromyelitis optica: proposito de 2 casos. Neurologia 21:314–317

# Index

# Current Topics in Microbiology and Immunology

## Volumes published since 1989

Vol. 271: **Koehler, Theresa M. (Ed.):**
Anthrax. 2002. 14 figs. X, 169 pp.
ISBN 3-540-43497-6

Vol. 272: **Doerfler, Walter; Böhm, Petra
(Eds.):** Adenoviruses: Model and Vectors in
Virus-Host Interactions. Virion and Structure,
Viral Replication, Host Cell Interactions.
2003. 63 figs., approx. 280 pp.
ISBN 3-540-00154-9

Vol. 273: **Doerfler, Walter; Böhm, Petra
(Eds.):** Adenoviruses: Model and Vectors in
VirusHost Interactions. Immune System,
Oncogenesis, Gene Therapy. 2004. 35 figs.,
approx. 280 pp. ISBN 3-540-06851-1

Vol. 274: **Workman, Jerry L. (Ed.):** Protein
Complexes that Modify Chromatin. 2003.
38 figs., XII, 296 pp. ISBN 3-540-44208-1

Vol. 275: **Fan, Hung (Ed.):** Jaagsiekte Sheep
Retrovirus and Lung Cancer. 2003. 63 figs.,
XII, 252 pp. ISBN 3-540-44096-3

Vol. 276: **Steinkasserer, Alexander (Ed.):**
Dendritic Cells and Virus Infection. 2003.
24 figs., X, 296 pp. ISBN 3-540-44290-1

Vol. 277: **Rethwilm, Axel (Ed.):** Foamy
Viruses. 2003. 40 figs., X, 214 pp.
ISBN 3-540-44388-6

Vol. 278: **Salomon, Daniel R.; Wilson,
Carolyn (Eds.):** Xenotransplantation. 2003.
22 figs., IX, 254 pp. ISBN 3-540-00210-3

Vol. 279: **Thomas, George; Sabatini, David;
Hall, Michael N. (Eds.):** TOR. 2004. 49 figs.,
X, 364 pp. ISBN 3-540-00534X

Vol. 280: **Heber-Katz, Ellen (Ed.):**
Regeneration: Stem Cells and Beyond. 2004.
42 figs., XII, 194 pp. ISBN 3-540-02238-4

Vol. 281: **Young, John A. T. (Ed.):** Cellular
Factors Involved in Early Steps of Retroviral
Replication. 2003. 21 figs., IX, 240 pp.
ISBN 3-540-00844-6

Vol. 282: **Stenmark, Harald (Ed.):**
Phosphoinositides in Subcellular Targeting
and Enzyme Activation. 2003. 20 figs., X,
210 pp. ISBN 3-540-00950-7

Vol. 283: **Kawaoka, Yoshihiro (Ed.):**
Biology of Negative Strand RNA Viruses:
The Power of Reverse Genetics. 2004. 24
figs., IX, 350 pp. ISBN 3-540-40661-1

Vol. 284: **Harris, David (Ed.):** Mad Cow
Disease and Related Spongiform
Encephalopathies. 2004. 34 figs., IX, 219 pp.
ISBN 3-540-20107-6

Vol. 285: **Marsh, Mark (Ed.):** Membrane
Trafficking in Viral Replication. 2004. 19 figs.,
IX, 259 pp. ISBN 3-540-21430-5

Vol. 286: **Madshus, Inger H. (Ed.):** Signalling
from Internalized Growth Factor Receptors.
2004. 19 figs., IX, 187 pp. ISBN
3-540-21038-5

Vol. 287: **Enjuanes, Luis (Ed.):** Coronavirus
Replication and Reverse Genetics. 2005. 49
figs., XI, 257 pp. ISBN 3-540- 21494-1

Vol. 288: **Mahy, Brain W. J. (Ed.):** Foot-and-
Mouth-Disease Virus. 2005. 16 figs., IX, 178
pp. ISBN 3-540-22419X

Vol. 289: **Griffin, Diane E. (Ed.):** Role of
Apoptosis in Infection. 2005. 40 figs., IX, 294
pp. ISBN 3-540-23006-8

Vol. 290: **Singh, Harinder; Grosschedl,
Rudolf (Eds.):** Molecular Analysis of B
Lymphocyte Development and Activation.
2005. 28 figs., XI, 255 pp. ISBN 3-540-23090-4

Vol. 291: **Boquet, Patrice; Lemichez
Emmanuel (Eds.):** Bacterial Virulence
Factors and Rho GTPases. 2005. 28 figs., IX,
196 pp. ISBN 3-540-23865-4

Vol. 292: **Fu, Zhen F. (Ed.):** The World of
Rhabdoviruses. 2005. 27 figs., X, 210 pp.
ISBN 3-540-24011-X

Vol. 293: **Kyewski, Bruno; Suri-Payer,
Elisabeth (Eds.):** CD4+CD25+ Regulatory
T Cells: Origin, Function and Therapeutic
Potential. 2005. 22 figs., XII, 332 pp.
ISBN 3-540-24444-1

Vol. 294: **Caligaris-Cappio, Federico, Dalla
Favera, Ricardo (Eds.):** Chronic
Lymphocytic Leukemia. 2005. 25 figs.,
VIII, 187 pp. ISBN 3-540-25279-7

Vol. 295: **Sullivan, David J.; Krishna Sanjeew (Eds.):** Malaria: Drugs, Disease and Post-genomic Biology. 2005. 40 figs., XI, 446 pp. ISBN 3-540-25363-7

Vol. 296: **Oldstone, Michael B. A. (Ed.):** Molecular Mimicry: Infection Induced Autoimmune Disease. 2005. 28 figs., VIII, 167 pp. ISBN 3-540-25597-4

Vol. 297: **Langhorne, Jean (Ed.):** Immunology and Immunopathogenesis of Malaria. 2005. 8 figs., XII, 236 pp. ISBN 3-540-25718-7

Vol. 298: **Vivier, Eric; Colonna, Marco (Eds.):** Immunobiology of Natural Killer Cell Receptors. 2005. 27 figs., VIII, 286 pp. ISBN 3-540-26083-8

Vol. 299: **Domingo, Esteban (Ed.):** Quasispecies: Concept and Implications. 2006. 44 figs., XII, 401 pp. ISBN 3-540-26395-0

Vol. 300: **Wiertz, Emmanuel J.H.J.; Kikkert, Marjolein (Eds.):** Dislocation and Degradation of Proteins from the Endoplasmic Reticulum. 2006. 19 figs., VIII, 168 pp. ISBN 3-540-28006-5

Vol. 301: **Doerfler, Walter; Böhm, Petra (Eds.):** DNA Methylation: Basic Mechanisms. 2006. 24 figs., VIII, 324 pp. ISBN 3-540-29114-8

Vol. 302: **Robert N. Eisenman (Ed.):** The Myc/Max/Mad Transcription Factor Network. 2006. 28 figs., XII, 278 pp. ISBN 3-540-23968-5

Vol. 303: **Thomas E. Lane (Ed.):** Chemokines and Viral Infection. 2006. 14 figs. XII, 154 pp. ISBN 3-540-29207-1

Vol. 304: **Stanley A. Plotkin (Ed.):** Mass Vaccination: Global Aspects – Progress and Obstacles. 2006. 40 figs. X, 270 pp. ISBN 3-540-29382-5

Vol. 305: **Radbruch, Andreas; Lipsky, Peter E. (Eds.):** Current Concepts in Autoimmunity. 2006. 29 figs. IIX, 276 pp. ISBN 3-540-29713-8 '

Vol. 306: **William M. Shafer (Ed.):** Antimicrobial Peptides and Human Disease. 2006. 12 figs. XII, 262 pp. ISBN 3-540-29915-7

Vol. 307: **John L. Casey (Ed.):** Hepatitis Delta Virus. 2006. 22 figs. XII, 228 pp. ISBN 3-540-29801-0

Vol. 308: **Honjo, Tasuku; Melchers, Fritz (Eds.):** Gut-Associated Lymphoid Tissues. 2006. 24 figs. XII, 204 pp. ISBN 3-540-30656-0

Vol. 309: **Polly Roy (Ed.):** Reoviruses: Entry, Assembly and Morphogenesis. 2006. 43 figs. XX, 261 pp. ISBN 3-540-30772-9

Vol. 310: **Doerfler, Walter; Böhm, Petra (Eds.):** DNA Methylation: Development, Genetic Disease and Cancer. 2006. 25 figs. X, 284 pp. ISBN 3-540-31180-7

Vol. 311: **Pulendran, Bali; Ahmed, Rafi (Eds.):** From Innate Immunity to Immunological Memory. 2006. 13 figs. X, 177 pp. ISBN 3-540-32635-9

Vol. 312: **Boshoff, Chris; Weiss, Robin A. (Eds.):** Kaposi Sarcoma Herpesvirus: New Perspectives. 2006. 29 figs. XVI, 330 pp. ISBN 3-540-34343-1

Vol. 313: **Pandolfi, Pier P.; Vogt, Peter K. (Eds.):** Acute Promyelocytic Leukemia. 2007. 16 figs. VIII, 273 pp. ISBN 3-540-34592-2

Vol. 314: **Moody, Branch D. (Ed.):** T Cell Activation by CD1 and Lipid Antigens, 2007, 25 figs. VIII, 348 pp. ISBN 978-3-540-69510-3

Vol. 315: **Childs, James, E.; Mackenzie, John S.; Richt, Jürgen A. (Eds.):** Wildlife and Emerging Zoonotic Diseases: The Biology, Circumstances and Consequences of Cross-Species Transmission. 2007. 49 figs. VII, 524 pp. ISBN 978-3-540-70961-9

Vol. 316: **Pitha, Paula M. (Ed.):** Interferon: The 50th Anniversary. 2007. VII, 391 pp. ISBN 978-3-540-71328-9

Vol. 317: **Dessain, Scott K. (Ed.):** Human Antibody Therapeutics for Viral Disease. 2007. XI, 202 pp. ISBN 978-3-540-72144-4